Acute Cardiac Care

A Practical Guide for Nurses

Edited by

Angela M. Kucia
PhD, BN, MA, Grad. Cert. Ed.

Clinical Practice Consultant, Acute Cardiac Assessment, Lyell McEwin Hospital and The Queen Elizabeth Hospital, Adelaide, South Australia.

Tom Quinn
MPhil, RN, FESC, FRCN

Professor of Clinical Practice, Faculty of Health and Medical Sciences, University of Surrey, UK.

WILEY-BLACKWELL

A John Wiley & Sons, Ltd., Publication

This edition first published 2010
© 2010 Blackwell Publishing Ltd

Blackwell Publishing was acquired by John Wiley & Sons in February 2007. Blackwell's publishing programme has been merged with Wiley's global Scientific, Technical, and Medical business to form Wiley-Blackwell.

Registered office
John Wiley & Sons Ltd, The Atrium, Southern Gate, Chichester, West Sussex, PO19 8SQ, United Kingdom

Editorial offices
9600 Garsington Road, Oxford, OX4 2DQ, United Kingdom
2121 State Avenue, Ames, Iowa 50014-8300, USA

For details of our global editorial offices, for customer services and for information about how to apply for permission to reuse the copyright material in this book, please see our website at www.wiley.com/wiley-blackwell

Wiley also publishes its books in a variety of electronic formats. Some content that appears in print may not be available in electronic books.

Designations used by companies to distinguish their products are often claimed as trademarks. All brand names and product names used in this book are trade names, service marks, trademarks or registered trademarks of their respective owners. The publisher is not associated with any product or vendor mentioned in this book. This publication is designed to provide accurate and authoritative information in regard to the subject matter covered. It is sold on the understanding that the publisher is not engaged in rendering professional services. If professional advice or other expert assistance is required, the services of a competent professional should be sought.

Library of Congress Cataloging-in-Publication Data
Acute Cardiac Care: A Practical Guide for Nurses/edited by Angela M. Kucia, Tom Quinn.
    p. ; cm.
  Includes bibliographical references and index.
  ISBN 978-1-4051-6361-3 (pbk.: alk. paper)
1. Heart—Diseases—Nursing.   I. Kucia, Angela M.   II. Quinn, Tom, 1961–
  [DNLM: 1. Heart Diseases—nursing.   2. Critical Care. WY 152.5 A189 2010]
RC674.A28 2010
616.1′20231—dc22   2009006627

A catalogue record for this book is available from the British Library.

Set in 9.5/11.5 pt Palatino by Macmillan Publishing Solutions, Chennai, India

Printed in Singapore by Ho Printing Singapore Pte Ltd

1   2010

Contents

Contributors

D. Barrett, RN, BA (Hons), PG Dip., PG Cert., is a Lecturer in Nursing in the Faculty of Health and Social Care, University of Hull, UK.

J.F. Beltrame, BSc, BMBS, PhD, FRACP, is Associate Professor and a National Heart Foundation Research Fellow at The University of Adelaide and a Senior Consultant Cardiologist at The Queen Elizabeth Hospital and Lyell McEwin Health Service, Adelaide, South Australia.

L. Belz, RN, Grad. Dip. Health Sc., is the Charge Nurse of the Coronary Care Unit at Auckland City Hospital, Auckland, New Zealand.

E. Birchmore, BN, MNP, Grad. Dip. Coronary Care, MRCNA, MACNP, is a Heart Failure Nurse Practitioner at The Queen Elizabeth Hospital, Adelaide, South Australia.

P. Davidson, RN, BA, MEd, PhD, is Professor and Director of the Centre for Cardiovascular & Chronic Care, Curtin University of Technology and St Vincent's Hospital, Sydney, New South Wales.

A. Day, RN (USA), RGN (UK), MSc, PGCE, BSc (Hons), is a Senior Lecturer in Emergency Nursing, and a member of the Applied Research Group on Pre-hospital, Emergency and Cardiovascular Care in the Faculty of Health and Life Sciences at Coventry University, UK.

D. Evans, MNS, PhD, is a Senior Lecturer and Program Director for Higher Degrees by Research in the School of Nursing and Midwifery, University of South Australia in Adelaide, South Australia.

B. Greaney, RGN, PG Dip., PGCE, MA(Ed), is a Senior Lecturer in Critical Care Nursing, and a member of the Applied Research Group on Pre-hospital, Emergency and Cardiovascular Care in the Faculty of Health and Life Sciences at Coventry University, UK.

P. Gregory, BSc (Hons), PGCE, Paramedic, is a Senior Lecturer in Paramedic Science, and a member of the Applied Research Group on Pre-hospital, Emergency and Cardiovascular Care in the Faculty of Health and Life Sciences, Coventry University, UK.

J.D. Horowitz, MBBS, BMedSci (Hons), PhD, FRACP, is Professor and Director of Cardiology at The Queen Elizabeth Hospital, and a Professor of Cardiology at the University of Adelaide, Adelaide, South Australia.

L. Jesuthasan, MBBS, BMedSci, FRACP, is a Staff Specialist in Cardiology at the Queen Elizabeth Hospital, Adelaide, South Australia.

K. Mishra, MBBS, MD, MRCP (UK), FRACP (Cardiology), is a Staff Specialist in Cardiology at the Lyell McEwin Hospital, Adelaide, South Australia.

C. Oldroyd, RGN, PGCE, RNT, Bsc (Hons), MSc, is a Senior Lecturer in Cardiac Nursing, and a member of the Applied Research Group on Pre-hospital, Emergency and Cardiovascular

Care in the Faculty of Health and Life Sciences, Coventry University, UK.

C. Ryan, BN, MNSc, is an Emergency Nurse Practitioner at The Queen Elizabeth Hospital, Adelaide, South Australia.

J. Smith, RN, BA (JUr), MHSc, is a Senior Project Officer in the Aboriginal and Torres Strait Islander Program with the National Heart Foundation of Australia, Adelaide, South Australia.

S.A. Unger, MBBS, FRACP, PhD, is a Staff Cardiologist and the Director of Nuclear Medicine at The Queen Elizabeth and Lyell McEwin Hospitals and as Senior Lecturer at the University of Adelaide, Adelaide, South Australia.

T. Wachtel, RN, MN, Grad. Cert. HD Nursing, MRCNA, is a Lecturer in Nursing and Clinical Coordinator in the School of Nursing and Midwifery, Flinders University, Renmark Campus, South Australia.

R. Webster, RN, BSc (Hons), MSc, is a Senior Nurse for Education and Practice Development for the Cardio-Respiratory Directorate, University Hospitals of Leicester, UK.

P. Whiston, RN, Grad. Dip. Coronary Care, is a Clinical Practice Consultant in the Coronary Care Unit at The Queen Elizabeth Hospital, Adelaide, South Australia.

B.F. Williams, NZRGON MHSc (Hons), is a Research Manager, Pacific Clinical Research Group (PCRG), Sydney, Australia.

C.J. Zeitz, MBBS, PhD, FRACP, OstJ, is Co-Director of Medicine and Emergency Clinical Services, and Director of Interventional Cardiology at the Queen Elizabeth Hospital in Adelaide, and Associate Professor of Rural and Indigenous Cardiovascular Health at the Spencer Gulf Rural Clinical School in Whyalla, South Australia.

Foreword

As the editors of this book cogently remind us, cardiovascular disease touches the lives of virtually everyone. Nurses are invariably at the forefront, working in collaboration with doctors and other health professionals, in providing acute cardiac care, including prevention and rehabilitation, to patients and their families. They have a professional duty to ensure that the care they give is safe and of a high quality and is informed by the best evidence. This requires them keeping up to date with the rapid developments in science and technology, changes in health policy and planning and increased expectations of the profession and the public whom they serve: a major challenge to busy nurses working in cardiac care settings.

Acute Cardiac Care, edited by two authorities in the field, with contributions from recognised experts (nurses, doctors and a paramedic) from both sides of the world, is therefore a welcome resource that will help meet this challenge. It is certainly a practical guide for nurses, presenting in a highly readable way, the essential topics that pertain to acute cardiac care. Each chapter begins with an overview, learning objectives and key concepts, is interspersed with key points and concludes with learning activities, pertinent references and resources and suggested further reading. It deserves to be in the library of every clinical setting where nurses care for patients with acute cardiac conditions.

David R Thompson BSc, MA, PhD, MBA, RN, FRCN, FAAN, FESC
Professor of Cardiovascular Nursing
School of Medicine
University of Leicester
Leicester
UK

July 2009

Preface

Cardiovascular diseases touch the lives of millions of people – patients, their families and friends, together with those who provide and plan care, and those responsible for planning and funding care: in essence, all members of society.

Great advances in scientific knowledge have accumulated since the advent of the cardiac care unit (CCU) in the 1960s, stimulated by the work of a British cardiologist, Professor Desmond Julian, who undertook pioneering work in the UK and Australia that changed the paradigm of care for patients with acute myocardial infarction. Much literature has accumulated on the key role nurses played in the development of the CCU in its formative years, and continue to do so in the present day.

But cardiac nursing is not solely about what happens on the CCU. We believe that nurses are crucial to improved prevention, care and rehabilitation of cardiovascular disease. Whether in the emergency department, cardiac care unit, catheter laboratory, cardiac surgical ward, or in the community setting, or as researchers, managers or policy makers, nurses have opportunities to make a real difference.

As two cardiac nurses with a combined total of more than half a century of experience in acute care, research and policy, we have worked with colleagues with a wide range of experience and knowledge from across our two countries to produce what we hope will be a key resource for nurses embarking on studies of this exciting and constantly evolving arena of practice, and serve as a stimulating source of continuing professional development for more experienced colleagues.

We are grateful to all our contributors for their expertise and commitment, and to Magenta Lampson, Senior Commissioning Editor and Rachel Coombs, Development Editor, Nursing, for their invaluable assistance in bringing this project to fruition.

We dedicate this book to our partners, with thanks for their love and support, and look forward to spending more time with them than we have had in the past 2 years while we've been nursing this book!

Angela Kucia
Adelaide, South Australia

Tom Quinn
Surrey, UK.

1 Mechanics of the Cardiovascular System

B. Greaney & A.M. Kucia

Overview

The cardiovascular system consists of two primary components: the heart and blood vessels. The lymphatic system also has a cardiovascular exchange function but does not contain blood. This chapter will highlight the mechanics of the cardiovascular system and present an overview of the essential elements and structures involved in the flow of blood through the venous and arterial systems. It will also highlight how abnormalities in the mechanics of the cardiovascular system can result in degrees of cardiac disease states.

Learning objectives

After reading this chapter, you should be able to:

- Identify the anatomical location of the heart and its basic function.
- Identify the key structures within the heart, which are involved in the flow of blood through the heart and identify their specific function.
- Define the term 'cardiac cycle' and explain the key physiological changes that occur in the heart during this process.
- Define the terms 'cardiac output' (CO) and 'stroke volume' (SV), and explain their physiological significance in relation to the cardiac cycle.
- Define the terms 'preload', 'afterload' and 'contractility', and explain their physiological impact upon myocardial contraction.

Key concepts

Cardiac cycle; cardiac output; cardiac chambers; cardiac valves; layers of the heart

Basic heart anatomy

The human heart is essentially a muscular pump which delivers blood containing oxygen, nutrients and other vital elements to the body tissues and major organs. The structure and location of the heart was described by Henry Gray in 1918. It is conical in shape, about the size of a human fist and weighs between 230 and 340 g in an adult. The heart is located in the mediastinum, with one-third lying to the right of the sternum and two-thirds to the left. The top of the heart is known as the base, and this is located behind the sternum; the bottom of the heart, known as the apex, is located in the fifth intercostal space in the mid-clavicular line. The heart is a four-chambered structure – the upper chambers known as the right and left atria, the lower two chambers known as the right and left ventricles, with right and left-sided chambers divided by the septum.

The bulk of the heart's wall is the myocardium, which is a thick contractile mass of cardiac muscle cells. It is the myocardium that provides the force of contraction to move blood out of the ventricles at the end of each cardiac cycle. The heart is surrounded by the pericardium, which is comprised of two principal layers that surround and protect the heart. The outer layer is known as the fibrous pericardium, which is made up of tough and fibrous connective tissue. This layer provides both protection and anchorage for the heart. The second layer, the serous pericardium, is a thinner, more delicate layer and forms two distinct layers around the heart. The outer parietal layer is adhered to the inner side of the fibrous pericardium, whilst the inner visceral layer, also known as the epicardium, is adhered tightly to the myocardium. Between these two layers there exists a potential space termed the pericardial cavity. Within this cavity is a very thin film of serous fluid known as pericardial fluid, which is normally between 15 and 35 mL in volume (Spodick 1997). The key function of this fluid is to reduce friction between the pericardial layers as the heart contracts. The inner layer lining the heart is a continuous sheet of squamous epithelium, continuing into the tunica intima of blood vessels, and is known as the endocardium.

The heart is divided into four chambers: two upper atria and two lower ventricles. These chambers are separated by a set of heart valves termed the atrioventricular (AV) valves; the tricuspid valve separates the right atrium (RA) and right ventricle (RV) and the bicuspid valve or mitral valve separates the left atrium (LA) and left ventricle (LV) (Figure 1.1a). Attached to each AV valve are two structures: the chordae tendinae and the papillary muscles. These two structures are adhered to the walls of each ventricle (Figure 1.1a). Their function is to prevent the valve cusps inverting or swinging upward into the atria during ventricular systole. The key function of the heart valves is to permit the flow of blood in one direction only as it flows through the heart.

The heart can be viewed functionally as two pumps serving the pulmonary and systemic circulations. The pulmonary circulation refers to the flow of blood within the lungs that is involved in the exchange of gases between the blood and the alveoli. Deoxygenated blood returns to the RA via the inferior and superior vena cavae. It then passes through the tricuspid valve to the RV before entering the pulmonary circulation via the pulmonary artery, where gases are exchanged. The pulmonary artery has a pulmonary valve or semilunar valve which opens and closes during contraction and relaxation of the heart, again having a similar function to the AV valves, allowing the flow of blood in one direction only (Figure 1.1). The systemic circulation consists of all the blood vessels within and outside of all organs excluding the lungs. Once oxygenated, the blood returns to the LA via the pulmonary veins and then passes through the mitral valve into the thicker-walled left ventricle, which ejects the oxygenated blood through the aortic valve into the aorta and into the systemic circulation. The aorta also has a valve, the aortic valve, which prevents the backflow of blood during myocardial contraction (Figure 1.1a).

The cardiac cycle

In simple terms, the heart is a pump that receives blood from the venous system at low pressure and generates pressure through contraction to eject the blood into the arterial system. The mechanical action of the heart is created by a synchronised contraction and relaxation of the cardiac muscle, referred to as systole and diastole. The actual mechanical function of the heart is influenced by pressure, volume and flow changes that occur within the heart during one single cardiac cycle.

When the heart muscle contracts (systole) and relaxes (diastole), sequential changes in pressure are produced in the heart chambers and blood vessels, which result in blood flowing from areas of high pressure to areas of lower pressure. The valves prevent backflow of blood. Under normal conditions, this cycle will take place in the human heart between 60 and 100 times per minute.

Figure 1.2a demonstrates the seven phases of the cardiac cycle.

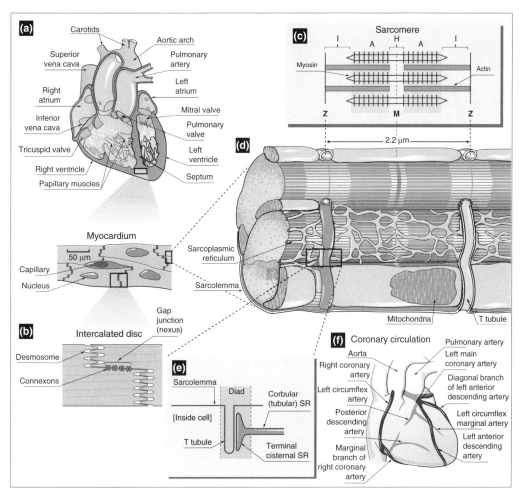

Figure 1.1   Gross anatomy of the heart.
Source: From Aaronson and Ward (2007).

Phase 1: Atrial systole

Atrial systole begins after a wave of depolarisation passes over the atrial muscle. Atrial depolarisation is represented by the P wave on the electrocardiograph (ECG). As the atria contract, pressure builds up inside the atria forcing blood through the tricuspid and mitral valves into the ventricles. Atrial contraction causes a small increase in proximal venous pressure (in the pulmonary veins and vena cavae). This is represented by the 'a' wave of the jugular venous pulse, which is used to measure jugular venous pressure (JVP) (Klabunde 2005).

- Blood flows from the RA across the tricuspid valve into the RV.
- Blood flows from the LA through the mitral valve into the LV.

Pressure in the atria falls and the AV valves float upward. Ventricular volumes are now at their maximum (around 120 mL) and this is known as end diastolic volume (EDV). Left ventricular end diastolic pressure (LVEDP) is approximately 8–12 mmHg; right ventricular end diastolic pressure (RVEDP) is usually around 3–6 mmHg. A fourth heart sound (S4) may be heard in this phase if ventricular compliance is reduced, such

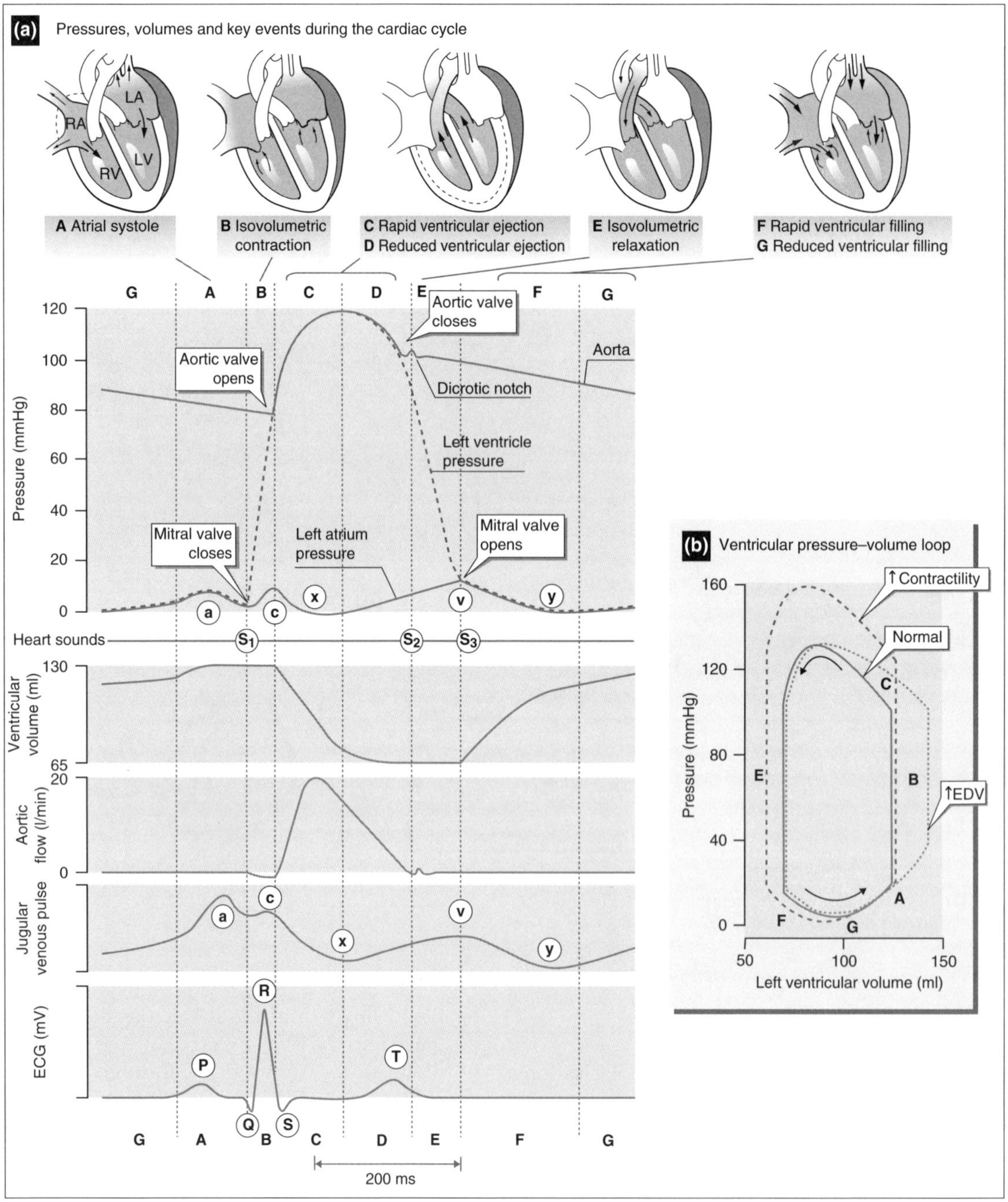

Figure 1.2   Cardiac cycle.
Source: From Aaronson and Ward (2007).

as happens with ventricular hypertrophy, ischae-mia or as a common finding in older individuals.

> ## Key point
>
> Ventricular filling occurs passively before the atria contract and depends upon venous return. Atrial contraction normally accounts for only around 10% of ventricular filling, when the body is at rest. However, at high heart rates (such as during exer-cise), there is a shortened period of diastole where passive filling normally occurs. Under these con-ditions, atrial contraction is more important and can contribute up to 40% of ventricular filling. Enhanced ventricular filling due to atrial contrac-tion is sometimes referred to as the 'atrial kick' (Klabunde 2005).

Phase 2: Isovolumetric contraction

This phase is represented by the QRS complex on the ECG. The ventricle depolarises and initiates contraction of the myocytes, resulting in a rapid increase in ventricular pressure. This rise in pres-sure causes the AV valves to close. Closure of the AV valves generates the first heart sound (S1). A split S1 may be heard as mitral valve closure precedes tricuspid valve closure by around 0.04 of a second, although usually only one sound can be heard through a stethoscope. The time between closure of the AV valves and opening of the semi-lunar valves is known as isovolumetric contrac-tion because there is no change in the volume of blood in the ventricle at this stage, although the ventricle contracts and becomes more spheroid in shape. The pressure in the LV becomes maximal at this stage and is termed dp/dt (maximal slope of the ventricular pressure tracing/time) (Klabunde 2005).

Phase 3: Rapid ventricular ejection

When the ventricular pressure exceeds that of the aorta (around 80 mmHg) and pulmonary arter-ies (around 10 mmHg) the aortic and pulmonary valves open and blood is ejected out of the ventri-cles. The LV has a thick muscular wall that allows it to generate high pressures during ventricular

contraction. Maximal outflow velocity occurs early in the ejection phase, so the highest aortic and pul-monary artery pressures are reached at this time (Klabunde 2005).

- Blood is ejected from the RV across the pulmo-nic valve and into the pulmonary artery to the pulmonary circulation.
- Blood is ejected from the LV across the aor-tic valve and into the aorta to the systemic circulation.

Between 70 and 90 mL of blood is ejected with each stroke (stroke volume), but about 50 mL remains in each ventricle. The residual amount of blood left in the ventricle is known as the end-systolic volume (ESV). Stroke volume thus is the difference between EDV and ESV. Around 60% of the total volume of the ventricle is ejected in each cycle. To work out the ejection fraction of the ven-tricle, divide the stroke volume by the EDV. The normal left ventricular ejection fraction (LVEF) is above 55% (Klabunde 2005).

> ## Key point
>
> In the healthy heart, no heart sounds should be heard during the ejection phase of the cardiac cycle. The presence of sounds during ejection indicates valvular disease or intracardiac shunts (Klabunde 2005).

Phase 4: Reduced ventricular ejection

The ventricle relaxes and the rate of ejection begins to fall, although kinetic or inertial energy continues to propel the blood forward into the aorta. This phase coincides with ventricular repo-larisation, which occurs approximately 150–200 ms after the QRS complex and appears as the T wave on the ECG. Atrial pressure starts to rise during this phase due to venous return (Klabunde 2005).

- The RA receives blood from the systemic circu-lation via the inferior and superior vena cavae at a low pressure (approximately 0–4 mmHg).
- After circulating through the lungs, blood returns to the heart via the four pulmonary veins into the LA. The pressure in the LA is usually between 8–12 mmHg.

Phase 5: Isovolumetric relaxation

In this phase, the pressure in the ventricles continues to fall and when the point is reached where the pressure is less in the ventricles than that in the outflow tracts (aorta and pulmonary veins), the aortic and pulmonary valves close abruptly, causing a second heart sound (S2). Aortic and pulmonary artery pressures fall slowly due to a combination of stored energy in the elastic walls of these vessels which controls pressure and flow, and because forward flow is impeded by systemic and pulmonic vascular resistance as blood is distributed through the systemic and pulmonary circulations (Klabunde 2005).

Key point

As the aortic valve closes before the pulmonic valve, there is a physiological splitting of the S2 sound and this may be heard with a stethoscope. Closure of the aortic and pulmonary valves result in a characteristic notch in aortic and pulmonary artery pressure tracings (Figure 1.2a). The aortic notch is important in setting timing for intra-aortic balloon counterpulsation.

Phase 6: Rapid ventricular filling

Low pressures in the heart allow blood to passively return to the atria. When the ventricular pressure falls below the atrial pressure, the AV valves open and the ventricles fill quickly. Blood flows into the atria and ventricles throughout diastole with the rate of filling decreasing as the amount of blood in the chambers distends the walls. About 70% of ventricular filling occurs passively at this time.

Key point

No prominent heart sounds should be heard at this time. If a third heart sound (S3) is heard during ventricular filling in adults, it may indicate tensing of the chordae tendinae and AV ring, often associated with ventricular dilation. It is a normal finding in children.

Phase 7: Reduced ventricular filling

There is no clear demarcation as to when this phase begins, but this is a stage during diastole when passive ventricular filling is near completion. As the ventricles fill, they become less compliant, causing intraventricular pressure to rise and the rate of ventricular filling starts to fall. Immediately following this phase, atrial systole occurs following firing of the sino-atrial node.

Key point

At slow heart rates, diastole is lengthened, resulting in increased filling time. In rapid heart rates, there is less filling time. This would compromise CO, if not for compensatory mechanisms.

Cardiac output

CO is an important index of cardiac function, and refers to the amount of blood that is ejected with each contraction (stroke volume) multiplied by heart rate (HR):

$$CO = SV \times HR$$

At typical resting values, if the heart rate is 75 beats/min and the stroke volume is 70 mL/beat, the CO should equal 5.25 L/min. Therefore the body's total volume of blood (4–6 L/min) passes through the body each minute (Saladin 2001).

CO never remains at a constant rate: any factor that alters stroke volume or heart rate will alter CO and it can vary significantly according to normal physical exercise as well as impaired cardiac function. Other factors such as preload, afterload and contractility (inotropy) will indirectly affect CO.

Preload is defined as the actual stretch or tension on the ventricular myocardium prior to contraction (Totora & Gabowski 2002). The greater the preload on the myocardium (the larger the amount of blood that has filled the heart during diastole), the greater the contraction will be. A simple analogy to explain this concept is that the further you stretch an elastic band prior to releasing it, the further it will recoil. The same principle applies here: the greater the stretch or tension on the myocardium, the greater the force of contraction. When venous return to the heart increases, ventricular filling and preload also increase. The Frank Starling Law of the Heart (Starling's Law) asserts that the more the ventricle is filled with blood during diastole (EDV), the greater the volume of blood that will be ejected (stroke volume) during the ensuing systolic contraction. Thus, altered preload is a mechanism by which the force of contractility can be affected (Klabunde 2005).

Contractility, also known as inotropy, is the ability of a cardiac myocyte to alter its tension development independently of preload changes (Klabunde 2005). Contractility is affected by autonomic innervation and circulating catecholamines (adrenaline, noradrenaline), and additionally changes in afterload and heart rate can augment contractility. A number of pharmacological agents positively or negatively affect contractility. Agents that affect contractility are called positive or negative inotropes, depending upon whether they increase or decrease contractility. Loss of myocardial contractility results in heart failure.

Afterload is defined as the force or pressure against which the ventricular myocardium must push prior to contraction (Totora & Grabowski 2003). This force or pressure is constantly present in the arteries as arterial blood pressure. Therefore, any increase in systemic blood pressure will result in the left ventricular myocardium having to contract more forcefully to eject its volume of blood. Any increase in the pressure of the pulmonary circulation, such as pulmonary oedema, or the presence of any physical obstruction to the pulmonary circulation, such as lung scar tissue, will result in the right ventricular myocardium having to contract more forcefully. In the long term, this increased workload for the myocardium will eventually result in the abnormal enlargement of the myocardium (hypertrophy), which may in turn lead to heart failure.

Key point

The myocardium requires oxygen to regenerate adenosine triphosphate (ATP) that is hydrolysed to produce energy during contraction and relaxation. Any change to the force or frequency of contraction will have an effect on myocardial oxygen consumption (MVO_2). Imbalances in the supply and demand of oxygen to the myocardium may result in myocardial ischaemia or infarction.

Conclusion

This chapter has provided you with an overview of anatomical and physiological underpinnings underlying much of the assessment and nursing care of the patient with a cardiovascular disorder. When next you check a patient's heart rate or blood pressure, or listen to their heart sounds, consider in detail the anatomical and physiological determinants of those measures.

Learning activities

There are a number of interactive online websites where you can test your knowledge of cardiac anatomy and physiology. The Columbia University Medical Center Department of Surgery in New York has some great heart animations and information at http://www.columbiasurgery.org/pat/cardiac/anatomy.html

The Texas Heart Institute at St Luke's Episcopal Hospital Heart Information Center likewise has some good cardiovascular information and animations at http://texasheart.org/HIC/Anatomy/index.cfm

---

References

Aaronson, P.I. & Ward, J.P.T. (2007). *The Cardiovascular System at a Glance3E*. Wiley Blackwell, Oxford.

Gray, H. (1918). *Anatomy of the Human Body*. Lea & Febiger, Philadelphia.

Klabunde, R. (2005). *Cardiovascular Physiology Concepts*. Lippincott Williams & Wilkins, Philadelphia.

Saladin, K.S. (2001). *Anatomy & physiology: The Unity of Form & Function*. McGraw Hill, New York.

Spodick, D.H. (1997). Pericardial macro- and micro-anatomy: A synopsis. In: D.H. Spodick, (ed.), *The Pericardium: A Comprehensive Textbook*. Marcel Dekker, New York, pp. 7–14.

Totora, G.J. & Grabowski, S.R. (2003). *Principles of Anatomy and Physiology*, 10th edn. John Wiley & Sons, New Jersey.

Useful Websites and Further Reading

Klabunde, R.E. (2007). Cardiovascular physiology concepts. Retrieved online 4th October 2007 from http://www.cvphysiology.com/

Rogers, J. (1999). Cardiovascular physiology. Retrieved online 4th October 2007 from http://www.nda.ox.ac.uk/wfsa/html/u10/u1002_01.htm

2 Regulation of Cardiac and Vascular Function

B. Greaney & A.M. Kucia

Overview

Regulation of cardiac and vascular function is somewhat complex and involves autonomic nerves and circulating hormones. You will hear this referred to as 'neurohumoral control of the cardiovascular system'. These mechanisms control cardiac output, blood pressure and local control of blood flow in response to physiological requirements and in the setting of an adverse clinical event such as trauma, disease or stress. In turn, neurohumoral control is influenced by sensors that monitor blood pressure (baroreceptors), blood volume (volume receptors), blood chemistry (chemoreceptors) and plasma osmolarity (osmoreceptors). These sensors work together to maintain arterial pressure at a level that is adequate for organ perfusion (Klabunde 2005). This chapter reviews the mechanisms involved in neurohumoral controls of the cardiovascular system.

Learning objectives

After reading this chapter, you should be able to:

- Describe the components of the autonomic nervous system that relate to cardiac function.
- Describe the effects of sympathetic and parasympathetic stimulation on the cardiovascular system.

- Discuss the function of baroreceptors in the regulation of arterial pressure.
- Discuss the function of chemoreceptors in the regulation of respiratory activity and arterial pressure.
- List the chemicals that can stimulate the heart and cardiovascular system and describe their negative and positive effects.

Key concepts

Neurohumoral control; sympathetic and parasympathetic nervous system; baroreceptors; chemoreceptors; blood pressure regulation

Central nervous system regulation of the cardiovascular system

The central nervous system (CNS) controls the autonomic regulation of cardiovascular function. Autonomic refers to functions of the nervous system that are not under voluntary control (such as regulation of heart rate). The heart is innervated by both parasympathetic and sympathetic nerve fibres. These fibres together play a vital role in the control of heart rate and contractility, as well as regulation of blood pressure. These nerve fibres are conveyed directly to the heart from the cardiovascular centre located in the medulla oblongata of the brain, which is the main region for nervous system regulation of the heart and blood vessels (Totora & Grabowski 2003). Parasympathetic innervation is associated with the cardioinhibitory centre of the cardiovascular centre, and sympathetic innervation is associated with the cardioacceleratory centre (also known as cardiostimulatory centre) of the cardiovascular centre.

The cardioinhibitory centre sends signals via parasympathetic fibres in the vagus nerve to the sino-atrial (SA) and atrio-ventricular (AV) nodes, conduction pathways, myocytes and coronary vasculature. The right vagus nerve predominantly innervates the SA node, and the left vagus nerve innervates the AV node and ventricular conduction system. Nerve fibres in the parasympathetic nervous system are cholinergic, which means they release acetylcholine. Acetylcholine binds to muscarinic receptors which are specifically associated with vagal nerve endings in the heart, resulting in negative chronotropy (decreased heart rate); negative inotropy (decreased contractility, more so in the atria than the ventricles) and negative dromotropy (decreased conduction velocity).

The cardioacceleratory centre sends signals by way of the thoracic spinal cord and sympathetic cardiac accelerator nerves to the SA node, AV node and myocardium. These nerves secrete norepinephrine, which binds to β-adrenergic receptors in the heart. The term 'pressor' is sometimes used to describe the responses associated with sympathetic stimulation on the heart, which are positive chronotropy (increased heart rate); positive inotropy (increased contractility, more so in the atria than the ventricles) and positive dromotropy (increased conduction velocity).

Key point

It is important to note that despite this continual regulation of the heart, the SA and AV nodes are autorhythmic: they fire at their own intrinsic rate (see Chapter 3 for further detail). Therefore, if parasympathetic and sympathetic nerve fibres to these nodes were severed, the heart would continue to

---

beat at its own intrinsic rate. Parasympathetic activity, or vagal tone, is the dominant controlling factor of heart rate and it inhibits the nodes to a normal rate of 70–80 beats per minute (bpm). Maximum vagal stimulation can reduce the heart rate to as low as 20 bpm (Saladin 2001). In clinical situations, where a patient's heart rate has become dangerously low due to myocardial infarction, ischaemia or other reasons, the drug atropine, a vagal nerve blocker, may be used to block vagal stimulation on the heart, allowing sympathetic nerve fibres to be the dominant nervous stimulus, producing an increase in the heart rate. Parasympathetic activity in the heart inhibits sympathetic activity and vice versa (Klabunde 2005).

The cardiovascular centre receives both neural and chemical input from many sources. Stimuli such as exercise, anxiety, fear, pyrexia and pain will act upon the cardiovascular centre via higher centres in the brain such as the cerebral cortex, the limbic system and the hypothalamus. A number of specific mechanisms exist at various locations in the body which control and regulate the heart and vascular system in response to such factors. Sudden fear or emotion, for example, may cause vagal stimulation resulting in bradycardia, loss of vascular tone and fainting (vasovagal syncope) (Klabunde 2005).

Vasomotor control

As described, the CNS plays an important role in regulating systemic vascular resistance (SVR) and cardiac function which in turn influence arterial blood pressure. The distribution of blood, as well as the control of arterial blood pressure, can be influenced by factors that control changes in the diameter of blood vessels. The vasomotor centre controls sympathetic activation of the vascular system and is located in the medulla of the brain. Sympathetic activation causes an impulse outflow via sympathetic fibres that terminate in the smooth muscle tissue of both resistance (arteries and arterioles) and capacitance (veins and venules) vessels, causing constriction. This increases SVR and thus arterial blood pressure.

Baroreceptors

Arterial blood pressure is regulated through a negative feedback system which uses pressure sensors, known as baroreceptors, located in the carotid sinus and aortic arch and the bifurcation of the subclavian artery (Bridges 2005). These baroreceptors are sensitive to changes in pressure or stretch in the vessels walls where they are located. They are also sensitive to the rate of pressure change and to a steady (mean) pressure.

To understand how baroreceptors function, let us consider what happens in the physiologic circumstance of when a person suddenly changes from a reclining position to one of standing as in Figure 2.1.

In addition to arterial baroreceptors, there are stretch receptors located at the veno-atrial junctions of the heart that respond to atrial filling and contraction (Klabunde 2005). Low-pressure baroreceptors are located in the atria, ventricles, pulmonary artery and veins that are sensitive to changes in transmural pressure in these chambers or vessels.

Standing (from reclining position)

⇩

Gravity causes blood pooling below the heart

⇩

Decreased venous return

Decreased central venous pressure

Decreased ventricular preload

⇩

Decreased cardiac output

Decreased arterial blood pressure

Reduced stretching of arterial baroreceptors

⇩

The cardiovascular centre in the medulla responds by:

increasing sympathetic activity

⇩

increased cardiac output

⇩

increased arterial blood pressure

⇩

increased stretching of arterial baroreceptors

Figure 2.1   Physiological changes to cardiac output associated with body position change.

Learning activity

Carotid sinus massage is sometimes used to abort some forms of supraventricular tachycardia. Considering the action of baroreceptors, how do you think this works?

Clinical states such as hypovolaemia may result in the vascular system recruiting blood from the reservoirs found in the venous plexuses and sinuses in the skin and abdominal organs, especially the liver and spleen (Thibodeau & Patton 2007). Blood can be shifted quickly out of these reservoirs to arteries that supply heart and skeletal muscles when increased activity demands.

Key point

Stimulation of certain mechanoreceptors (sensory receptors that respond to mechanical pressure or distortion), and chemoreceptors in the heart and coronary arteries can result in a vagally mediated triad of bradycardia, apnoea and hypotension (Bridges 2005) known as the Bezold–Jarisch reflex. This happens commonly when dye is injected into the coronary arteries during coronary angiography or during ischaemia/reperfusion involving the infero-posterior wall of the left ventricle.

Chemoreceptors

Chemoreceptors are specialised cells that have a significant role in the regulation of respiratory activity to maintain arterial blood PO_2, PCO_2 and pH within a physiologic range (Klabunde 2005). These receptors are sensitive to small changes in oxygen levels but are more sensitive to abnormal carbon dioxide and hydrogen ion levels in the blood plasma. Abnormal levels of any of these substances trigger the chemoreceptors to send impulses to the cardiovascular centre. In response, the cardiovascular centre increases sympathetic stimulation to the smooth muscle of arterioles and veins, bringing about vasoconstriction and a subsequent increase in arterial blood pressure and heart rate, thus improving tissue perfusion. Peripheral chemoreceptors are located in the aortic arch (known as the aortic bodies) and in the carotid arteries (known as the carotid bodies), and are responsive to hypoxaemia (decreased arterial PO_2), hypercapnia (increased arterial PCO_2) and hydrogen ion concentration (acidosis). Central chemoreceptors are located within the medulla of the brain (central chemoreceptors) and are responsive to hypercapnia and acidosis but not directly to hypoxia (Klabunde 2005). Stimulation of these receptors leads to hyperventilation and sympathetic activation causing vasoconstriction in most vascular beds except those of the brain and heart (Bridges 2005). Although the chemoreceptor reflex results in an increase in arterial blood pressure, this rise will be mediated by the baroreceptor response.

Key point

Central and peripheral chemoreceptor responses may be enhanced in heart failure patients, resulting in increased sympathetic activation which may contribute to sleep apnoea in those patients and is associated with a poor prognosis (Javaheri 2003; Narkiewicz & Somers 2003).

Humoral control

There are a number of naturally produced chemicals (humoral substances) in the body that significantly effect the action of the heart and vascular system. These can have both positive and negative effects. These include circulating catecholamines, the renin-angiotensin-aldosterone system (RAAS), atrial natriuretic peptide (ANP) and antidiuretic

hormone (ADH) (vasopressin). Other substances such as thyroxine, oestrogen, insulin and growth hormone also have direct or indirect effects on the cardiovascular system (Klabunde 2005).

Epinephrine (adrenalin) and norepinephrine (noradrenalin) are classed as non-steroid hormones called catecholamines and are particularly potent cardiac stimulants. They are secreted by the adrenal medulla and cardiac accelerator nerves in response to arousal, stress (physical or emotional) and exercise (Saladin 2001) and are associated with the body's 'fight and flight' reflex. Epinephrine accounts for about 80% of the adrenal medullas secretion, the other 20% is norepinephrine (Thibodeau & Patton 2007). When secreted into the bloodstream, epinephrine prepares the body to respond to an acute stressor by increasing the supply of oxygen and glucose to the brain and muscles, while suppressing other non-emergency bodily processes such as digestion (fight or flight mechanism). It binds to numerous adrenergic receptors (β_1, β_2, α_1 and α_2) throughout the body, although it has a greater affinity for β-adrenoreceptors than α-adrenoreceptors. Therefore, when plasma levels of epinephrine are low, it will bind preferentially to β-adrenoreceptors. This is important to know because heart rate, inotropy and dromotropy are mainly mediated by β_1-adrenoreceptors (Klabunde 2005). Low dose epinephrine binds to β_2-adrenoreceptors in skeletal muscle and splanchnic arterioles, triggering vasodilation. However, when epinephrine binds with α-adrenergic receptors that are found in smooth muscle in the walls of blood vessels, it causes vasoconstriction. Blood pressure is increased due to the resulting increase in cardiac output and SVR.

Key point

When epinephrine is administered exogenously, its effects are dose related. Low dose epinephrine stimulates the β-adrenoreceptors resulting in vasodilation and increased heart rate and contractility. Higher doses stimulate the α-adrenoreceptors, increasing vascular resistance and blood pressure. Thus, if the intent of epinephrine administration is vasoconstriction, it is important to administer a large enough dose to achieve this effect (Bridges 2005).

Circulating norepinephrine transiently increases heart rate and increases β_1-adrenoreceptor-mediated inotropy. It causes vasoconstriction in most systemic arteries and veins (α_1 and α_2 adrenoreceptors). The overall effect is increased cardiac output and SVR leading to an increase in arterial blood pressure. The initial increase in heart rate is not sustained due to activation of baroreceptors which cause vagal-mediated slowing of heart rate (Klabunde 2007).

Learning activity

β-blockers are drugs that bind to β-adrenoceptors, blocking the ability of norepinephrine and epinephrine to bind to these receptors. The first generation of β-blocking drugs were 'non-selective' – what does this mean and what disadvantage does this have?

Second generation β-blockers are said to be more 'cardioselective' – what does this mean and which beta blockers are 'cardioselective'?

Third generation β-blockers have vasodilator actions through blockade of α-adrenoreceptors. Which drugs are included in this class?

Arginine vasopressin (AVP), commonly known as antidiuretic hormone (ADH), is a peptide hormone produced in the hypothalamus and stored in the posterior pituitary gland, and is mainly released into the bloodstream (and some directly into the brain) in response to increased plasma osmolality (detected by osmoreceptors in the hypothalamus). AVP may also be secreted in response to decreased blood volume or blood pressure (detected by baroreceptors), but this is a less sensitive mechanism than osmolality. AVP causes the kidneys to conserve water (but not sodium) by concentrating the urine and reducing urine volume, and elevates blood pressure through vasoconstriction.

Natriuretic peptides are hormones that are involved in the homeostatic regulation of blood pressure, volume and electrolytes. Atrial natriuretic peptide (ANP) is released from the walls of the atria, and brain (B-type) natriuretic peptide (BNP) from the walls of the ventricles in response to increased stretch or hormonal stimuli (angiotensin II, catecholamines, glucocorticoids,

endothelin 1). C-type natriuretic peptide (CNP) is distributed throughout the heart, brain, lungs, kidneys and endothelin and is released in response to stress. Natriuretic peptides increase excretion of sodium and water and inhibit sodium reabsorption, thereby reducing blood pressure. They also inhibit activation of the RAAS.

Key point

Evidence from clinical trials suggests that short-term administration of intravenous BNP (nesiritide) may be effective in improving haemodynamic function and reducing symptoms of acute decompensated heart failure (Mills et al. 1999; Colucci et al. 2000; Keating & Goa 2003), although a trend towards an increase in early mortality in nesiritide-treated patients has raised some safety concerns (Aaronson & Sackner-Bernstein 2005).

The RAAS is a hormone system that has a role in regulating long-term blood pressure and extracellular fluid volume. A number of hormones and enzymes which are significant in the RAAS cause both vasodilation and vasoconstriction, and therefore influence arterial blood pressure in specific clinical and associated disease states.

The RAAS has a cascade effect (Figure 2.2) that is triggered by renin release from the kidney in response to sympathetic nerve activation (acting via β_1-adrenoceptors); renal artery hypotension (caused by systemic hypotension or renal artery stenosis) or decreased sodium delivery to the distal tubules of the kidney (Klabunde 2007). When renin is released into the bloodstream, it acts upon a circulating substrate, angiotensinogen, which through the process of proteolytic cleavage becomes angiotensin I. Angiotensin converting enzyme, found mainly in vascular endothelium in the lungs, converts angiotensin I to angiotensin II. Angiotensin II is a powerful substance that causes vasoconstriction in the resistance vessels leading to increased SVR and arterial pressure and stimulates the adrenal cortex to release aldosterone which acts on the kidneys to increase sodium and fluid retention. It also stimulates the posterior pituitary to release AVP (ADH) which acts on the kidneys to increase fluid retention, stimulates

Regulation of Cardiac and Vascular Function   13

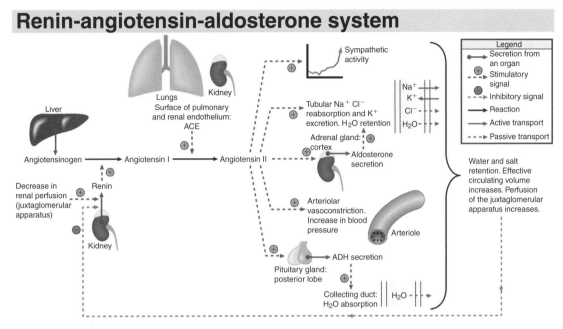

Figure 2.2   The renin-angiotensin-aldosterone system (RAAS).
Source: Reproduced from Rad (2006). Copyright 2006.

thirst centres within the brain and enhances sympathetic adrenergic function by facilitating the release of norepinephrine from sympathetic nerve endings and inhibiting its reuptake. The net effect of this cascade is to maintain blood pressure and volume. Natriuretic peptides modulate the function of the RAAS and have an important counter-regulatory influence (Klabunde 2007).

Learning activity

Knowledge of the RAAS pathway is necessary in understanding the action of drugs used to treat heart failure and hypertension, as the RAAS is often the target of therapeutic manipulation in treating these conditions. Review the drugs used to treat hypertension and heart failure and their actions on the RAAS.

Electrolytes

Potassium, sodium and calcium have an influence on heart rate and rhythm through their role in action potentials (see Chapter 3). Elevated blood levels of potassium and sodium decrease heart rate and the contractility of the heart, but a moderate increase in extracellular and intracellular calcium levels increases both heart rate and contractility (Totora & Grabowski 2003). Potassium also appears to induce vasodilation, though its specific role in vaso-regulatory processes has not yet been fully elucidated (Berne & Levy 2001).

Conclusion

This chapter has provided an overview of the regulation of cardiovascular function. The processes and mechanisms by which the cardiovascular system is regulated are many and complex. It is important for nurses to have a broad understanding of these mechanisms in order to recognise any disturbance in neurohumoral control that might compromise the patient, and also to understand the actions of a number of pharmacological substances that are utilised to therapeutically manipulate neurohumoral processes.

References

Aaronson, K.D. & Sackner-Bernstein, J. (2005). Risk of death associated with nesiritide in patients with acutely decompensated heart failure. *Journal of the American Medical Association*, **296**:1465.

Bridges, E.J. (2005). Regulation of cardiac output and blood pressure. In: S.L. Woods, E.S.S. Froelicher, S.U. Motzer & E.J. Bridges (eds), *Cardiac Nursing*, 5th edn. Lippincott Williams and Wilkins, Philadelphia, pp. 81–108.

Berne, R.M. & Levy, M.N. (2001). *Cardiovascular Physiology*, 8th edn. Mosby, Philadelphia.

Colucci, W.S., Elkayam, U., Horton, D.P., et al. (2000). Intravenous nesiritide, a natriuretic peptide, in the treatment of decompensated congestive heart failure. *The New England Journal of Medicine*, **343**:246–53.

Javaheri, S. (2003). Heart failure and sleep apnea: emphasis on practical therapeutic options. *Clinics in Chest Medicine*, **24**:207–22.

Keating, G.M. & Goa, K.L. (2003). Nesiritide: a review of its use in acute decompensated heart failure. *Drugs*, **63**:47–70.

Klabunde, R. (2005). *Cardiovascular Physiology Concepts*. Lippincott Williams & Wilkins, Philadelphia.

Klabunde, R.E. (2007). Cardiovascular physiology concepts. Retrieved online 12th October 2007 from http://www.cvphysiology.com/index.html

Mills, R.M., LeJemtel, T.H., Horton, D.P., et al. (1999). Sustained hemodynamic effects of an infusion of nesiritide (human b-type natriuretic peptide) in heart failure: a randomised, double-blind, placebo-controlled clinical trial. *Journal of the American College of Cardiology*, **34**:155–62.

Narkiewicz, K. & Somers, V.K. (2003). Sympathetic nerve activity in obstructive sleep apnoea. *Acta Physiologica Scandanavia*, **177**:385–90.

Rad, A. (2006). The renin-angiotensin system. Retrieved online 2nd February 2009 from http://en.wikipedia.org/wiki/Renin_angiotensin_aldosterone_system

Saladin, K.S. (2001). *Anatomy & Physiology: The Unity of Form & Function*. McGraw Hill, New York.

Thibodeau, G.A. & Patton, K.T. (2007). *Anatomy & Physiology*, 8th edn. Mosby, Philadelphia.

Totora, G.J. & Grabowski, S.R. (2003). *Principles of Anatomy and Physiology*, 10th edn. John Wiley & Sons, New Jersey.

Useful Websites and Further Reading

Klabunde, R.E. (2007). Cardiovascular physiology concepts. Retrieved online 12th October 2007 from http://www.cvphysiology.com/index.html

3 Cardiac Electrophysiology

B. Greaney & A.M. Kucia

Overview

This chapter outlines the anatomy and physiology of the conduction system of the heart and the vital role it plays in the overall function of the heart. An understanding of cardiac electrophysiology will provide a basis for interpretation of the 12-lead electrocardiogram (ECG), and the impact that myocardial ischaemia and other metabolic derangements have upon the 12-lead ECG. This chapter will also facilitate an understanding of the electrophysiological basis of arrhythmia generation, the pharmacological actions of certain classes of medications and the underlying physiological concepts related to defibrillation and cardioversion.

Learning objectives

After reading this chapter, you should be able to:

- Describe the structure and function of cardiac myocytes and autorhythmic cells.
- Describe the process of action potentials within the myocardium.
- Name the key components of the heart's conduction system.
- Describe the specific anatomical location of the key components of the heart's conduction system.
- Relate the specific electrophysiological events in the cardiac cycle to the generation of ECG waveforms.

Key concepts

Electrophysiology; automaticity; contractility; action potential; cardiac conduction system

Cardiac cells

When referring to the electrophysiology of the heart, we are describing the overall electrical activity within the myocardium, which plays a vital role in the overall effective function of the heart. The conduction system is made up of a series of specific structures within the myocardium, which are still essentially part of the cardiac muscle, but are modified enough in their structure and function to be significantly different from ordinary cardiac muscle (Thibodeau & Patton 2007). The main function of the cardiac cells is to contract. Contraction is initiated by electrical changes within the cardiac cells making up the cardiac muscle (myocardium). The myocardium is mainly composed of muscle cells that can be classified into two types: contractile cells that account for around 99% of cardiac cells, and autorhythmic cells that account for the remaining 1%.

Contractile cells (myocytes) have an elongated structure and are connected to adjacent cells by intercalated discs. Gap junctions between the cells allow electrical (ionic) conduction to pass between neighbouring cells, allowing the heart to contract as a single unit. The myocyte cell membrane (sarcolemma) contains long, tubular invaginations called transverse T tubules that extend in-between myofibrils to facilitate rapid calcium influx during depolarisation. Cardiac myocytes are composed of bundles of myofibrils that contain sarcomeres, the basic contractile units of the myocyte, which are aligned with each other and separated by Z lines. Sarcomeres are composed of thick and thin filaments – myosin and actin, respectively – which are important in myocardial contraction. Using adenosine triphosphate (ATP) for energy, filaments of actin chemically link and unlink with those of myosin, resulting in cardiac contraction and relaxation. Between the actin strands are rod-shaped proteins known as tropomyosin to which the troponin complex is attached at regular intervals (see Figure 1.1a). The troponin complex is responsible for the regulation of actin–myosin function and is made up of three subunits: troponin-T (TN-T), troponin-C (TN-C) and troponin-I (TN-I).

Key point

Troponin-I and troponin-T are released into the circulation when myocytes die – they are measured and used as diagnostic markers of myocardial infarction.

Autorhythmic cells have the ability to generate electrical activity without an external stimulus and are found in the sinoatrial (SA) node, atrioventricular (AV) node, bundles of His and Purkinje fibres.

The action potential

All living cells in the body have an electrical potential across the cell membrane. This can be measured by inserting a microelectrode into the cell and measuring the electrical potential in millivolts (mV) inside the cell relative to that outside the cell. At rest, a ventricular myocyte has a membrane potential of around $-90\,mV$, and this is known as the resting membrane potential (Em). Em is determined by a combination of the concentrations of

negatively and positively charged electrons across the cell membrane, the relative permeability of the cell membrane to these ions and the function of the ionic pumps that transport ions across the cell membrane (Klabunde 2005). The primary ions involved in the determination of cell membrane potential are sodium (Na^+), chloride (Cl^-), potassium (K^+) and calcium (Ca^{++}). The cardiac action potential is the electrical activity of the individual cells of the heart that occurs through changes in the cell membrane, permitting the inward and outward flow of ions, resulting in:

- depolarisation, which occurs when the interior of the cardiac cell is maximally charged with positive ions; and
- repolarisation, the process of restoration of a cell to its normal resting membrane polarity following depolarisation.

Cardiac action potentials act in a similar manner to other action potentials within the human body, excepting the extended contraction time requirement of the cardiac muscle to effectively move blood through the heart and lungs and into the systemic circulation. The duration of ventricular action potentials range from 200 to 400 ms, compared to 2–5 ms in skeletal muscle cells or 1 ms in a typical nerve cell (Klabunde 2005).

As outlined earlier in this chapter, there are two types of cells in the heart: myocytes (non-pacemaker cells) and autorhythmic (pacemaker) cells. These cells have different action potentials. Non-pacemaker action potentials are triggered by depolarisation currents from adjacent cells, whereas pacemaker action potentials are capable of spontaneous action potential generation, known as automaticity (Klabunde 2005).

Key point

The electrical activity of cardiac myocytes (non-pacemaker cells) is apparent on the ECG. The electrical activity of the specialized conduction tissues (pacemaker cells) are not apparent on the surface ECG because of the relatively small mass of these tissues compared to the myocardium. Pacemaker cells have no true resting potential; instead, they generate regular, spontaneous action potentials.

The action potential in non-pacemaker cells

The action potential in non-pacemaker cells (atrial and ventricular myocytes and Purkinje cells) has five phases, numbered 0–4 (Figure 3.1).

- Phase 0 represents the rapid depolarisation phase where the fast sodium channels open and there is a rapid influx of Na^+ into the cell. Calcium moves slowly but steadily into the cell. The membrane potential moves from the negative charge of 85–90 mV to +10–20 mV. This creates a gradient with the surrounding cell membranes, allowing the electrical current to flow from the depolarised cell to the surrounding cells, propagating the impulse.
- Phase 1 represents an initial repolarisation of the cell caused by opening of special transient outward K^+ channels and the inactivation of the Na^+ channels. Cl^- ions re-enter the cell.
- Phase 2 represents the plateau phase where repolarisation is delayed because of the slow inward movement of Ca^{++} through long lasting (L-type) calcium channels.

> ### Key point
>
> L-type calcium channels are blocked by pharmacological L-type calcium channel blockers such as verapamil, diltiazem and dihydropyradines such as nifedipine.

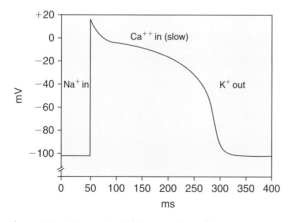

Figure 3.1   Action potential in a cardiac cell.

- Phase 3 is the final repolarisation phase. Ca^{++} channels close and K^+ flows rapidly out of the cell.
- Phase 4 refers to the phase where the cell is not stimulated (the resting membrane potential). This phase coincides with diastole. K^+ is restored to the inside of the cell and Na^+ to the outside by active transport through the sodium–potassium pump.

> ### Key point
>
> The ability of the cell to open fast Na^+ channels during phase 0 is related to the membrane potential at the moment of excitation. For the cell to be able to open the fast Na^+ channels, the resting membrane potential must be at baseline (85–90 mV) and all Na^+ channels closed. Excitation opens the Na^+ channels, causing a large influx of Na^+ ions. If, however, the membrane potential is less negative, some of the fast Na^+ channels will not open, resulting in a reduced response to excitation of the cell membrane. In some cases, the cell may not be excitable, and conduction through the heart may be delayed, which increases the risk of arrhythmias.

During phases 0, 1, 2 and part of phase 3, the cell is refractory (unexcitable, unresponsive) to the initiation of new action potentials. This is known as the effective refractory period (ERP). The ERP acts as a protective mechanism in the heart by limiting the frequency of action potentials (and therefore contractions) that the heart can generate, enabling the heart to have adequate time to fill and eject blood. At the end of ERP, the cell is in its relative refractory period, where suprathreshold depolarisation stimuli are required to elicit action potentials (Klabunde 2005).

> ### Learning activity
>
> Potassium is a most important ion in the cardiac action potential. What would you expect to happen to the action potential and heart rhythm in hyperkalaemia and hypokalaemia? You may find the

following clinical review from the *British Medical Journal* useful in answering these questions: He, J.F. & MacGregor, G.A. (2001). Beneficial effects of potassium. *British Medical Journal*, **323**:497–501. Retrieved online 17th October 2007 from http://www.bmj.com/cgi/content/full/323/7311/497

The cardiac conduction system

Cells within the cardiac conduction system are described as autorhythmic or self-excitable, that is to say that they are able to repeatedly and rhythmically generate their own electrical impulses. The conduction system therefore forms a route or pathway for electrical impulses to travel through the myocardium, which in turn will initiate the mechanical contraction of the heart.

The sinoatrial (SA) node is often described as the natural pacemaker of the heart, as this is where initial electrical impulses arise. It is located in the wall of the right atrium just below the opening of the superior vena cava. The SA node at rest generates impulses at an inherent rate of between 60 and 70 impulses per minute (Jones 2006). This rate will increase in response to specific stimuli including exercise, stimulant drugs such as epinephrine, and pyrexia. Additionally, there are specific structures that link the SA node to the left atrium and the atrioventricular (AV) node to ensure rapid propagation of the electrical impulse throughout the atria (Figure 3.2). These structures are termed the internodal tracts over which conduction proceeds more rapidly

than in other areas of the atrial myocardium. The conduction of the electrical impulse throughout the right and left atria is seen on the ECG as the P wave and stimulates atrial contraction (Figure 3.3).

Key point

If a rhythm originates from the sinus node at a rate less than 60 bpm, this is known as sinus bradycardia. If a rhythm originates from the sinus node at a rate greater than 100 bpm, this is known as sinus tachycardia.

Impulses from the SA node are received directly by the AV node via the internodal tracts. The AV node lies in the right atrium along the lower part of the interatrial septum and forms the only acceptable

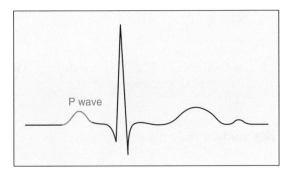

Figure 3.3   The P wave.
Source: Reproduced from Meek and Morris (2002). With permission from BMJ Publishing Group Ltd.

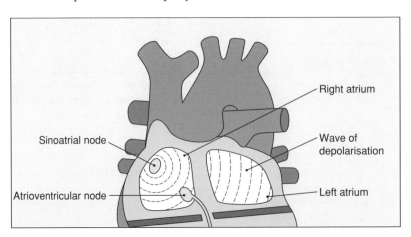

Figure 3.2   Atrial conduction.
Source: Reproduced from Meek and Morris (2002). With permission from BMJ Publishing Group Ltd.

pathway between the atria and the ventricles. It delays passage of the impulse to the ventricles to allow time for ventricular filling. This delay is represented on the ECG by the P–R interval. Like the SA node, the AV node is autorhythmic and therefore generates its own impulses. At rest, the AV node generates impulses of 40–60 per minute. From the AV node, the impulses pass down the bundle of His, which is a direct extension of the AV node and thus often referred to as the AV bundle. It is located at the top of the ventricular septum and separates within the ventricular septum into two distinct divisions, termed the left and right bundle branches. They course through the interventricular septum towards the apex of the heart (Figure 3.4). These branches allow impulses to pass equally through both ventricles. In contrast to the right ventricle, the left ventricle constitutes a larger mass of myocardium due to the increased workload that is demanded of it; thus, the left bundle branch separates into two distinct fascicles termed the anterior and posterior fascicles, allowing impulses to pass effectively and evenly throughout the left ventricle.

Learning activity

You will hear the term 'bundle branch block'. What do you think this phrase means in electrophysiological terms? The Texas Heart Institute's website may be useful to you in answering this question at http://www.texasheart.org/HIC/Topics/Cond/bbblock.cfm

At the apex of the ventricles, the left and right bundle branches separate further into a sheet of fibres termed the Purkinje fibres, or conduction myofibres which spread across the posterior of the left and right ventricles. These fibres come into contact with the myocardium at the subendocardial regions, depolarising the myocardium. The papillary muscles contract first, followed by a wave of excitation and contraction which proceeds from endocardium to epicardium, and travels from the apex of the heart to the ventricular outflow tract, causing the ventricle to contract and expel blood into the systemic and pulmonary circulations. This part of the electrical impulse is represented by the QRS complex on the ECG (Figure 3.5). Both the Purkinje fibres and the left and right bundle branches intrinsically fire impulses at a much lower rate than the SA node and AV node (approximately 20–40 impulses per minute). Normal passage of electrical impulses through the entire conduction system takes approximately 0.15–0.2 s (Totora & Grabowski 2003).

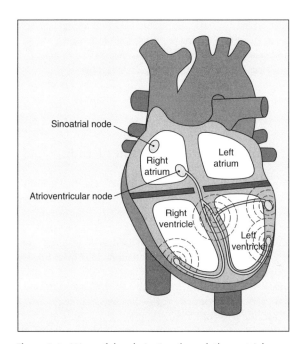

Figure 3.4 Wave of depolarisation through the ventricles giving rise to the QRS complex.
Source: Reproduced from Meek and Morris (2002). With permission from BMJ Publishing Group Ltd.

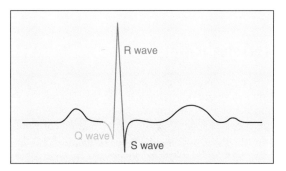

Figure 3.5 Components of the QRS complex.
Source: Reproduced from Meek and Morris (2002). With permission from BMJ Publishing Group Ltd.

The electrocardiogram

The ECG is separated into a series of three distinct waveforms: the P wave, the QRS complex and the T wave. Each of these waveforms represents a specific phase in the passage of electrical impulses through the heart's conduction system and subsequently atrial and ventricular depolarisation as well as ventricular repolarisation.

The P wave represents depolarisation of the atria which is a result of the passage of an electrical impulse from the SA node through the musculature of both atria (Thibodeau & Patton 2007). The QRS complex represents depolarisation of the ventricles. Depolarisation of the ventricles is a process involving depolarisation of the interventricular septum and the subsequent spread of depolarisation by the Purkinje fibres through the lateral ventricular walls (Thibodeau & Patton 2007). The T wave represents repolarisation of the ventricles and the return of the ventricles to the resting membrane potential (Jones 2006). Occasionally a U wave may be seen immediately following the T wave. The U wave it is believed results from late repolarisation of Purkinje fibres in the papillary muscle of the ventricular myocardium (Thibodeau & Patton 2007); however, there still remains some contention as to its true origin.

Learning activity

Can electrophysiological activity be seen in the heart in the absence of mechanical activity? Can mechanical activity be seen in the heart in the absence of electrophysiological activity? You may find the following eMedicine article useful: Verma, S. & Marks, D.S. (2005). Pulseless electrical activity. eMedicine. Retrieved online 17th October 2007 from http://www. emedicine.com/med/topic2963.htm Alternately, type 'pulseless electrical activity' into your web browser and have a look at the resulting information.

Conclusion

This chapter has provided an overview of the anatomy and physiology of the conduction system of the heart, and the complex way it interacts and augments mechanical function. Disturbances of the conducting system can result in arrhythmias, which may result in suboptimal mechanical function of the heart, and in some cases, death. It is therefore essential that nurses understand the principles of cardiac electrophysiology as a basis for early recognition and management of cardiac arrhythmias.

References

Jones, I. (2006). *Cardiac Care: An Introductory Text*. Whurr Publishers, Philadelphia.

Klabunde, R. (2005). *Cardiovascular Physiology Concepts*. Lippincott Williams & Wilkins, Philadelphia.

Thibodeau, G.A. & Patton, K.T. (2007). *Anatomy & Physiology*, 8th edn. Mosby, Philadelphia.

Totora, G.J. & Grabowski, S.R. (2003). *Principles of Anatomy and Physiology*, 10th edn. John Wiley & Sons, New Jersey.

Useful Websites and Further Reading

American Heart Association (2007). Cardiac conduction system. Retrieved online 17th October 2007 from http://www.americanheart.org/presenter.jhtml?identifier=68

Klabunde, R.E. (2007). Cardiovascular physiology concepts. Retrieved online 4th October 2007 from http://www.cvphysiology.com

Meek, S. & Morris, F. (2002). ABC of clinical electrocardiography: Introduction. II—Basic terminology. *British Medical Journal*, **324**:470–3.

Rogers, J. (1999). Cardiovascular physiology, Issue 10. Retrieved online 17th October 2007 from http://www.nda.ox.ac.uk/wfsa/html/u10/u1002_01.htm

4 The Coronary Circulation

B. Greaney & A.M. Kucia

Overview

This chapter will outline the structure and function of the coronary circulation, describing the key coronary arteries and the specific areas of the heart muscle supplied by each of these arteries. An understanding of the structure and function of the coronary circulation will be useful in the interpretation of cardiac catheterisation reports and assist the nurse in understanding the signs and symptoms that occur as a result of occlusion of a particular coronary artery, relative to the myocardial structures that it supplies.

Learning objectives

After reading this chapter, you should be able to:

- List the components of the coronary circulation.
- Name the specific areas of the heart supplied by each of the coronary arteries.
- Describe the structure and function of the coronary arterial and venous circulation.
- Discuss the function of collateral vessels.
- Describe the function of the coronary microvascular system.

Key concepts

Sub-epicardial arteries; collateral circulation; microvascular circulation; coronary dominance; coronary perfusion

The coronary circulation

In order to maintain the function of supplying all body organs and tissues with oxygen and nutrients, the heart requires an effective and reliable blood supply. Disruption to this blood supply has potentially catastrophic consequences. The coronary circulation has blood vessels that supply blood to, and remove blood from, the heart. The vessels that supply blood rich in oxygen to the heart are known as coronary arteries. The vessels that remove the deoxygenated blood from the heart are known as cardiac veins. When we think of the coronary arteries, we generally form a picture of the large arteries that run on the surface of the heart known as the epicardial or sub-epicardial arteries, which, in a healthy state, are capable of autoregulation to maintain coronary blood flow at levels appropriate to the needs of the myocardium at any given time. The other component to the normal coronary arterial circulation consists of high

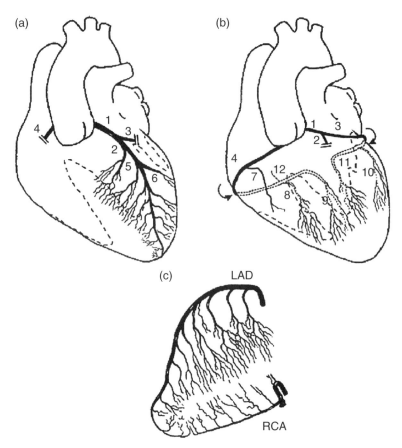

Figure 4.1   Coronary artery diagram.
Source: From Bayes De Luna et al. (2006).

resistance distal microvascular vessels that form the arteriolar–capillary network (Angelini et al. 2002).

The right and left coronary arteries originate from the aortic root, immediately above the aortic valve, and provide the entire blood supply to the myocardium (Berne & Levy 2001). The venous circulation returns to the right atrium through the coronary sinus, a large vein located on the posterior surface of the heart. The name and nature of a coronary artery is defined by the vessel's distal vascularisation pattern or territory rather than its origin (Pelech 2006). The exact anatomy of the myocardial blood supply varies considerably from person to person, but the common anatomical characteristics of the epicardial arteries are depicted in Figure 4.1.

The left main coronary artery

In the majority of people, there is a left main coronary artery (LMCA or LMA) that originates from the ostium of the left sinus of Valsalva. Typically, it is 1–2 cm in length and 5–10 mm in diameter. The LMCA courses between the left atrial appendage and the pulmonary artery, before reaching the left atrioventricular (AV) groove, where it bifurcates into the left anterior descending (LAD) and the left circumflex (LCX or CX) arteries. In some cases, an artery may arise from the LMCA between the LAD and LCX, and this may be referred to as the intermediate, ramus or optional diagonal coronary artery.

The LAD artery

The LAD artery continues directly from the bifurcation of the LMCA down the anterior interventricular groove, and its length is extremely variable. In most cases, it reaches the apex of the heart and supplies the anterolateral myocardium, apex and interventricular septum. Arteries branching from the LAD artery include the diagonals, septal perforators and right ventricular branches. There may be between two and six diagonals, which supply the anterior wall of the myocardium. The first diagonal is usually the largest of these vessels. The septal perforators are generally between two and six in number. The first of these vessels, the largest, originates just beyond the take-off of the first diagonal. The septal perforators supply the anterior two-thirds of the ventricular septum (Mill et al. 2003). In some cases, the LAD artery gives off right ventricular branches that supply the anterior surface of the right ventricle. The LAD artery may extend for several millimetres and wrap around the apex of the left ventricle to supply the apical portion of the inferior wall (Sadanandan et al. 2003). In rare cases it may replace the posterior descending artery (PDA) (Mill et al. 2003).

The LCX or CX artery

The LCX artery runs across the left AV groove and gives off obtuse marginal (OM) branches that supply blood to the lateral wall of the left ventricle and the posteromedial papillary muscle. In 10–15% of cases, the LCX artery continues to the crux of the heart and gives rise to the PDA and posterolateral artery (PLA). You may hear medical or nursing staff refer to a patient/client as being 'right or left dominant' in terms of their coronary blood supply. The artery that supplies the PDA and the PLA determines the coronary dominance. Thus, if the LCX artery supplies the PDA and PLA, the person is said to be 'left dominant'. When the LCX artery supplies the PDA, it also supplies the AV node. Additional branches supply blood to the left atrium and to the sinoatrial (SA) node in 40–50% of people (Mill et al. 2003).

The right coronary artery

The right coronary artery (RCA) originates from the aorta, above the right cusp of the aortic valve and travels down the right AV groove. In the majority of people, the RCA crosses to the crux and makes a characteristic 'U turn' before bifurcating into the PDA and right PLA. The RCA gives off the PDA and PLA in 85% of people (right dominance). The PDA runs along the posterior intraventricular groove towards the apex of the heart and gives off perpendicular branches, the posterior septal perforators, that supply the posterior third of the ventricular septum. The right PLA gives rise to branches that supply the posterior surface of the left ventricle.

The first branch arising from the RCA is the conal or infundibular branch which courses anteriorly to supply the right ventricular outflow tract (Pelech 2006). The atria are supplied by the RCA but the pattern of branches supplying them is highly variable. The RCA supplies the SA node in 50–60% of people. The acute marginal branches of the RCA supply the anterior wall of the right ventricle, and in 10–20% of people, one of the branches will course along the diaphragmatic surface of the right ventricle to supply the distal ventricular septum. The RCA supplies collaterals to the LAD artery through its septal perforators and additionally, the conus branch may serve as collateral to the LAD artery.

Collateral circulation

Blood flow to the myocardium can be influenced by the function of collateral vessels (Chilian 1997). These small, normally closed vessels connect two larger arteries or different parts of the same artery. When blood flow to one of the major vessels is obstructed, the collaterals enlarge and the blood flow through them increases, providing an alternate blood supply. In the setting of a coronary occlusion, collaterals may provide sufficient perfusion to limit myocardial damage, prevent myocardial infarction and/or sudden ischaemic death (Marcus 1983). Collaterals only become visible angiographically when coronary occlusion is complete or virtually complete (Chilian 1997). Collaterals may grow quite large in people with coronary artery disease. Although collaterals are present in all people, they do not necessarily open in all individuals (American Heart Association 2007).

Microvascular circulation

The microcirculation is comprised of arterioles, capillaries, venules and terminal lymphatic vessels. The vessels in this system have a much higher resistance to blood flow compared to the epicardial arteries (Klabunde 2005). The microvascular arterioles are very sensitive to agents causing vasoconstriction. Tissue perfusion is regulated at the microvascular level: thus, any downstream resistance to flow due to vasoconstriction, microemboli or inflammation will have a strong influence on coronary perfusion (Becker & Armani 2003).

Coronary venous circulation

The venous circulation of the heart is essentially a venous drainage system from the myocardial capillary bed. The source of this capillary network within the myocardial fibres stems from the coronary arteries, which penetrate the myocardium and proliferate in a rich network of capillaries (Little & Little 1989). The venous drainage system from the myocardial capillary bed is drained via three major systems:

1   The thespian veins, which empty into the right and left atrium and a limited amount into the right ventricle
2   The anterior cardiac veins, which empty into the right atrium
3   The coronary sinus and its connecting coronary veins, which return blood to the right atrium

Table 4.1 shows the regions of the heart that are supplied by the different coronary arteries in the majority of people. It is important to know this anatomic distribution because these cardiac regions are assessed by 12-lead ECGs to help localise ischaemic or infarcted regions. Although cardiac regions can be loosely correlated with

Table 4.1   Anatomical correlation between anatomical region of the heart and most likely associated coronary artery.

Anatomic region of the heart	Most likely associated coronary artery
Inferior	RCA
Antero-septal	LAD
Antero-apical	LAD (distal)
Lateral	LCX
Posterior	RCA

specific coronary vessels, because of variations (heterogeneity) in coronary vessels between people, actual vessel involvement in ischaemic conditions needs to be verified by coronary angiogram or other imaging techniques (Klabunde 2005).

Learning activity

Visit the radiology assistant at http://rad.desk.nl/en/48275120e2ed5 for further information and to view the coronary arteries in anterior, lateral and right anterior oblique (RAO) projection.

References

American Heart Association (2007). Collateral circulation. Retrieved online 17th October 2007 from http://www.americanheart.org/presenter.jhtml?identifier=4583

Angelini, P., Velasco, J.A. & Flamm, S. (2002). Coronary anomalies: incidence, pathophysiology, and clinical relevance. *Circulation*, **105**:2449–54.

Becker, R.C. & Armani, A. (2003). Linking biochemistry, vascular biology, and clinical events in acute coronary syndromes. In: C.P. Cannon (ed.), *Management of Acute Coronary Syndromes*, 2nd edn. Humana Press, New Jersey.

Bayes De Luna, A., Fiol-Sala, M. & Antman, E.M. (2006). *The 12 Lead ECG in ST Elevation Myocardial Infarction.* Blackwell Publishing. Oxford.

Berne, R.M. & Levy, M.N. (2001). *Cardiovascular Physiology*, 8th edn. Mosby, Philadelphia.

Chilian, W.M. (1997). Coronary microcirculation in health and disease: summary of an NHLBI workshop. *Circulation*, **95**:522–8.

Klabunde, R. (2005). *Cardiovascular Physiology Concepts*. Lippincott Williams & Wilkins, Philadelphia.

Little, R.C. & Little, W.C. (1989). *Physiology of the Heart and Circulation*, 4th edn. Year Book Medical Publishers Inc., Chicago.

Marcus, M.L. (1983). *The Coronary Circulation in Health and Disease*. McGraw-Hill, New York.

Mill, M.R., Wilcox, B.R. & Anderson, R.H. (2003). Surgical anatomy of the heart. In: L.H. Cohn & L.H.J. Edmunds (eds), *Cardiac Surgery in the Adult*. McGraw Hill, New York, p. 3152.

Pelech, A.N. (2006). Coronary artery anomalies. *eMedicine*, Retrieved online 20th August 2007 from http://www.emedicine.com/ped/topic2506.htm

Sadanandan, S., Hochman, J.S., Kolodziej, A., et al. (2003). Clinical and angiographic characteristics of patients with combined anterior and inferior ST-segment elevation on the initial electrocardiogram during acute myocardial infarction. *American Heart Journal*, **146**:653–61.

Useful Websites and Further Reading

American Heart Association (2007). Angiogenesis. Retrieved online 17th October 2007 from http://www.americanheart.org/presenter.jhtml?identifier=4435

Klabunde, R.E. (2005). Cardiovascular physiology concepts. Retrieved online 28th August 2007 from http://cvphysiology.com/index.html

5 Risk Factors for Cardiovascular Disease

A.M. Kucia & E. Birchmore

Overview

The development of cardiovascular disease is associated with a number of conditions and behaviours that collectively are known as "cardiovascular risk factors". These risk factors are targeted in both primary and secondary prevention strategies, but education and management often begins in the setting of an acute coronary syndrome presentation. Knowledge of cardiovascular risk factors and how they contribute to the development of cardiovascular disease is essential in the assessment and management of patients with acute coronary syndromes. This chapter discusses factors that are associated with increased cardiovascular risk and how they impact upon patients with acute coronary syndromes.

Learning objectives

After reading this chapter, you should be able to:

- Describe non-modifiable and modifiable behavioural and biomedical risk factors for CVD.
- Recognise the interplay of risk factors that result in an increased risk of developing CVD.
- Discuss the impact of psychosocial factors in risk of developing CVD.
- Discuss how risk factors for CVD are identified
- Recognise that risk of CVD is greater in some individuals than others

Key concepts

Behavioural risk; non-modifiable and modifiable risk; psychosocial risk factors; risk assessment; risk reduction.

Classification of risk factors for CVD

A number of risk factors for the development of CVD have been identified (Table 5.1). These risk factors can be classed as biomedical, behavioural and psychosocial. Biomedical risk factors can be further categorised as non-modifiable and modifiable. Non-modifiable risks are age, gender and family history, and modifiable risk factors include hypertension, dyslipidaemia, overweight/obesity, diabetes/insulin resistance and renal disease. Behavioural risk factors include tobacco smoking, physical inactivity, poor nutrition and excessive alcohol consumption.

Table 5.1   Risk factors for the development of CVD.

Biomedical		Behavioural	Psychosocial
Non-modifiable	Modifiable		
• age • gender • family history CVD	• hypertension • dyslipidae mia • overweight/ obesity • diabetes/insulin resistance • renal disease	• tobacco smoking • physical inactivity • poor nutrition • excessive alcohol consumption	• depression • anxiety • social isolation • stress

There is increasing evidence demonstrating strong links between psychosocial factors such as depression, stress, anxiety, social isolation and CVD. Modifiable and behavioural risk factors are themselves strongly influenced by factors such as personal economic resources, education, living and working conditions, access to health care and social services (Australian Institute of Health and Welfare [AIHW] 2004).

Biomedical risk factors

Non-modifiable risk factors are listed as age, gender and a family history of CVD. CVD predominantly affects middle-aged and older individuals. Traditionally it has been believed that men are at greater risk of CVD than women and this has been attributed to the protective effects of oestrogen, but by the age of 65, women have a risk equal to that of men, and it is important to note that mortality due to CVD in men and women 65 years and over is about the same. The risk of developing CVD is increased if a first-degree relative is diagnosed with heart or blood vessel disease before the age of 60 (Access Economics 2005). Although these risk factors cannot be modified, awareness of these risks and their interplay with other CVD risk factors may encourage clients to take positive steps in addressing risk factors that can be modified.

Modifiable biomedical risk factors include dyslipidaemia, hypertension, diabetes and renal failure.

Dyslipidaemia

Dyslipidaemia is a metabolic derangement resulting from elevation of plasma cholesterol and/or triglycerides (TG), or a low high-density lipid (HDL) level that contributes to the development of atherosclerosis. Whilst dyslipidaemia itself does not cause symptoms, it leads to symptomatic vascular disease. Dyslipidaemia may be a hereditary (primary) or acquired (secondary) disorder. Primary causes of dyslipidaemia are genetic mutations that result in either overproduction or defective clearance of TG and low-density lipid (LDL) cholesterol, or in underproduction or excessive clearance of HDL. Primary causes of dyslipidaemia are more common in children, but secondary causes are more common in adults, with the most common cause in developed countries being a sedentary lifestyle with excessive dietary intake of saturated fat, cholesterol and trans fatty acids (TFAs) (Merck Inc. 2005). Other causes include diabetes mellitus, alcohol overuse, chronic renal insufficiency and/or failure, hypothyroidism, primary biliary cirrhosis and other cholestatic liver diseases. Drugs such as thiazides, β-blockers, retinoids, highly active antiretroviral agents, oestrogen and progestins, and glucocorticoids may also cause, or contribute to, dyslipidaemia (Merck Inc. 2005).

Key point

Individuals at greater risk of dyslipidaemia include those with clinical evidence of vascular disease (including CVD, peripheral arterial disease or stroke); diabetes mellitus; chronic kidney disease and familial hypercholesterolaemia. Ethnic minority populations (South Asian and African) and indigenous (Maori and Australian Aboriginal and Torres Strait Islander) populations also have an increased risk of dyslipidaemia. Individuals who have been identified as having an absolute risk of ≥15% risk of a CVD event in the next 5 years using 1991 Framingham equation also have an increased risk of dys-lipidaemia (Cappuccio et al. 2002; National Heart Foundation of Australia [NHFA] and the Cardiac Society of Australia and New Zealand 2005).

Measuring lipids

Dyslipidaemia is diagnosed by measuring serum lipids. Lipids can be measured in the non-fasting state, but for consistency and accuracy, all patients should at some time have fasting serum lipids measured. Target lipid levels for those at high risk or known to have CVD are more aggressively managed than for individuals with no known risk for CVD. Target lipid levels vary slightly according to the information source and perceived disease risk. Table 5.2 lists suggested target lipid levels for those with known or at high risk of CVD.

Key point

In the context of considering lipid measurement in the setting of acute coronary syndromes (ACS), it should be known that TGs increase and cholesterol levels decrease in inflammatory states. Generally, lipid screens should be postponed until an acute illness has resolved, but there is a risk that patients with ACS may be lost to follow-up or that test-ing may be overlooked if it is not done during an admission for an acute event. Lipid profiles are generally reliable within the first 24 h following an acute myocardial infarction, and if testing can be done in this timeframe, that is the preferred option.

Management of dyslipidaemia

Lifestyle interventions, including dietary modifi-cation, should underpin management in all people with dyslipidaemia. Different types of fats found in food have different effects on the level of cho-lesterol in the blood. Fats that may help to lower cholesterol, if other food intake is low in saturated fat, are polyunsaturated fats found in foods such as fish, some nuts (walnuts, hazelnuts and brazil nuts) and polyunsaturated margarines and oils; and monounsaturated fats found in foods such

Table 5.2 Target lipid levels for those with known or at high risk of CVD.

Component	mmol/mL
LDL cholesterol	<2
HDL cholesterol	>1
Triglycerides	<1.5
Total cholesterol	<4

as avocado, plain nuts (peanuts, cashews and almonds) and monounsaturated margarine and oils. Fats that raise blood cholesterol are saturated fats found in many take-away meals, potato chips, commercial cakes, biscuits and pastries, butter and dairy products (full fat milk, cream, cheese); and trans fats found in foods that use hydrogenated or partially hydrogenated vegetable fats (baked products such as pies, pastries, cakes, biscuits and buns) (NHFA 2008a).

Learning activity

The management of lipids requires a collaborative approach between health care professionals and the client. Although clear guidelines for the man-agement of dyslipidaemia have been around for some years, many treated individuals do not meet target levels for lipids. In addition to pharmacologi-cal management, lipid management often requires extensive lifestyle which is best achieved through a collaboration of physicians, nurses and allied health professionals, including dietitians and exer-cise specialists (Fletcher et al. 2005). Visit the foun-dation or association that formulates the guidelines for lipid management in your country, and read the article by Fletcher and colleagues (listed under 'Useful Websites and Further Reading') to identify strategies that you may be able to employ in your own area of practice.

Statin therapy should be considered for those identified as being at high risk and should be com-menced in hospital for those admitted with ACS. If TG are markedly elevated, fibrates may be used. The combination of statin and fibrates, whilst effective, leads to an increased risk of myopathy and rhabdomyolysis and should only be used together under close supervision. Other agents that may be used with statins are ezetimibe, niacin and bile acid sequestrants (Thompson 2004).

Key point

People with diabetes (particularly type 2 diabetes) have a particularly atherogenic type of dyslipidaemia (diabetic dyslipidaemia or hypertriglyceridaemic hyperapo B), characterised by elevated TG which are thought to have atherogenic properties; low HDL cholesterol; shift in LDL particle density towards small, dense LDL (type B); and a tendency towards postprandial lipidaemia. Most patients with diabetes and dyslipidaemia will require pharmacological therapy to reach target lipid goals (WHO 2006a).

Hypertension

Hypertension has been identified as the first cause of death worldwide (Ezzati et al. 2002). It is estimated that hypertension is present in more than a quarter of the world's adult population and that this proportion will continue to rise (Kearney et al. 2005). Hypertension is a major risk factor for a number of cardiovascular and related diseases as well as for diseases leading to an increased cardiovascular risk (Mancia et al. 2007). Causes of hypertension are shown in Table 5.3. Hypertension usually occurs as primary (essential) hypertension, where the cause is not known. About 5–10% of cases occur as secondary hypertension where the cause is identifiable.

High blood pressure (BP) is a major cause of CVD and is more likely to occur in those who are physically inactive, overweight or have high sodium intakes (AIHW 2002). The risk of developing CVD due to hypertension is directly related to both elevated systolic and diastolic BP levels (Lewington et al. 2003), although systolic BP is a stronger and more consistent predictor of cardiovascular risk than diastolic BP, particularly in those aged 50 or over (Chobanian et al. 2003). Evidence suggests that in adults aged 40–69 years of age, each 20 mmHg increase in usual systolic BP, or 10 mmHg increase in usual diastolic BP, doubles the risk of death from CVD. Risk of death from CVD is also increased for those over 69 years with

Table 5.3   Causes of hypertension.

Primary (essential) hypertension	Secondary hypertension[a]
Cause unknown	Renal artery stenosis
	Chronic renal disease
	Primary hyperaldosterinism
	Hyperthyroidism
	Hypothyroidism
	Stress
	Sleep apnoea
	Pheochromocytoma
	Preeclampsia
	coarctation of the aorta

[a]From Klabunde (2007).

hypertension, although not as dramatically (British Heart Foundation [BHF] 2008).

Measuring BP

In non-acute situations, BP should be measured using standard measurement techniques on several occasions to obtain a realistic assessment and plan appropriate management of BP. For clients with unusual BP variability or a 'white coat' effect where BP becomes elevated primarily during visits to the health professional, it may be necessary to assess blood in the home or ambulatory setting.

Key point

Although automated non-invasive BP monitoring is widely used in the acute setting, a baseline measurement with a mercury sphygmomanometer and an appropriately sized cuff (with the bladder length at least 80% and the width at least 40% of the circumference of the mid-upper arm) is recommended to ensure accuracy.

Management of hypertension

The level at which BP is considered to change from normotensive to hypertensive is somewhat arbitrary, and international definitions of hypertension vary. The current definition of hypertension is based on the level of BP above which a therapeutic plan is recommended, and is influenced by an assessment of the patient's absolute risk for CVD,

Table 5.4 Classification and follow-up of BP in adults.

Diagnostic category[a]	Systolic (mmHg)	Diastolic (mmHg)	Follow-up
Normal	<120	<80	Recheck in 2 years (or earlier as guided by patient's absolute cardiovascular risk)[b]
High-normal	120–139	80–89	Recheck in 1 year (or earlier as guided by patient's absolute cardiovascular risk)[b]
Grade 1 (mild) hypertension	140–159	90–99	Confirm within 2 months. See *When to intervene*
Grade 2 (moderate) hypertension	160–179	100–109	Reassess or refer within 1 month. See *When to intervene*
Grade 3 (severe) hypertension	≥180	≥110	Reassess or refer within 1–7 days as necessary. See *When to intervene*
Isolated systolic hypertension	≥140	<90	As for category corresponding to systolic BP.
Isolated systolic hypertension with widened pulse pressure	≥160	≤70	As for grade 3 hypertension[c]

Source: From National Heart Foundation of Australia, Heart Foundation Guide to Management of Hypotension (2008).
[a]When a patient's systolic and diastolic BP levels fall into different categories, the higher diagnostic category and recommended action's apply.
[b]See *Absolute cardiovascular risk assessment in hypertension management.*
[c]In middle-aged and elderly patients with cardiovascular risk factors or associated clinical conditions, isolated systolic hypertension with large pulse pressure indicates high absolute risk for CVD.

according to the presence and magnitude of other risk factors. BP management is determined in the context of other existing cardiovascular risk factors. For those at higher absolute risk of CVD and those that have already had a coronary event, BP will be managed more aggressively. As BP may have large spontaneous variations, the diagnosis of hypertension should be based on multiple BP measurements taken on several separate occasions (NHFA 2008b). See Table 5.4 for definitions, classification and follow-up of BP levels in adults.

Primary prevention target BP levels are ≤140/90 mmHg, but ≤130/80 mmHg is suggested as a reasonable target BP for individuals with demonstrated coronary artery disease (CAD) or with CAD risk equivalents, including carotid artery disease, peripheral arterial disease, abdominal aortic aneurysm, diabetes mellitus or chronic renal disease (Rosendorff et al. 2007). For adults with proteinuria >1 g/day (with and without diabetes), a target BP of <125/75 may be more appropriate (NHFA 2008b). As with hyperlipidaemia, hypertension management is underpinned by lifestyle modifications including weight control, increased physical activity, alcohol moderation, sodium reduction and emphasis on increased consumption of fresh fruits, vegetables and low-fat dairy

products (Rosendorff et al. 2007). Patients should also be counselled to quit smoking – smoking causes vasoconstriction which may result in acute increases in BP, and in combination with increased alcohol intake and body mass index (BMI) can also exert chronic effects on BP (Primatesta et al. 2001).

Pharmacotherapy used in the management of hypertension includes angiotensin-converting enzyme inhibitors, low-dose thiazide diuretics, calcium channel blockers angiotensin II receptor antagonists and beta blockers. Combination drug therapy will often be required to control BP, and the choice of drugs used is often influenced by co-existing conditions that contribute to cardiovascular risk (NHFA 2008b).

Key point

In the setting of ACS, severe uncontrolled hypertension on presentation (>180 mmHg systolic or >110 mmHg diastolic) is a contraindication for fibrinolytic therapy and may limit use of other agents such as glycoprotein IIb/IIIa inhibitors, antithrombin and antiplatelet therapies.

Diabetes mellitus

Diabetes has been described as a current world-wide epidemic. CVD is the leading cause of death in people with diabetes, and despite advances in current therapies for ACS, diabetes confers an adverse prognosis in ACS (Donahoe et al. 2007). The risk of developing CVD increases along a spectrum of blood glucose concentrations even at levels that are regarded as normal. Abnormal glucose tolerance is almost twice as common amongst patients with a myocardial infarction as in population-based controls (Bartnik et al. 2007). Both type 1 and type 2 diabetes mellitus are independent risk factors for CVD (McGill & McMahan 1998; Wilson et al. 1998) but the most prevalent form is type 2, which typically manifests later in life and is associated with obesity and physical inactivity (see Table 5.5). Type 2 diabetes is often preceded by insulin resistance and accompanied by dyslipidaemia, hypertension and prothrombotic factors, with the common clustering of these risk factors in a single individual known as the metabolic syndrome (Grundy et al. 1999).

Testing for diabetes

The fasting blood glucose (FBG) and oral glucose tolerance test (OGTT), also referred to as the glucose tolerance test, are blood tests used in the diagnosis of diabetes. The OGTT measures the body's ability to metabolise glucose, or clear it out of the bloodstream, and although it is more time consuming than the FBG, it is a more sensitive measure and can be used to diagnose diabetes, gestational diabetes (diabetes during pregnancy) or pre-diabetes.

Management of diabetes

For patients with CVD and diabetes, the gold standard in treatment is intensified insulin therapy with appropriate nutrition and self-monitoring

Table 5.5   Diabetes mellitus classifications.

Diabetes mellitus		
Type 1	Type 2	Pre-diabetes
Occurs due to pancreas being unable to produce insulin because the pancreatic b-cells that make the insulin have been destroyed by the body's own immune system	Occurs when the body does not produce enough insulin or when the insulin that is produced is not effective (insulin resistance)	Also known as impaired glucose tolerance (IGT) or impaired fasting glucose (IFG) Diagnosed when the blood glucose level (BGL) is higher than normal but not high enough to be classed as diabetes. Occurs as a result of insulin resistance.
Accounts for 10–15% of all cases of diabetes	Accounts for 85–90% of all cases of diabetes	
Previously known as juvenile onset or insulin-dependent diabetes	May be referred to as mature onset or non-insulin-dependent diabetes	
Is not caused by lifestyle factors	Being overweight and physically inactive are contributors to diabetes development	
Requires insulin injections	May require pharmacotherapy to keep BGLs in the ideal range	
One of the most common chronic childhood diseases in developed nations	Modifications to lifestyle such as improved levels of physical activity and diet are needed	

Source: Diabetes Australia – NSW (2008).

of blood glucose levels (BGLs), aiming for a HbA$_{Ic}$ <7%. A common pharmacological approach for type 2 diabetes is not as well agreed upon, although the use of polypharmacy appears to be an accepted practice that maximises efficacy and reduces some of the side effects experienced with higher doses of single agents (Rydén et al. 2007). There are a number of pharmacological agents used in the management of type 2 diabetes including sulfonylureas, biguanides, thiazolidinediones, alpha-glucosidase inhibitors meglitinides, dipeptidyl peptidase IV (DPP-IV) inhibitors and combination therapies that combine two medications in one tablet.

Nutritional and lifestyle modification, including exercise and weight loss, can reduce progression to type 2 diabetes (Knowler et al. 2002; Tuomilehto et al. 2002; Wadden et al. 2005) and should be strongly encouraged.

Key point

For patients with ACS, the glucose level on admission to the hospital is a significant predictor of 1-year mortality (Capes et al. 2000) and among patients with diabetes, hyperglycaemia on arrival and hypoglycaemia during hospitalisation are both independently associated with worse adjusted all-cause 2-year mortality risk (Svensson et al. 2005). Aggressive management of hyperglycaemia with insulin infusion in the first few days of ACS may offer improved clinical outcomes but there is no current consensus on the range of glucose values that should be considered abnormal or the method of measurement and management of hyperglycaemia in the acute setting of ACS, and the benefits of treating hyperglycaemia has not been definitively established (Deedwania et al. 2008).

Renal failure

Renal failure can be either a cause or a consequence of CVD. Increased serum creatinine levels and microalbuminuria are independent risk factors for CVD. Microalbuminuria is a recognised early sign of kidney disease; it can occur as a long-term complication of diabetes (diabetic nephropathy),

and can be detected using a simple urine dipstick test. Renal disease can also contribute to hypertension and adversely alter plasma lipid profiles. CVD is the major cause of death in people with end-stage renal failure (ESRD), and mortality from CVD is 30 times greater in people with ESRD than the general population (American Heart Association 2008).

Behavioural risk factors

A number of risk factors for CVD may have biomedical consequences but are often due to behavioural factors. Included in this group are obesity/overweight (which may be due to biomedical or behavioural factors), tobacco use, physical inactivity and alcohol use at harmful levels.

Overweight/obesity

The WHO (2006b) defines overweight and obesity as 'abnormal or excessive fat accumulation that presents a risk to health'. Overweight and obesity is related to greater cardiovascular risk in a number of observational studies (Wilson et al. 2002). The number of overweight adults and children are increasing worldwide.

Overweight and obesity is caused by an energy imbalance between calories consumed and calories expended. Globally, overweight and obesity is influenced by a shift in diet towards increased intake of energy-dense foods that are high in fat and sugars but low in vitamins, minerals and other micronutrients; and a trend towards decreased physical activity due to the increasingly sedentary nature of many forms of work, changing modes of transportation and increasing urbanisation (WHO 2008b).

Measuring overweight and obesity

Body mass index, an index of weight-for-height that is calculated by dividing weight in kilograms by height in metres squared (kg/m^2), is the usual measure used to define obesity (Table 5.6). Overweight is defined by the WHO (2008c) as a BMI equal to or more than 25 and obesity as a BMI equal to or more than 30, although these cut-off points may differ slightly in some populations.

Table 5.6 The International classification of adult underweight, overweight and obesity according to BMI.

	BMI(kg/m^2)	
Classification	Principal cut-off points	Additional cut-off points
Underweight	<18.50	<18.50
Severe thinness	<16.00	<16.00
Moderate thinness	16.00–16.99	16.00–16.99
Mild thinness	17.00–18.49	17.00–18.49
Normal range	18.50–24.99	18.50–22.99
		23.00–24.99
Overweight	≥25.00	≥25.00
Pre-obese	25.00–29.99	25.00–27.49
		27.50–29.99
Obese	≥30.00	≥30.00
Obese class I	30.00–34.99	30.00–32.49
		32.50–34.99
Obese class II	35.00–39.99	35.00–37.49
		37.50–39.99
Obese class III	≥40.00	≥40.00

Source: From World Health Organization, The International Classification of Adult Underweight, Overweight and Obesity according to BMI.

There is evidence that the risk of chronic disease increases progressively from a BMI of 21.

Another measure that may be used is waist circumference, which is an approximate index of intra-abdominal fat mass and total body fat and correlates closely with BMI. Men with a waist circumference ≥102 cm and women with a waist circumference ≥88 cm are at increased risk of CVD, although this risk can vary in different populations (WHO 2008c).

Management of overweight and obesity

Management of overweight and obesity is aimed at achieving a balance between energy intake and healthy weight. This can be achieved through improved diet and physical activity. Patients should be educated about limiting energy intake from total fats and replacing foods high in saturated fats with those containing unsaturated fats. Consumption of fruits and vegetables, legumes, whole grains and nuts should be increased and sugar intake limited. Physical activity should include at least 30 min of regular, moderate-intensity activity on most days (WHO 2008a).

Tobacco use

There are more than one billion smokers in the world, and whilst tobacco use is decreasing in high income countries, overall global use of tobacco is increasing due to increased use in developing countries. Tobacco is one of the main risk factors for a number of chronic diseases, including CVD, and kills around half of those who use it (WHO 2008b). It is one of the most important causes of acute myocardial infarction globally, especially in men (Teo et al. 2006).

Although no direct dose-dependent relationship between cigarette smoke exposure and CVD risk has been identified (Ambrose & Barua 2004), it is clear that cigarette smoke has both long- and short-term effects on the cardiovascular system and impacts upon the development of atherosclerosis, inflammation, vascular dysfunction and thrombosis via a number of mechanisms (Table 5.7) (Ambrose & Barua 2004).

All forms of tobacco use (inhalation or ingestion) are harmful (Teo et al. 2006), and both active and passive (environmental or secondhand) cigarette smoke exposure increases cardiovascular risk (Ambrose & Barua 2004; Barnoya & Glantz 2005).

Table 5.7 Cardiovascular effects of cigarette smoke.

Atherogenic effects
  Inflammation
  Modification of lipid profile (Ambrose & Barua 2004)
Increased blood viscosity
  Increased red blood cell count
  Increased haematocrit (Ambrose & Barua 2004)
Thrombotic effects
  Platelet activation and aggregation (Fusegawa et al. 1999)
  Alterations in antithrombotic and prothrombotic factors
  Alterations in fibrinolysis (Barua et al. 2002)
Coronary flow reduction (Czernin et al. 1995)
  Endothelial dysfunction
  Coronary vasospasm (Sugiishi & Takatsu 1993)
Autonomic effects
  Increased heart rate
  Increased BP
  Increased stroke volume
  Increased cardiac output (Smith & Fischer 2001)
  Increased myocardial workload
Increased carbon monoxide levels
  Decreased oxygen delivery to the heart

Key point

Patients are often highly motivated to quit smoking following an acute cardiac event, but may require assistance with nicotine withdrawal (Willmer & Bell 2003; Hubbard et al. 2005). Nicotine replacement therapy (NRT) includes nicotine gum, transdermal patches, nicotine nasal spray and nicotine inhalers. NRT does not have the prothrombotic effects of cigarette smoke and has less sympathetic stimulatory effects than cigarette smoking in long-term smokers (Blann et al. 1997; Lucini et al. 1998; Zevin et al. 1998) due to the development of nicotine tolerance (Palmer et al. 1992; Zevin et al. 1998). Studies suggest that early introduction of smoking cessation counselling and NRT may be effective in smoking cessation in both short and long terms (Willmer & Bell 2003; Ford & Zlabek 2005).

Physical inactivity

Physical inactivity is estimated to cause 2 million deaths worldwide annually. It is estimated that 60% of the world's population fails to achieve the minimum recommendation of 30 min moderate-intensity physical activity on most days (WHO 2008c). Physical inactivity is a major risk factor for developing CVD and contributes to other CVD risk factors including obesity, hypertension, elevated TG, decreased levels of HDL and diabetes.

Learning activity

The primary focus in the acute setting of ACS for physically inactive individuals is on education in hospital and referral to exercise programmes on discharge. A number of organisations produce guidelines for physical activity. Visit:
  Australian Government's Department of Health and Ageing at http://www.health.gov.au/internet/wcms/Publishing.nsf/Content/phd-physical-activity-adults-pdf-cnt.htm/$FILE/adults_phys.pdf
  United States Government Centers for Disease Control and Prevention at http://www.cdc.gov/nccdphp/dnpa/physical/health_professionals/promotion/community_guide.htm

Alcohol consumption

Light to moderate alcohol consumption has been associated with lower risk of CVD and overall mortality (Djoussé et al. 2005). The beneficial effects are probably due to increased HDL cholesterol, inhibition of platelet aggregation, improved fibrinolysis (Rimm et al. 1999) and anti-inflammatory effects (Imhof et al. 2001) seen with light to moderate alcohol intake. Heavy alcohol consumption, on the other hand, is associated with an increased risk of CVD but this risk is only similar to that of non-drinkers (Emberson et al. 2005). Alcohol may impact upon other risk factors for CVD as it can contribute to elevation of TG, BP and body weight.

Psychosocial risk factors

There is increasing recognition of the role of psychosocial risk factors in promotion of atherosclerosis and subsequent development of CVD. Psychosocial risk factors can be divided into emotional factors and chronic stressors. Emotional factors include major depression and anxiety disorders, as well as hostility and anger. Examples of chronic stressors are low social support, low socioeconomic status, work stress, marital stress and caregiver strain (Rozanski et al. 2005).

Emotional factors and chronic stressors tend to cluster: for example, people with chronic job strain often are depressed (Mausner-Dorsch & Eaton 2000). Any life situation that results in stress and has the capacity to provoke negative emotional responses may contribute to CVD (Rozanski et al. 2005).

Emotional disturbance and chronic stress can result in increased output from the sympathetic nervous system and hypothalamic-pituitary-adrenal axis (HPA axis) responses, resulting in a range of pathophysiologic responses such as autonomic nervous system dysfunction, hypertension, inflammation, platelet activation, insulin resistance, endothelial dysfunction and central obesity (Rozanski et al. 2005).

Psychosocial risk factors can also impact upon other risk factors for CVD. Individuals with anxiety and depression are more likely to have a poor diet with increased dietary cholesterol and total energy intake, an increased prevalence of smoking and a sedentary lifestyle than non-anxious or non-depressed subjects (Bonnet et al. 2005).

Individuals who have mental illness are also at increased risk of CVD. Those with severe mental illness are more likely to have diabetes, low amounts of HDL cholesterol and raised Framingham risk scores (a composite of risk for coronary heart disease) compared with those without severe mental illness (Osborn et al. 2006). Individuals with mental illness are more likely to smoke, and those with schizophrenia may have a genetic disposition to nicotine addiction (Ho & Rumsfeld 2006). Mental illness is also associated with a high rate of medication non-compliance, and so individuals with mental illness and risk factors for CVD are less likely to comply with therapies to reduce risk (Marder 2003). Furthermore, evidence has recently emerged to suggest that new generation antipsychotic medications may be the cause of metabolic syndrome in this group of individuals (Melkersson & Dahl 2004). Many characteristics of people with schizophrenia, such as sedentary behaviour, may also contribute to the higher prevalence of metabolic abnormalities in people with this disorder.

Conclusion

This chapter has outlined the common risk factors for CVD. Risk for CVD rises progressively according to the number of risk factors present in an individual. Individuals with CVD often have multiple risk factors which elevate their risk of an acute event exponentially. The application of risk assessment tools and identifying those individuals at greatest risk of CVD is dealt with in the next chapter. We do know that people with existing CVD are in the highest risk group for future cardiac events; so a stringent approach to risk factor management through pharmacological and lifestyle interventions will be required. Secondary interventions to reduce risk of further cardiac events will be covered in Chapter 27.

Learning activity

Think about the patient/client population that you work with. Are there any particular social demographics that put these individuals at risk of psychosocial distress? What strategies are in place to identify emotional factors and chronic stress as potential contributors to ACS in your workplace? If this aspect of risk assessment is overlooked, what strategies could you introduce to ensure that these risk factors are recognised?

References

ACC/AHA (2007). Guidelines for the management of patients with unstable angina/non-ST-elevation myocardial infarction: a report of the American College of Cardiology/American Heart Association Task Force on Practice Guidelines (Writing Committee to revise the 2002 Guidelines for the Management of Patients with Unstable Angina/Non-ST-elevation Myocardial Infarction): developed in collaboration with the American College of Emergency Physicians, the Society for Cardiovascular Angiography and Interventions, and the Society of Thoracic Surgeons: endorsed by the American Association of Cardiovascular and Pulmonary Rehabilitation and the Society for Academic Emergency Medicine. *Circulation*, **116**:e148–304.

Access Economics (2005). The shifting burden of cardiovascular disease. National Heart Foundation of Australia. Retrieved online 16th June 2008 from http://www.heartfoundation.org.au/document/NHF/cvd_shifting_burden_0505.pdf

Ambrose, J.A. & Barua, R.S. (2004). The pathophysiology of cigarette smoking and cardiovascular disease: an update. *Journal of the American College of Cardiology*, **43**:1731–7.

American Heart Association (2008). An overview of the kidney in cardiovascular disease (CVD). Retrieved online 18th July 2008 from http://www.american-heart.org/presenter.jhtml?identifier=681

Australian Institute of Health and Welfare (AIHW) (2002). Epidemic of coronary heart disease and treatment in Australia (No. AIHW cat. No. CVD 21). Canberra, Australia.

Australian Institute of Health and Welfare (AIHW) (2004). Australia's health 2004 (No. AIHW cat. no. AUS 44), Australian Institute of Health and Welfare. Retrieved online 16th June 2008 from http://www.aihw.gov.au/publications/index.cfm/title/10014

Barnoya, J. & Glantz, S.A. (2005). Cardiovascular effects of secondhand smoke: nearly as large as smoking. *Circulation*, **111**:2684–98.

Bartnik, M., Norhammar, A. & Ryden, L. (2007). Hyperglycaemia and cardiovascular disease. *Journal of Internal Medicine*, **262**:145–56.

Barua, R.S., Ambrose, J.A., Saha, D.C. & Eales-Reynolds, L. (2002). Smoking is associated with altered endothelial-derived fibrinolytic and antithrombotic factors: an in vitro demonstration. *Circulation*, **106**:905–8.

Blann, A.D., Steele, C. & McCollum, C.N. (1997). The influence of smoking and of oral and transdermal nicotine on blood pressure, and haematology and coagulation indices. *Thrombosis and Haemostasis*, **78**:1093–6.

Bonnet, F., Irving, K., Terra, J.-L., Nony, P., Berthezène, F. & Moulin, P. (2005). Anxiety and depression are associated with unhealthy lifestyle in patients at risk of cardiovascular disease. *Atherosclerosis*, **178**:339–44.

British Heart Foundation (BHF) (2008). Blood pressure. Retrieved online 18th July 2008 from http://www.heartstats.org/topic.asp?id=881

Capes, S.E., Hunt, D., Malmberg, K. & Gerstein, H.C. (2000). Stress hyperglycaemia and increased risk of death after myocardial infarction in patients with and without diabetes: a systematic overview. *The Lancet*, **355**:773–8.

Cappuccio, F.P., Oakeshott, P., Strazzullo, P. & Kerry, S.M. (2002). Application of Framingham risk estimates to ethnic minorities in United Kingdom and implications for primary prevention of heart disease in general practice: cross sectional population based study. *British Medical Journal*, **325**:1271.

Chobanian, A.V., Bakris, G.L., Black, H.R., et al. (2003). Seventh report of the joint national committee on prevention, detection, evaluation, and treatment of high blood pressure. *Hypertension*, **42**:1206–52.

Czernin, J., Sun, K., Brunken, R., Bottcher, M., Phelps, M. & Schelbert, H. (1995). Effect of acute and long-term smoking on myocardial blood flow and flow reserve. *Circulation*, **91**:2891–7.

Deedwania, P., Kosiborod, M., Barrett, E., et al. (2008). Hyperglycemia and acute coronary syndrome: a scientific statement from the American Heart Association diabetes committee of the council on nutrition, physical activity, and metabolism. *Circulation*, **117**:1610–9.

Diabetes Australia – NSW (2008). Types of diabetes. Retrieved online 15th May 2008 from http://www.diabetesnsw.com.au/about_diabetes/overview.asp

Djoussé, L., Levy, D., Herbert, A.G., et al. (2005). Influence of alcohol dehydrogenase 1C polymorphism on the alcohol–cardiovascular disease association (from the Framingham Offspring Study). *American Journal of Cardiology*, **96**:227–32.

Donahoe, S.M., Stewart, G.C., McCabe, C.H., et al. (2007). Diabetes and mortality following acute coronary syndromes. *JAMA: The Journal of the American Medical Association*, **298**:765–75.

Emberson, J.R., Shaper, A.G., Wannamethee, S.G., Morris, R.W. & Whincup, P.H. (2005). Alcohol intake in middle age and risk of cardiovascular disease and mortality: accounting for intake variation over time. *American Journal of Epidemiology*, **161**:856–63.

Ezzati, M., Lopez, A.D., Rodgers, A., Vander Hoorn, S. & Murray, C.J. (2002). Selected major risk factors and global and regional burden of disease. *The Lancet*, **360**:1347–60.

Fletcher, B., Berra, K., Ades, P., et al. (2005). Managing abnormal blood lipids: a collaborative approach. *Circulation*, **112**:3184–209.

Ford, C.L. & Zlabek, J.A. (2005). Nicotine replacement therapy and cardiovascular disease. *Mayo Clinic Proceedings*, **80**:652–6.

Fusegawa, Y., Goto, S., Handa, S., Kawada, T. & Ando, Y. (1999). Platelet spontaneous aggregation in platelet-rich plasma is increased in habitual smokers. *Thrombosis Research*, **93**:271–8.

Grundy, S.M., Benjamin, I.J., Burke, G.L., et al. (1999). Diabetes and cardiovascular disease: a statement for healthcare professionals from the American Heart Association. *Circulation*, **100**:1134–46.

Ho, P.M. & Rumsfeld, J.S. (2006) Cardiac risk management in severe mental illness. *The Lancet*, **367**:1469–71.

Hubbard, R., Lewis, S., Smith, C., et al. (2005). Use of nicotine replacement therapy and the risk of acute myocardial infarction, stroke and death. *Tobacco Control*, **14**:416–21.

Imhof, A., Froehlich, M., Brenner, H., Boeing, H., Pepys, M.B. & Koenig, W. (2001). Effect of alcohol consumption on systemic markers of inflammation. *The Lancet*, **357**:763–67.

Kearney, P.M., Whelton, M., Reynolds, K., Muntner, P., Whelton, P.K. & He, J. (2005). Global burden of hypertension: analysis of worldwide data. *The Lancet*, **365**:217–23.

Klabunde, R. (2007). Primary (essential) hypertension. Cardiovascular physiology concepts. Retrieved online 11th May 2008 from http://www.cvphysiology.com/Blood%20Pressure/BP024.htm

Knowler, W.C., Barrett-Connor, E., Fowler, S.E., et al. (2002). Diabetes prevention program research group: reduction in the incidence of type 2 diabetes with lifestyle intervention or metformin. *New England Journal of Medicine*, **346**:393–403.

Lewington, S., Clarke, R., Qizilbash, N., Peto, R. & Collins, R. (2003). Age-specific relevance of usual blood pressure to vascular mortality. *The Lancet*, **361**:1391–2.

Lucini, D., Bertocchi, F., Malliani, A. & Pagani, M. (1998). Autonomic effects of nicotine patch administration in habitual cigarette smokers: a double-blind, placebo-controlled study using spectral analysis of RR interval and systolic arterial pressure variabilities. *Journal of Cardiovascular Pharmacology*, **31**:714–20.

Mancia, G., De Backer, G., Dominiczak, A., et al. (2007). Guidelines for the management of arterial hypertension. *European Heart Journal*, **28**:1462–536.

Marder, S.R. (2003). Overview of partial compliance. *Journal of Clinical Psychiatry*, **64**(Suppl. 16):3–9.

Mausner-Dorsch, H. & Eaton, W. (2000). Psychosocial work environment and depression: epidemiologic assessment of the demand-control model. *American Journal of Public Health*, **90**:1765–70.

McGill, H.C. Jr. & McMahan, C.A. (1998). Determinants of atherosclerosis in the young: Pathobiological Determinants of Atherosclerosis in Youth (PDAY) Research Group. *American Journal of Cardiology*, **82**:30T–36T.

Melkersson, K. & Dahl, M. (2004). Adverse metabolic effects associated with atypical antipsychotics: literature review and clinical implications. *Drugs*, **64**:701–23.

Merck & Co., Inc. (2005). Dyslipidemia. The Merck Manuals. Retrieved online 10th May 2008 from http://www.merck.com/mmpe/sec12/ch159/ch159b.html

National Heart Foundation of Australia (NHFA) (2008a). Fats and cholesterol. Retrieved online 11th May 2008 from http://www.heartfoundation.org.au/Healthy_Living/Eating_and_Drinking/Fats_and_Cholesterol.htm

National Heart Foundation of Australia (NHFA) (2008b). Guide to management of hypertension. Retrieved online 18th July 2008 from http://www.heartfoundation.org.au/document/NHF/Hypertension_Management_QRG_2008_FINAL.pdf

National Heart Foundation of Australia and the Cardiac Society of Australia and New Zealand (2005). Position statement on lipid management. *Heart, Lung and Circulation*, **14**:275–91.

Osborn, D.P., Nazareth, I. & King, M.B. (2006). Risk for coronary heart disease in people with severe mental illness: cross-sectional comparative study in primary care. *British Journal of Psychiatry*, **188**:271–7.

Palmer, K.J., Buckley, M.M. & Faulds, D. (1992). Transdermal nicotine: a review of its pharmacodynamic and pharmacokinetic properties, and therapeutic efficacy as an aid to smoking cessation. *Drugs*, **44**:498–529.

Primatesta, P., Flaschetti, E., Gupta, S., Marmot, M.G. & Poulter, N.R. (2001). Association between smoking and blood pressure: evidence from the health survey for England. *Hypertension*, **37**:187–93.

Rimm, E.B., Williams, P., Fosher, K., Criqui, M. & Stampfer, M.J. (1999). Moderate alcohol intake and lower risk of coronary heart disease: meta-analysis of effects on lipids and haemostatic factors. *British Medical Journal*, **319**:1523–8.

Rosendorff, C., Black, H.R., Cannon, C.P., et al. (2007). Treatment of hypertension in the prevention and management of ischemic heart disease: a scientific statement from the American Heart Association council for high blood pressure research and the councils on clinical cardiology and epidemiology and prevention. *Circulation*, **115**:2761–88.

Rozanski, A., Blumenthal, J.A., Davidson, K.W., Saab, P.G. & Kubzansky, L. (2005). The epidemiology, pathophysiology, and management of psychosocial risk factors in cardiac practice: the emerging field of behavioral cardiology. *Journal of the American College of Cardiology*, **45**:637–51.

Rydén, L., Standl, E., Bartnik, M., et al. (2007). Guidelines on diabetes, pre-diabetes, and cardiovascular diseases: executive summary: the task force on diabetes and cardiovascular diseases of the European Society of Cardiology (ESC) and the European Association for the Study of Diabetes (EASD). *Revista Española De Cardiología*, **60**:525.

Smith, C.J. & Fischer, T.H. (2001). Particulate and vapor phase constituents of cigarette mainstream smoke and risk of myocardial infarction. *Atherosclerosis*, **158**:257–67.

Sugiishi, M. & Takatsu, F. (1993). Cigarette smoking is a major risk factor for coronary spasm. *Circulation*, **87**:76–9.

Svensson, A.-M., McGuire, D.K., Abrahamsson, P. & Dellborg, M. (2005). Association between hyper- and hypoglycaemia and 2 year all-cause mortality risk in diabetic patients with acute coronary events. *European Heart Journal*, **26**:1255–61.

Teo, K.K., Ounpuu, S., Hawken, S., et al. (2006). Tobacco use and risk of myocardial infarction in 52 countries in the INTERHEART study: a case-control study. *The Lancet*, **368**(9536):647–58.

Thompson, G.R. (2004). Management of dyslipidaemia. *Heart*, **90**:949–55.

Tuomilehto, J., Lindstrom, J. & Eriksson, J.G. for the Finnish Diabetes Prevention Study Group (2002). Prevention of type 2 diabetes mellitus by changes in lifestyle among subjects with impaired glucose tolerance. *New England Journal of Medicine*, **344**:1343–50.

Wadden, T.A., Berkowitz, R.I., Womble, L.G., et al. (2005). Randomized trial of lifestyle modification and pharmacotherapy for obesity. *The New England Journal of Medicine*, **353**:2111–20.

Willmer, K.A. & Bell, B. (2003). Use of nicotine replacement therapy early in recovery post-acute myocardial infarction to aid smoking cessation. *British Journal of Cardiology*, **10**:212–3.

Wilson, P.W.F., D'Agostino, R.B., Levy, D., Belanger, A.M., Silbershatz, H. & Kannel, W.B. (1998). Prediction of coronary heart disease using risk factor categories. *Circulation*, **97**:1837–47.

Wilson, P.W.F., D'Agostino, R.B., Sullivan, L., Parise, H. & Kannel, W.B. (2002). Overweight and obesity as determinants of cardiovascular risk: the Framingham experience. *Archives of Internal Medicine*, **162**:1867–72.

World Health Organization (WHO) (2006a). Guidelines for the management of dyslipidaemia in patients with diabetes mellitus. Retrieved online 18th July 2008 from http://whqlibdoc.who.int/emro/2006/9789290215677_eng.pdf

World Health Organization (WHO) (2008b). Obesity and overweight. Retrieved online 16th May 2008 from http://www.who.int/mediacentre/factsheets/fs311/en/index.html

World Health Organization (WHO) (2006c). BMI classification. Retrieved online 15th May 2008 from http://www.who.int/bmi/index.jsp?introPage=intro_3.html

World Health Organization (WHO) (2008a). General strategies for obesity prevention. Retrieved online 16th May 2008 from http://www.who.int/nutrition/topics/5_population_nutrient/en/index5.html

World Health Organization (WHO) (2008b). Tobacco key facts. Retrieved online 15th May 2008 from http://www.who.int/topics/tobacco/facts/en/index.html

World Health Organization (WHO) (2008c). Physical activity facts. Retrieved online 18th May 2008 from http://www.who.int/dietphysicalactivity/publications/facts/pa/en/index.html

Zevin, S., Jacob, P. III, Benowitz, N.L. (1998). Dose-related cardiovascular and endocrine effects of transdermal nicotine. *Clinical Pharmacology and Therapeutics*, **64**:87–95.

Useful Websites and Further Reading

Adamopoulos, D., van de Borne, P. & Argacha, J.F. (2008). New insights into the sympathetic, endothelial and coronary effects of nicotine. *Clinical and Experimental Pharmacology and Physiology*, **35**:458–63.

American Heart Association: http://www.american-heart.org/presenter.jhtml?identifier=1200000

Australian Government Department of Health and Ageing's webpage on Alcohol and other drugs: http://www.aodgp.gov.au/

British Heart Foundation: http://www.bhf.org.uk/default.aspx

Gupta, R., Gurm, H. & Bartholomew, J.R. (2004). Smokeless tobacco and cardiovascular risk. *Archives of Internal Medicine*, **164**:1845–9.

European Society of Cardiology: http://www.escardio.org/Pages/index.aspx

Ezzati, M., Henley, S.J., Thun, M.J. & Lopez, A.D. (2005). Role of smoking in global and regional cardiovascular mortality. *Circulation*, **112**:489–97.

National Heart Foundation of Australia: http://www.heartfoundation.org.au/index.htm

National Institute for Health and Clinical Excellence (NICE): http://www.nice.org.uk/

The Merck Manuals: http://www.merck.com/pubs/

World Health Organization: http://www.who.org

Whooley, M.A. (2006). Depression and cardiovascular disease: Healing the broken-hearted. *JAMA: The Journal of the American Medical Association*, **295**:2874–81.

6

Populations at Risk

T. Wachtel, R. Webster & J. Smith

Overview

Cardiovascular disease (CVD) is a major source of disease burden in Western nations and is increasing in developing countries. The prevalence and economic impact of CVD is likely to be significant and ongoing and thus we must continue to explore opportunities to improve prevention strategies and reduce risk for CVD in both primary and secondary settings. In this chapter, population groups that are at increased risk of developing CVD are identified. Reducing risk in this population requires comprehensive and ongoing management of all lifestyle, biomedical and psychosocial risk factors.

There is a role for both primary and secondary prevention in addressing risk. Individuals with existing disease have the highest absolute risk for subsequent events. Recognition of factors associated with high risk of CVD may also influence clinician's decision-making in the management of individuals who present with possible acute coronary syndrome.

Clinical practice should include the use of absolute risk assessment tools; however, care providers must be aware of the limited predictive ability of these tools within the population groups identified in this chapter and adjust their assessment accordingly.

Learning objectives

After reading this chapter, you should be able to:

- Define absolute and relative risk and how these can be applied to CVD.
- Identify populations who are at particular risk from CVD.
- Discuss the reasons why certain populations are at increased risk of development and recurrence of CVD-related illness.
- Describe the role of risk assessment tools.
- Use a risk assessment tool to calculate absolute risk.

Key concepts

Relative risk; absolute risk; risk assessment tools; at-risk populations; guideline implementation

Risk factors for CVD

The previous chapter outlines factors that are associated with a higher likelihood of developing CVD. The link between having a risk factor for coronary heart disease and the development of clinical manifestations of the disease is complex and not uniform. The risk of developing CVD is greater in some populations than others, and this is known as the relative risk. The relative risk is the ratio of the incidence of CVD among individuals who have one or more risk factors compared with those who do not have any risk factors. This chapter aims to build on the knowledge of individual risk factors and consider populations who are at particular risk of CVD. An appreciation of these population groups is important, particularly when considering treatment and the targeting of preventative strategies, as the greatest absolute benefits of treatment are in those at highest risk.

Individuals most at risk from coronary heart disease are:

- Those with established atherosclerotic coronary artery disease
- Those who after appropriate screening are identified as being at high risk of developing symptomatic atherosclerotic coronary heart disease

The reasons why individuals from certain population groups exhibit higher risk of coronary heart disease than those from other population groups is not always known, but some proposed explanations include:

- A high occurrence of particular risk factors within individuals from that population. It is estimated that 75% of coronary heart disease cases can be predicted by established risk factors such as tobacco use, physical inactivity and inappropriate diet (as expressed through elevated blood pressure, overweight and unfavourable lipid levels) and that increases to over 85% if diabetes is added (Magnus & Beaglehole 2001).
- A tendency for individuals from within that population group to have several risk factors. This is known as 'clustering' of risk factors. One risk factor will multiply the risk of another, and an asymptomatic individual with a number of slightly abnormal risk factors is likely to be more at risk from a cardiovascular event than an individual with just one highly elevated risk factor. For example, three risk factors (high cholesterol, high blood pressure and

smoking) account for 80% of the attributable risk for CVD in middle age (National Health Priority Action Council 2006).
- Particular risk factors carrying a higher weighting for the development of CVD within certain population groups.
- The prevalence of as yet unknown risk factors within certain population groups.
- Inequalities in access to services for primary prevention, diagnosis and treatment for particular population groups. This is particularly evident in indigenous populations.

Clarifying risk

Strategies for the treatment of coronary heart disease are linked to the probability or risk of individuals from within population groups developing symptomatic CVD or sustaining a cardiovascular event over a defined period of time. This risk is referred to as the 'absolute' risk and is informed by recording the incidence of cardiovascular events in particular groups over time and subsequently using this information to quantify the likelihood of future events in similar population groups. Absolute risk equations acknowledge the multi-factorial causation of CVD, the gender difference in risk and the steep increase in risk with ageing (Tonkin et al. 2003).

Risk assessment tools

The accurate estimation of cardiovascular risk is essential in order to calculate the benefit–risk ratio and the most effective and cost-effective use of preventative therapies. Information on cardiovascular risk in studied population groups has led to the development of multiple cardiovascular risk assessment tables, equations, charts and computer programs designed to inform assessment of overall risk of CVD (Sheridan et al. 2003). The European Systemic Coronary Risk Estimation (SCORE) for example is designed as a framework that can be adapted to the different regions of Europe. It is based on data from a prospective study of almost 3 million people from 12 European countries and is used to estimate fatal cardiovascular events over a period of 10 years in European populations with either a high or low background risk (Conroy et al. 2003).

Risk assessment tools take into account the multi-factorial causation of CVD and use variables including age, sex, smoking history and the measurement of blood cholesterol, blood glucose and blood pressure to quantify the overall risk of developing CVD over a particular time period. As they use data from studies of particular population groups, these tools are limited in that this data cannot always be accurately extrapolated for use with other populations such as ethnic minority groups (Brindle et al. 2006). The fact that the relationship between risk factors and CVD is different across populations also needs to be considered. Using a value of estimated risk that is too high or too low will result in the proportion of treated patients being incorrect. To be inclusive and to remain relevant, the studies on which subsequent risk assessment tools are based need to record a comprehensive range of variables including data on emerging risk factors and risk factors that apply exclusively to particular groups, such as women. Box 6.1 describes several well-known cardiovascular risk assessment tools from different countries that focus on different populations.

Many of the risk assessment tools available use data taken from a series of longitudinal studies of the predominately white middle-class population of the small American town of Framingham beginning in the late 1940s. Framingham risk equations have been used for several decades to estimate the risk of coronary heart disease over periods of time. The equation was derived from calculations based on age, sex, smoking status, diabetes status, and blood pressure, cholesterol and high density lipoprotein (HDL) cholesterol levels (Tonkin et al. 2003). The Joint British Societies (JBS) representing the British Hypertension Society, the British Cardiac Society, Diabetes UK, HEART UK, the Primary Care Cardiovascular Society and the Stroke Association, continue to use risk assessment based on the Framingham data despite the fact that this does not take into account obesity or impaired glucose tolerance and underestimates risk in population sub-groups such as the most economically disadvantaged (Chauhan 2007). The Framingham risk equations are also not applicable to people less than 35 years old and have limited

Box 6.1   Cardiovascular risk assessment tools

- ASSIGN (Assessing cardiovascular risk using SIGN) – estimates a 10-year risk percentage of developing CVD in disease-free men and women aged 30–74, developed in Scotland and includes an index of social deprivation and family history. Available at http://assign-score.com/
- European Systemic Coronary Risk Estimation (SCORE) – used to estimate fatal cardiovascular events over 10 years in low- and high-risk people. Available at http://www.escardio.org/initiatives/prevention/prevention-tools/SCORE-Risk-Charts.htm
- Joint British Coronary Risk Prediction Charts – used to identify people at high risk (JBS2 2005). Available from http://www.bmj.com/cgi/content/full/320/7236/705
- New Zealand Cardiovascular Risk Calculator – where the results are presented as a 5-year risk of CVD. Available at http://www.nps.org.au/resources/Health_Professional_Tools/nz_cardiovascular_risk_calculator.pdf
- Reynolds Risk Score – provides a greater accuracy for assessment of cardiovascular risk in women. Available at http://www.reynoldsriskscore.org/
- UK PDS (Prospective Diabetes Study) Risk Engine for people with type 2 diabetes provides risk estimates and 95% confidence intervals, in individuals with type 2 diabetes not known to have heart disease. Available at http://www.dtu.ox.ac.uk/

applicability to indigenous populations such as Māori and Pacific People in New Zealand (New Zealand Guidelines Group 2003). They have also been shown to substantially underestimate the actual risk of coronary heart disease in Australian Aboriginals, particularly women and younger adults (Wang & Hoy 2005).

Populations at increased risk

Some of the population groups with increased risk of coronary heart disease are discussed below. It is of course possible for individuals to belong to more than one of these groups.

People with established CVD

People with established atherosclerotic disease are at high risk for recurrent events. Any symptomatic manifestation of atherosclerosis in any vascular territory puts a person at risk of dying from CVD (JBS2 2005).

People with a strong family history

A family history of coronary heart disease becomes significant when an individual has a parent, sibling or child with the disease (the more family members with the disease, the greater the risk for the individual), or when an individual has a family member who has developed the disease at a young age. If a first-degree blood relative has had coronary heart disease or stroke before the age of 55 years (for a male relative) or 65 years (for a female relative), then the risk of developing coronary heart disease is increased by a factor of 1.5 (Shah 2003) . If both parents have suffered from heart disease before the age of 55 then the risk of developing heart disease can rise up to 50% compared to the general population (World Heart Federation 2008).

Families are likely to have similar geographical and socioeconomic backgrounds and comparable lifestyles and it is difficult to tease out the relative influences of nature versus nurture. Families will certainly have the same ethnicity and related genetic profiles. Modifiable risk factors for coronary heart disease such as diabetes, hypertension and hyperlipidaemia tend to run through families, and it is likely that genetic factors influence susceptibility to these risk factors particularly as several regions of the human genome have been found to be associated with coronary heart disease (Broeckel et al. 2002). There is also evidence of a genetic link with vessel wall proteins, coagulation factors and growth factors, the insulin receptor gene and the angiotensin-converting enzyme gene. Although the population attributable risk for any gene linked to coronary heart disease is limited at present, with no one gene having been identified for coronary artery disease, it is likely that this area of work will be of importance in the future, particularly with regard to susceptibility to myocardial infarction (Topol et al. 2006).

People with a high incidence of significant risk factors

A history of any of the following conditions places people at high risk of coronary heart disease: diabetes, familial hypercholesterolaemia, raised total cholesterol to HDL cholesterol ratio of more than 6 mmol/L, or severe hypertension, where systolic blood pressure is greater than 180 mmHg and/or diastolic blood pressure is greater than 100 mmHg.

Advancing age

Advancing age is the most powerful independent risk factor for CVD, with the risk of stroke doubling for every decade after the age of 55 (Mackay & Mensah 2004). The absolute risk of CVD is higher in the elderly and the mortality from coronary heart disease almost doubles with every additional 5 years of life. This is probably due to the cumulative effect of longer exposure to the known, modifiable risk factors such as smoking, hypertension and hyperlipidaemia, rather than simple degeneration resulting from the ageing process. The magnitude of risk factors is also linked to age with blood pressure, cholesterol and glucose rising and HDL cholesterol falling with advancing age and therefore exacerbating the risk. Physical activity and formal exercise also decline with age, along with any preventative effects gained from this activity.

Women

Nearly one out of three women worldwide dies due to CVD. This disease afflicts more women than any other and there is a steep increase in the incidence of CVD with age (World Heart Federation 2008). Many of the risk factors for coronary heart disease, such as hypertension, dyslipidaemia, unhealthy diet, physical inactivity and stress, are the same for women as they are for men. However, there is a higher prevalence of some modifiable risk factors in women, such as diabetes, obesity and depression. In addition, the relative weighting of several risk factors is different, with smoking, hypertension and hyper-triglyceridaemia being more significant for women than for men.

Women smokers for example are at higher risk of heart attack than male smokers, with their risk of heart attack doubling with the consumption of 3–5 cigarettes per day compared to men who double their risk at 6–9 cigarettes per day. The female sex hormone oestrogen tends to raise HDL cholesterol levels, which may help explain why pre-menopausal women are relatively protected from developing coronary heart disease (Mackay & Mensah 2004). However, diabetes negates the protective effects that the pre-menopausal state confers on women (Abramason 2004). Blood cholesterol levels among women increase with age. After menopause, women's cholesterol levels are on average higher than those of men the same age (World Heart Federation 2008). While menopause has no direct affect on risk, hormone replacement therapy increases the risk of CVD (Mackay & Mensah 2004). Other risk factors applicable only to women include oral contraceptive use and polycystic ovary syndrome (Mackay & Mensah 2004).

Ethnic populations

Different ethnic groups have different incidences of coronary heart disease within their populations. Whilst cardiovascular risk factors are the same in all nationalities, the metabolic response to various risk factors may differ in different populations (Yusuf et al. 2004). Populations at particular risk include Hispanics, Asians, Arabs, Africans, Pacific Islanders and indigenous (American, Canadian, Australian, Māori) populations (World Heart Federation 2008).

The incidence of coronary heart disease is changing in many populations influenced by globalisation, shifts in lifestyle caused by economic growth, affluence, urbanisation, industrialisation and adoption of a Western diet. For those who migrate, the process of moving and assimilation into a different culture may contribute to ethnic differences. Factors such as access to services and uptake of treatment strategies are also important. Many indigenous communities are subject to geographical isolation as well as dealing with limited availability and affordability of health services.

South Asians have an unusually high tendency to develop coronary heart disease with mortality rates of south Asians in the UK being approximately 40% higher when compared to the white population (Balarajan 1991). This is thought to be influenced by a tendency for the clustering of cardiovascular risk factors (McKeigue et al. 1992) including diabetes mellitus, insulin resistance, adiposity (abdominal obesity), high triglycerides, low HDL and increased lipoprotein (a) levels within this population group (Pinto 1998). Adding 10 years to the age of south Asian people is thought to be a reliable way of calculating coronary heart disease risk using current charts (Aarabi & Jackson 2005). There are also an increased number of deaths from CVD among African Americans in comparison with whites, and an increased prevalence of stroke is also noted for African Americans, some Hispanic Americans, Chinese and Japanese populations (Mackay & Mensah 2004).

In Australia, the 15–20 year lower life expectancy among Aboriginal and Torres Straight Islander (ATSI) people is largely due to coronary heart disease (National Health and Medical Research Council 2005). Indigenous Australians experience higher rates of death and illness from CVD, with death rates 2.6 times higher than those of non-indigenous Australians (National Health Priority Action Council 2006), and they have greater difficulty accessing health services (National Health and Medical Research Council 2005). ATSI people have 3 times the rate of major coronary events such as heart attacks and 1.4 times the out-of-hospital death rate from coronary heart disease (Mathur et al. 2006). This may be explained by the fact that when compared to other Australians, ATSI people are more likely to smoke, have high blood pressure, be obese and drink alcohol at harmful levels (National Heart Foundation Australia 2004). ATSI populations are also almost 4 times more likely than non-indigenous populations to have diabetes and tend to have diabetes at a younger age (National Health Priority Action Council 2006).

Death rates from CVD for Caribbeans and West Africans are comparatively low. The premature mortality for these groups in England and Wales is reported to be about half the rate of that in the general population for men and about two-thirds of the rate found in women (British Heart Foundation 2007). It is not clear why this difference exists, although genetic factors may be significant.

Low socioeconomic populations

The link between socioeconomic factors and risk of developing coronary heart disease is complex. Studies have identified that risk factors are distributed differently between socioeconomic groups with a larger risk factor burden being found in those in lower socioeconomic positions (Ljung & Hallqvist 2006). It is thought that socioeconomic status affects coronary heart disease through a combination of lifestyle and behavioural patterns (such as smoking, heavy alcohol consumption, physical inactivity and obesity), ease of access to health care and chronic stress (Mackay & Mensah 2004). A lower level of health literacy (the ability to understand and use information to promote and maintain good health) is also often present in lower socioeconomic groups (National Health Priority Action Council 2006). While men and women from lower socioeconomic groups tend to have multiple risk factors more often than those from higher socioeconomic groups, this difference cannot always explain the socioeconomic gradient in coronary heart disease (Kivimaki et al. 2007).

Socioeconomically disadvantaged populations in Australia experience higher rates of CVD than other Australians, and there is evidence that the differential has widened. A similar trend of widening socioeconomic inequalities in CVD mortality is also evident in other countries (Australian Institute of Health and Welfare 2006a).

Geographical population distributions

Major geographical variations in the incidence of coronary heart disease are apparent and are ever changing. In recent years, it is the populations of the countries of Eastern Europe where there has been much political and social unrest and moves towards Western culture where the death rates for coronary heart disease are rising (World Health Organization 2004). Even a land mass the size of Great Britain demonstrates regional variability in terms of death rates from coronary heart disease with the premature death rate for men living in Scotland being 50% higher than it is in East Anglia (British Heart Foundation 2007).

In Australia, rural and remote populations have a significantly higher incidence of cardiac mortality and morbidity than metropolitan areas (Access Economics 2005; Australian Institute of Health and Welfare 2006), yet they have poorer access to cardiac services (Dollard et al. 2004; Clark et al. 2005) and are prescribed cardiovascular medications at half the rate of people living in major cities (Australian Institute of Health and Welfare 2006b). Men and women living in rural and remote areas have poorer access to health care due to transport issues, distance, financial reasons and lack of resources (National Health Priority Action Council 2006).

Individuals with poor psychosocial health

Psychosocial factors are associated with the development and progress of CVD. The pathological mechanisms underpinning these associations remain unclear although it is likely that there are important links between psychosocial state and physiological functioning. Patients with similar psychosocial profiles may be exposed to similar stressors putting them more at risk from CVD and/or they may have genetically determined methods of coping with stressors that influence their predisposition to developing the disease. There is also strong evidence to suggest a causal association between social isolation and lack of quality social support, and the causes and prognosis of CVD (Bunker & Goble 2003).

It is also possible that those with psychosocial problems are also disadvantaged by inequalities in primary prevention and access to services thereby increasing their risk. A specific example of this is people with a diagnosis of schizophrenia have a significantly elevated 10-year risk of coronary heart disease based on Framingham predictor variables (Goff et al. 2005). It is also known that the presence of concurrent psychiatric disorder, such as depression, increases the rates of death from myocardial infarction (Van Melle et al. 2004). There is likely to be a complex relationship between behaviour, environment, symptoms and psychosocial state (Everson-Rose & Lewis 2005; Steptoe & Whitehead 2005). Patients with mental health problems may be less compliant with treatment regimes, less likely to consent for interventional procedures and have negative home circumstances and other socioeconomic factors (Goldbloom & Kurdyak 2007). Psychosocial factors also play a part in behaviours linked to cardiovascular risk including smoking, physical activity and alcohol intake. Smoking rates may be as high as 60% in those diagnosed with depression or bipolar disorder (Kalman et al. 2005).

Attention is turning to the possible effects of psychological factors on biological precursors of CVD. For example, depression, chronic stress and cynical distress have been linked to higher concentrations of the inflammatory markers associated with atherosclerosis (Ranjit et al. 2007). Stress causes physiological changes in the cardiovascular system which can have negative affects on heart health. Acute stress reduces blood flow to the heart, promotes irregular heart beats and increases the likelihood of blood clotting; all of which can contribute to the development of CVD (World Heart Federation 2008).

Targeting treatment

While knowledge of the risk for coronary heart disease for different population groups is informative, it is the appropriate treatment of individuals from within populations that is important. Historically, patients were managed based on the presence or absence of individual cardiovascular risk factors. This approach does not take into account the fact that CVD is generally the result of a combination of several risk factors and the complex interaction between the different risk factors that comprise total CVD risk. Interventions based on elevated levels of a single risk factor may result in treatment being allocated to individuals with little chance of gain because of a low absolute risk and conversely neglect those with an overall higher cardiovascular risk. Treatment guidelines have been designed to follow on from the risk assessment process with preventative treatment and intervention being recommended if a patient's absolute risk exceeds a certain cut-off point (Diverse Populations Collaborative Group 2002). These cut-off points have been defined to focus finite resources on the care of high-risk individuals.

The Joint British Society Guidelines (2005) recommend that clinical practice should focus equally on people with established atherosclerotic (cardiovascular) disease, people with diabetes

and asymptomatic individuals at high total risk (a 10-year absolute cardiovascular risk equal to or greater than 20%).

A significant challenge is identifying those asymptomatic and apparently healthy individuals who are at highest risk of developing CVD. European guidelines on CVD prevention in clinical practice (De Backer et al. 2003) have defined 'high risk' in asymptomatic individuals in three ways:

1. Individuals with type 2 diabetes or with type 1 diabetes with microalbuminuria
2. People with a markedly elevated single risk factor, including;
    *   cholesterol greater than 8 mmol/L (320 mg/dL)
    *   low density lipoprotein (LDL) cholesterol greater than 6 mmol/L (240 mg/dL)
    *   blood pressure greater than 180/ 110 mmHg
3. People identified at high risk using total risk assessment tools

The Joint British Society Guidelines (2005) recommend that all those identified as being at high risk are treated to the same lifestyle objectives and targets for lipids, blood pressure and glucose. These include total cholesterol less than 4.0 mmol/L (less than 155 mg/dL) and LDL cholesterol less than 2.0 mmol/L (less than 78 mg/dL). The National Institute for Health and Clinical Excellence (NICE) guidance on statins for the prevention of cardiovascular events recommend that statins be used where the risk of an individual developing CVD within 10 years is estimated to be 20% or greater (NICE 2006).

Care providers need to appraise the systems they have in place to ensure individuals identified as being at risk from coronary heart disease receive this appropriate treatment. Population-based risk assessment as part of a coordinated vascular disease control programme, for example inviting all individuals for risk assessment at certain memorable landmarks such as their 45th birthday, encourages a coordinated approach (Department of Health 2006). Integrating this with self-assessment and opportunistic screening would add to the current focus on 'individuals at risk strategy' (Chauhan 2007). The JBS2 (2005) guidelines advocate that all adults aged 40 and above, who have no history of coronary heart disease, and who are not already on treatment for raised blood pressure or lipids, should be considered for an opportunistic comprehensive cardiovascular risk assessment. The New Zealand Guidelines Group (2003) recommend cardiovascular risk assessment at the age of 35 years for men and 45 years for women for the following populations: Māori, Pacific Peoples, people from the Indian subcontinent and all people with known cardiovascular risk factors or at high risk of developing diabetes.

Ideally there should be an incremental association between an individual's risk for coronary heart disease and their level of treatment. Populations with specific risks such as those discussed within this chapter need to be targeted with strategies designed for their specific circumstances. It is of course possible that there will be some patients where the level of required risk reduction is considerably greater than what is achievable with treatment. The value of any intervention is dependent on the extent to which it reduces the absolute rather than relative risk (Smith et al. 2004). Linking estimates of the likely absolute benefit of interventions with calculation of absolute risk should reinforce the rationale for lifestyle measures for all individuals and pharmacological treatment for those at higher risk. Absolute risk assessment will not only optimise health gains, but will result in more cost-effective treatment and prevention (Tonkin et al. 2003).

A comprehensive CVD risk-management programme relies on individual patient adherence to daily drug treatments, accepting and implementing lifestyle advice and returning for follow-up assessments. Patients, their families and communities need to be empowered to actively participate in patient care through health education and through community mobilisation programs (World Health Organization 2002).

Identifying those who benefit from treatment does not necessarily lead to more people being treated. Consensus as to the level of risk at which to initiate treatment is influenced by financial and political as well as clinical criteria. Populations with high-risk patients may be the very populations where resources for appropriate intervention are limited. Offering treatment does not always lead to this treatment being followed, and tailoring care to the specific cultural, social, educational and emotional needs of population groups remains a challenge.

Using what we know

The importance of early recognition and identification of CVD risk factors has been highlighted throughout this chapter, and risk calculators have been identified as a useful method of achieving this. Early risk factor management is essential for patients to regain optimal function and reduce the risk of further cardiovascular events and death (Dalal & Evans 2003; Giannuzzi et al. 2003).

Early identification, however, must precede the timely and effective implementation of proven therapies to ensure optimal patient outcomes (Chew et al. 2005). Clinical guidelines exist to facilitate the delivery of effective and consistent therapeutic interventions (National Health Priority Action Council 2006); however, this alone is not sufficient to influence clinical practice (Euroaspire II Study Group 2001). Despite significant increases in the use of cardiovascular medicines over the past decade, secondary prevention targets are not being met. These poor outcomes have been linked to a failure to address underlying lifestyle issues such as obesity and smoking (Euroaspire II Study Group 2001). For primary and secondary CVD prevention to be successful, a paradigm shift is required away from the treatment of risk factors in isolation to a comprehensive cardiovascular risk management approach (WHO 2002), and pharmacological interventions must be combined with the assessment of biomedical, and lifestyle and behavioural assessment and interventions to address identified risk factors (Aroney et al. 2006).

The wide gap that exists in the implementation of evidence-based medicine in both primary and secondary care needs to be urgently addressed at both National and local levels to ensure continuity of risk factor management and to ensure long-term compliance with evidence-based therapies (Euroaspire II Study Group 2001).

Conclusion

The enormity of CVD is never more apparent then when trying to determine who would most benefit from intervention. Preventing cardiovascular deaths and avoiding unnecessary treatment in those at lower risk of CVD is the goal of pragmatic health systems. For the care providers within health systems being able to identify who is at the highest risk of developing CVD is therefore critical.

Population groups who are at high risk of CVD have been identified in this chapter. For clinicians, a critical understanding is that those individuals with existing CVD have the highest absolute risk for subsequent events. Comprehensive treatment guidelines that provide management goals for this high-risk population are available and they support systematic interventions to address the ongoing management of risk.

Population-based risk assessment is the key to determining other individuals who are at high risk, and systematic approaches including absolute risk assessment are required to support high risk identification. Clinical practice should therefore include the use of absolute risk assessment tools. It has been clearly identified in this chapter, however, that care providers must be aware of the limited predictive ability of these tools with some population groups. For individuals found to be at high risk of CVD, the same treatment guidelines as for those with CVD should be applied.

Learning activities

Compare three of the risk assessment models/risk calculators in Box 6.1. What are the benefits of calculating a patient's absolute risk of CVD?

What are the limitations of these risk calculators?

What other resources could you use to determine a person's risk of developing CVD?

Visit three of the online risk calculators listed in Box 6.1 and type your own details to calculate your cardiovascular risk.

Were there questions in the calculator/tool that you were not able to answer?

Did at least two calculators/tools predict the same level of risk?

Can you identify any specific population groups for which these tools would not be appropriate?

References

Aarabi, M. & Jackson, P.R. (2005). Predicting coronary risk in UK South Asians: an adjustment method for Framingham based tools. *European Journal of Cardiovascular Prevention and Rehabilitation*, **12**:46–51.

Abramason, B.L. (2004). Women and cardiovascular disease: update 2004. *Patient Care*, **5**:33–8.

Access Economics (2005). The shifting burden of cardiovascular disease: a report prepared for the National Heart Foundation of Australia. Retrieved online 6th May 2006 from http://www.heartfoundation.com.au/media/nhfa.pdf

Aroney, C., Aylward, P., Kelly, A., Chew, D. & Clune, E. (2006). Guidelines for the management of acute coronary syndromes 2006: on behalf of the Acute Coronary Syndrome Guidelines Working Group. *Medical Journal of Australia*, **184**:S1–30.

Australian Institute of Health and Welfare (2006a). Socioeconomic inequalities in cardiovascular disease in Australia: current picture and trends since 1992. *Bulletin*, **37**. Retrieved online 5th September 2008 from http://www.aihw.gov.au/publications/aus/bulletin37/bulletin37.pdf

Australian Institute of Health and Welfare (2006b). Rural, regional and remote health: mortality trends 1992–2003. Retrieved online 5th September 2008 from http://www.aihw.gov.au/publications/index.cfm/title/10276

Balarajan, R. (1991). Ethnic differences in morality from ischaemic heart disease and cerebrovascular disease in England and Wales. *British Medical Journal*, **302**:560–4.

British Heart Foundation (2007). Coronary heart disease statistics database. British Heart Foundation, London. Retrieved online 5th September 2008 from http://www.heartstats.org/uploads/documents%5C48160_text_05_06_07.pdf

Brindle, P., Beswick, A., Fahey, T. & Ebrahim, S. (2006). Accuracy and impact of risk assessment in the primary prevention of cardiovascular disease: a systematic review. *Heart*, **92**:1752–9.

Broeckel, U., Hengstenberg, C., Mayer, B., et al. (2002). A comprehensive linkage analysis for myocardial infarction and its related risk factors. *Nature Genetics*, **30**:210–4.

Bunker, S. & Goble, A. (2003). Cardiac rehabilitation: under-referral and underutilization. *The Medical Journal of Australia*, **179**:332–5.

Chauhan, U. (2007). Cardiovascular disease prevention in primary care. *British Medical Bulletin*, **81 & 82**:65–9.

Chew, D., Allan, R., Aroney, C. & Sheerin, N. (2005). National data elements for the clinical management of acute coronary syndromes. *Medical Journal of Australia*, **182**:S1–15.

Clark, A.L., Hartling, L., Vandermeer, B. & McAllister, A. (2005). Meta-analysis: secondary prevention programs for patients with coronary artery disease. *Annals of Internal Medicine*, **143**:659–72.

Conroy, R.M., Pyorala, K., Fitzgerald, A.P., et al. (2003). Estimation of the 10 year risk of fatal cardiovascular disease in Europe: the ACORE project. *European Heart Journal*, **24**:987–1003.

Dalal, H.M. & Evans, P.H. (2003). Achieving national service framework standards for cardiac rehabilitation and secondary prevention, *British Medical Journal*, **326**:481.

De Backer, G., Ambrosioni, E., Borch-Johnsen, K., et al. (2003). European guidelines on cardiovascular disease prevention in clinical practice. Third Joint Task Force of European and Other Societies on Cardiovascular Disease Prevention in Clinical Practice, *European Heart Journal*, **24**:1601–10.

Department of Health (2006). Our health, our care, our say: a new direction for community services', The Stationary Office. Retrieved online 5th September 2008 from http://www.dh.gov.uk/en/Healthcare/Ourhealthourcareoursay/index.htm

Diverse Populations Collaborative Group (2002). Prediction of mortality from coronary heart disease among diverse populations: is there a common predictive function? *Heart*, **88**:222–8.

Dollard, J., Smith, J., Thomson, D. & Stewart, S. (2004). Broadening the reach of cardiac rehabilitation to rural and remote Australia. *European Journal of Cardiovascular Nursing*, **3**:27–42.

Euroaspire II Study Group (2001). Lifestyle and risk factors management and use of drug therapies in coronary patients from 15 countries; principle results from Euroaspire II Euro Heart Survey Programme. *European Heart Journal*, **22**:554–72.

Everson-Rose, S.A. & Lewis, T.T. (2005). Psychosocial factors and cardiovascular diseases. *Annual Review of Public Health*, **26**:469–500.

Giannuzzi, P., Saner, H., Bjornstad, H., et al. (2003). Secondary prevention through cardiac rehabilitation: position paper of the working group on cardiac rehabilitation and exercise physiology of the European Society of Cardiology. *European Heart Journal*, **24**:1273–8.

Goff, D.C., Sullivan, L.M., McEvoy, J.P., et al. (2005). A comparison of ten year cardiac risk estimates in schizophrenic patients from the CATIE study and matched controls. *Schizophrenic Research*, **80**:45–53.

Goldbloom, D.S. & Kurdyak, P. (2007). Mental illness and cardiovascular mortality: searching for the links. *Canadian Medical Association Journal*, **176**:787–9.

Joint British Societies (JBS2) (2005). Guidelines on prevention of cardiovascular disease in clinical practice. *Heart*, **91**(Suppl. 5):v1–52.

Kalman, D., Morisette, S.B. & George, T.P. (2005). Co-morbidity of smoking and patients with psychiatric and substance use disorders, *American Journal of Addiction*, **14**:106–23.

Kivimaki, M., Lawlor, D.A., Davey-Smith, G., et al. (2007). Socioeconomic position, co-occurrence of behaviour related risk factors and coronary heart disease: the Finnish Public Sector study. *American Journal of Public Health*, **97**:874–9.

Ljung, R. & Hallqvist, J. (2006). Accumulation of adverse socioeconomic position over entire life course and the risk of myocardial infarction among men and women: results from the Stockholm Heart Epidemiology Program (SHEEP). *Journal of Epidemiology and Community Health*, **60**:1080–4.

Mackay, J. & Mensah, G. (2004). The atlas of heart disease and stroke. World Health Organization. Retrieved online 5th September 2008 from http://www.who.int/cardiovascular_diseases/resources/atlas/en/

Magnus, P. & Beaglehole, R. (2001). The real contribution of the major risk factors to the coronary epidemics: time to end the "Only-50%" Myth. *Archives of Internal Medicine*, **161**:2657–60.

Mathur, S.L., Moon, L. & Leigh, S. (2006). Aboriginal and Torres Straight Islander people with coronary heart disease – summary report. Australian Institute of Health and Welfare, Canberra, AIHW cat. no. CVD 34. Retrieved online 5th September 2008 from http://www.aihw.gov.au/publications/index.cfm/title/10364

McKeigue, P.M., Pierpoint. T., Ferrie, J.E. & Marmot, M.F. (1992). Relationship of glucose tolerance and hyperinsulinaemia to body fat pattern in South Asians and Europeans. *Diabetologia*, **35**:785–91.

National Health and Medical Research Council (2005). Strengthening cardiac rehabilitation and secondary prevention for Aboriginal and Torres Straight Islander peoples: a guide for health professionals. Australian Government Department for Health and Ageing. Retrieved online 5th September 2008 from http://www.nhmrc.gov.au/publications/synopses/ind1syn.htm

National Health Priority Action Council (2006). National service improvement framework for heart, stroke and vascular disease. Australian Government Department for Health and Ageing, Canberra. Retrieved online 5th September 2008 from http://www.health.gov.au/internet/main/publishing.nsf/content/pq-ncds-cardio

National Heart Foundation Australia (2004). Heart, stroke and vascular disease. Australian facts 2004, National Heart Foundation Australia. Retrieved online 5th September 2008 from http://www.aihw.gov.au/publications/index.cfm/title/10005

New Zealand Guidelines Group (2003). Assessment and management of cardiovascular risk – evidence-based practice guidelines, December. Wellington, New Zealand.

National Institute for Health and Clinical Excellence (NICE) (2006). Statins for the prevention of cardiovascular events, Technology Appraisal Guidance no. 94, London, UK. Retrieved online 5th September 2008 from http://www.nice.org.uk/nicemedia/pdf/TA094guidance.pdf#null

Pinto, R. (1998). Risk factors for coronary heart disease in Asian Indians: clinical implications for prevention of coronary heart disease. *Indian Journal of Medical Sciences*, **52**:49–54.

Ranjit, N., Diez-Rouz, A.V., Shea, S., et al., (2007). Psychosocial factors and inflammation in the multi-ethnic study of atherosclerosis. *Archives of Internal Medicine*, **167**:177.

Shah, R. (2003). Assessment tools to identify CHD risk. *GP*, **65**:1.

Sheridan, S., Pignone, M. & Mulrow, C. (2003). Framingham-based tools to calculate the global risk of coronary heart disease: a systematic review of tools for clinicians. *Journal of General Internal Medicine*, **18**:1039–52.

Smith, S.C., Jr., Jackson, R., Pearson, T., et al. (2004). Principles for national and regional guidelines on cardiovascular disease prevention. A scientific statement from the world heart and stroke forum. *Circulation*, **109**:3112–21.

Steptoe, A. & Whitehead, D.L. (2005). Depression, stress and coronary heart disease: the need for more complex models. *Heart*, **91**:419–20.

Tonkin, A., Lim, S. & Schirmer, H. (2003). Cardiovascular risk factors: when should we treat? *The Medical Journal of Australia*, **178**:101–2.

Topol, E.J., Smith, J., Plow, E.F. & Wang, Q.K. (2006). Genetic susceptibility to myocardial infarction and coronary artery disease, *Human Molecular Genetics*, **15**: R117–23.

Van Melle, J.P., De Jonge, P., Spijkerman, T.A., et al. (2004). Prognostic association of depression following myocardial infarction with mortality and cardiovascular events: a meta-analysis. *Psychosomatic Medicine*, **66**:814–22.

Wang, Z. & Hoy, W.E. (2005). Is the Framingham coronary heart disease absolute risk function applicable to Aboriginal people? *Medical Journal of Australia*, **182**:66–9.

World Health Organization (2002). Integrated management of cardiovascular risk. Report of a WHO Meeting 9–12 July, Geneva. Retrieved online 5th September 2008 from http://whqlibdoc.who.int/publications/9241562242.pdf

World Health Organization (2004). WHO Statistics Annual, Geneva. Retrieved online 5th September 2008 from http://www.who.int/en/

World Heart Federation (2008). Cardiovascular disease risk factors, World Heart Federation. Retrieved online 5th September 2008 from http://www.world-heart-federation.org/cardiovascular-health/cardiovascular-disease-risk-factors/

Yusuf, S., Hawken, S, Ounpuu, S. on behalf of the INTERHEART Study Investigators (2004). Effect of potentially modifiable risk factors associated with myocardial infarction in 52 countries (the INTERHEART study): case-control study. *The Lancet*, **364**:937–52.

Useful Websites and Further Reading

American Heart Association: http://www.americanheart.org/

British Heart Foundation: http://www.bhf.org.uk/

Cardiac Society of Australia and New Zealand: http://www.csanz.edu.au/

European Society of Cardiology: http://www.escardio.org/

Joint British Society Guidelines of the Prevention of CVD in Clinical Practice: http://heart.bmj.com/cgi/content/extract/91/suppl_5/v1

National Heart Foundation Australia: http://www.heartfoundation.org.au/index.htm

WHO CVD Risk Management Package for low and medium resource settings: http://www.who.int/cardiovascular_diseases/priorities/management/package/en/

World Heart Federation: http://www.world-heart-federation.org/

7 Evidence-Based Practice

D. Evans & T. Quinn

Overview

In recent times, there has been a gradual transformation in the way in which health care is delivered, with a shift from a system focusing on individual expertise to one that is based on a common body of scientific knowledge. This body of knowledge is the evidence that informs the many decisions that guide practice. This shift to a practice based on the best available evidence has been fuelled by such things as the growing expectations of consumers, rising costs of service delivery, the many new health technologies and the significant developments in information technology. At the same time, there has been a growing awareness of the limitations of existing research evidence and recognition of the difficulties of implementing change in health care.

This health care environment saw the emergence of the evidence-based practice (EBP) movement. It started first in Canada and the United Kingdom (UK), but quickly spread to have a major influence on health care internationally. This chapter explores the nature of EBP and its implications for the cardiovascular nurse.

Learning objectives

After reading this chapter, you should be able to:

- Explain the principles of EBP.
- Relate EBP to contemporary cardiovascular care.
- Provide worked examples of EBP applied to acute cardiac care.
- Develop a critical approach to appraising the literature.
- Identify key EBP resources for the cardiovascular nurse.

Key concepts

Literature review; level of evidence; evidence-based guidelines; change implementation

The need for change

The changing nature of modern society has placed additional expectations on health systems struggling to keep pace with demand. The pressure from many interrelated factors has increased the complexity of health care decision-making, and fuelled interest in EBP. While it is beyond the scope of this chapter to address all of the factors, some of those considered most influential are summarised below.

- Consumer factors
  An ageing population, particularly in the developed countries, has resulted in an increased burden on health of long-term conditions. In addition, consumers have a better understanding of illness and treatment, and as a

result have much higher expectations regarding the standard of care and their right of access to these services. Health expenditure has increased dramatically in response to this greater demand.

- Health service delivery factors
Health care is dynamic and is currently at the crest of a wave of new technology. The rapid development of many new drugs, devices and procedures presents a significant challenge, particularly when widespread use of these technologies seems to happen almost overnight (Ley 2001) and where clinicians and patients often forget that a new technique is not necessarily a better one (Wilson 2006).
- Public scrutiny
Health care is delivered under a watchful media and public scrutiny, with adverse outcomes and therapeutic or system errors quickly open to public debate, and increasingly politicised.
- Increased complexity of health care
Deciding which of a growing range of new and expensive technologies to implement, and meeting the demand for high quality care within budgetary constraints common to all health care systems, underscores the complexity of modern health care. Determining what best practice *is*, and setting priorities for funding and implementation, has never been more difficult.

The above challenges are compounded by difficulties in identifying the best evidence for practice. Despite attempts to reduce the gap between research and practice, the evidence base of large components of health care remains limited. Some of the difficulties facing nurses, physicians, policy makers and patients include:

- Volume of literature
The volume of health information increases daily. An online search using the single term 'cardiovascular', undertaken by one of the authors of this chapter, yielded almost 120,000 published papers in the last 5 years alone. This growing volume of literature, with more than two million clinical research articles published each year (Breen & Feder 1999) has simply become too great for any single clinician to be able to keep up to date with all new research in their field of practice (Antman et al. 1992).

- Poor quality research
A significant proportion of published research is of poor quality, containing errors or has vital information omitted from the report (Mills 1993; Altman 2002), especially if the results are subject to publication bias (Liebeskind et al. 2006). This has made it very difficult to know which research to implement into practice.
- Internet
In more recent times, the rise to prominence of the Internet has resulted in a large volume of readily accessible information. However, the quality of this information is often poor (Powell & Clarke 2002), further threatening the evidence on which health care decisions are based.

Added to these many challenges, implementing research evidence and changing the practice of health professionals have proven to be very difficult. Reasons for this have included:

- Research literacy
Some nurses have suboptimal reading habits, and so are not aware of changes in their field of practice (Hutchinson & Johnson 2004). In addition, research reports are complex documents, and many clinicians lack the necessary appraisal skills to identify high quality research.
- Implementing change
Health professionals, like all other people, get comfortable in their routine practices and habits, and so implementing change can be very difficult (Grol & Grimshaw 2003). When change is implemented, there is a risk that the practice will eventually revert to the original practice.

Given these many challenges, there remains considerable variability in the way health services are delivered and in the outcomes that are achieved. This variability is observed between different health systems and organisations and also between different units within an organisation. The recognition of the complexities surrounding health care, health care decisions and change management provides impetus for the continuing growth in the evidence-based health care (EBHC) movement.

Evidence-based practice

Evidence-based practice is an approach to health care to ensure that it is based on the best available evidence. It has been described in many different ways, but one of the most commonly used definitions is:

> Evidence based medicine is the conscientious, explicit, and judicious use of current best evidence in making decisions about the care of individual patients. The practice of evidence based medicine means integrating individual clinical expertise with the best available external evidence from systematic research (Sackett et al. 1996, p. 71).

One of the major aims of EBP is to promote effective clinical practice by ensuring it is based on the best available evidence. However, EBP is also concerned with cost containment, clinical efficiency and change management. It differs from earlier research utilisation models because of its more explicit integration of research evidence with patient preferences and available resources (DiCenso et al. 1998).

The EBP process is summarised in Figure 7.1. The process starts with the development of an answerable question; collecting, appraising and implementing the best evidence; and then evaluating the impact of the change in practice (Newman et al. 2000). It is a cyclical process, because the evaluation phase may necessitate beginning again as new issues/questions, and indeed new evidence, are identified.

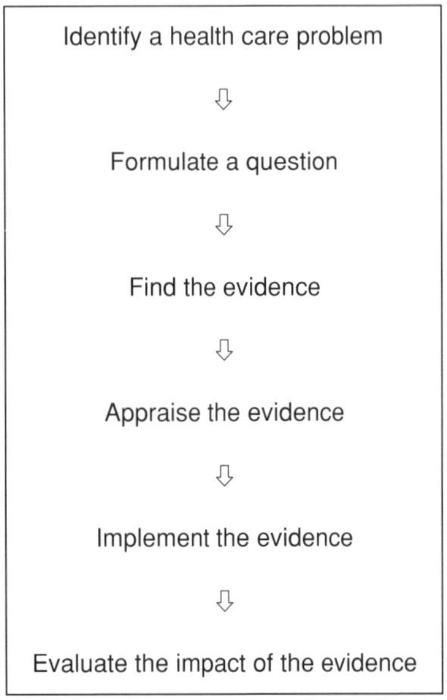

Identifying a problem

The starting point for EBP is when the practitioner observes, questions and reflects on care provided, increasingly in collaboration with a patient or caregiver. While often overlooked in the literature, these activities help identify the opportunities for practice improvement and development. Observation in this context entails observing and monitoring the processes and outcomes of care. It also entails 'benchmarking': comparing practice and outcomes against those of other similar areas, to identify areas for improvement. While reflective practice may seem at odds with some tenets of EBP, it helps bridge the theory/practice gap by facilitating evaluation and improvement of practice (Wilson et al. 2007). Given the complex reality of clinical practice, it is important to embrace the principles of being critical and to reflect on the effectiveness of decision-making (McCormack 2006). These activities form the starting point of the EBP process.

Formulating a question

When a clinical problem has been identified, the first activity in the evidence-based process is to develop a question. This is important because a well-formulated question gives the subsequent activities a clear focus and direction. The process of developing a question also helps to define the boundaries of the problem, which is important given the large volume of health care information that must be searched.

The clear direction provided by the question comes from the identification of the key components of the problem (Counsell 1997). The most common approach to developing a question is the PICO format:

- **Population** and health problem being investigated
- **Intervention** or phenomena of interest
- **Comparator** (control) against which the practice is being compared
- **Outcomes** of concern

Identify a health care problem

⇩

Formulate a question

⇩

Find the evidence

⇩

Appraise the evidence

⇩

Implement the evidence

⇩

Evaluate the impact of the evidence

Figure 7.1   Evidence-based practice.

The population component of the question defines the specific participants, setting or condition that is of interest, for example, people diagnosed with ischaemic heart disease. The intervention defines the treatment, and is therefore important in defining the scope of the problem; for example, conducting an education programme that helps people to adopt a healthier lifestyle and minimise risk factors. When the problem concerns a form of treatment, then a comparison may also need to be identified. The comparison in the question enables the effect of the intervention to be measured alongside another treatment option. In this example, the comparison may simply be not to receive an education programme. The final component of the question is the outcome of interest, which will help determine the effectiveness of the intervention. For example, the short-term outcome of interest for an education programme might be that participants adopt a healthier lifestyle. However, longer-term outcomes would more likely focus on the prevention of heart disease. Using these four components, the question in this example might be formulated as follows:

> Are [people with ischaemic heart disease] who [participate in a health promoting education programme] more likely to [adopt a healthier lifestyle] than [those who do not participate] in the programme?

Question formulation assists the nurse in identifying the nature of a problem. A well-formulated question is just as important when the problem does not concern the effectiveness of a treatment, because it is still necessary to define the area of interest and to ensure the boundaries of the problem have been identified. For example:

> What are the educational needs of people being discharged home following angiography, to minimise the risk of post-procedure complications?

Finding the evidence

There are two issues to be considered when contemplating the evidence to support practice. Firstly we will have to determine what might constitute the best evidence for our clinical practice and then we must search for this evidence.

Best evidence

The definition of EBHC by Sackett et al. (1996) suggests that it is the integration of clinical expertise with the best external evidence. Therefore, what constitutes this external evidence is critical. However, the term 'evidence' is quite ambiguous and is used to designate research knowledge as well as other types of knowledge (Egerod & Hansen 2005).

When deciding what evidence to use, it is important to recognise that not all research designs are equal in terms of their risk of error and bias in their results, and that some research methods provide better evidence than others (Evans 2003). For questions concerning the effectiveness of a treatment or intervention, the most reliable source of evidence is from systematic reviews and randomised controlled trials (RCTs). However, other types of evidence are also used, depending on the nature of the question being investigated. For example, the use of clinical practice guidelines has increased in recent years.

Systematic reviews

A systematic review is a rigorous approach to summarising and communicating findings of research, using explicit methods to identify, appraise and synthesise relevant studies (Evans & Kowanko 2000). These methods are pre-planned and on completion of the review, the methods used are reported in the same manner as for any other type of research. Systematic reviews are considered to provide the highest level of evidence and are increasingly used to inform decisions and underpin the development of clinical practice guidelines. As part of systematic reviews, a meta-analysis is often undertaken. Meta-analysis is a method that is used to combine the results of studies to produce a conclusion about a body of research. Meta-analysis can only be undertaken when studies address the same question, use a similar population, administer the intervention in a similar manner, measure the same outcomes for all participants and use the same research design (Jones & Evans 2000). Meta-analysis is an important component of the systematic review because it seeks to estimate the average effect of an intervention across a range of different studies.

Randomised controlled trials

Randomised controlled trials are used to evaluate the effectiveness of health care interventions. They are considered to provide rigorous evidence because they utilise methods that minimise the risk of bias or error. But RCTs are not infallible, and in one recent report, as many as 16% of the findings were contradicted by subsequent studies (Ioannidis 2005).

Clinical practice guidelines

Clinical practice guidelines are increasingly being used as the basis for clinical decision-making. Guidelines are systematically developed statements that aim to assist clinicians by identifying what is considered to be best practice, and have become an important way of implementing research findings and helping to standardise clinical practice.

Despite the large volume of literature and research, many areas still lack rigorous evidence. This lack of evidence is reflected in uncertainty that surrounds decisions about what is the most effective treatment. This uncertainty is one of the factors contributing to variability in practice. When clinical practice guidelines are being developed, these gaps in the evidence are addressed through consensus by experts. That is, experts in the field meet and discuss what they believe to be the best approach based on their experience. However, a recent strategy to address this problem has been through the formation of a specialist database that focuses on these gaps in the knowledge. The Database of Uncertainties about the Effects of Treatments (DUETs) (NHS 2008) seeks to identify and publish unanswered questions about the effects of treatments which have been asked by patients and clinicians.

Searching for the evidence

Identifying all the relevant publications on a topic of interest is challenging because of the large volume of journals that must be searched. It is increasingly likely that many published papers will quickly be lost to the intended readership, hidden in the vast and ever-increasing volume of health care literature. To try and overcome this problem, publications are listed in databases, and there are now hundreds of different databases that record the health care literature. While there is considerable overlap of coverage between databases, each has its own specific focus. The two most common databases used by nurses are MEDLINE for the medical literature and CINAHL for the nursing literature. However, in recent times, the Cochrane Library has emerged as a very important database because of its comprehensive listing of well-conducted systematic reviews.

To increase the likelihood that all relevant papers are identified, a search strategy is essential. This outlines the intended approach and documents the sources to be searched. One of the main challenges during this search of databases is not to retrieve every single paper written on a subject, but rather to filter only those considered most relevant (Booth 1996). Developing a database search strategy involves the identification of the most appropriate terms related to the topic. It is common to combine these terms with methodological search filters, such as 'randomised controlled trial', 'RCT', 'systematic review' or 'clinical guidelines' and to restrict to a pre-defined time period (e.g. within the past 5 years).

Appraising the evidence

While the aim of EBP is to implement the best available evidence into practice, the quality of research is highly variable because of a range of factors including the use of inappropriate research methods, poor conduct of research and inappropriate data analysis. At times, because of poor research methods, the research findings can provide misleading or incorrect information. To minimise the risks, studies are normally critically appraised before their findings are used to guide practice. Even when a systematic review or clinical practice guideline is being used, it is still considered good practice to evaluate quality. This 'critical appraisal' aims to discover if the methods and results of research are sufficiently valid for the findings to be considered useful information (Fowkes and Fulton 1991). Critical appraisal is important because, despite the peer review process of health care journals, a good proportion of the published research is invalid (Rosenberg & Donald 1995). A large range of tools have been developed to aid in the appraisal of research. These tools focus on the critical stages of the research or systematic review process to ensure that the processes that were used minimised the risk of bias and error. See Figure 7.2 for an example of a critical appraisal tool that is used to appraise systematic reviews.

Implementing the evidence

Clinical expertise is increasingly seen as the ability to integrate research evidence and patients' circumstances and preferences to help patients arrive at optimal decisions (Guyatt et al. 2004). But key challenges remain in ensuring that the best evidence is implemented to benefit patients and provide optimal value for finite resources. It is clear in cardiovascular care that while there is an abundance of evidence, this is not universally implemented. For example, the use of evidence-based therapies for managing patients with acute coronary syndromes varies depending on country or region (Kramer et al. 2003), as does the use of invasive

treatments for the elderly (Alexander et al. 2006). Such differences are also apparent within individual countries as shown by national registries such as the UK Myocardial Infarction National Audit Project (Birkhead et al. 2004) and the US National Cardiovascular Data Registry and National Registry of Myocardial Infarction (ACCF 2008).

At the 'macro' level, evidence-based policy making sets the context for which evidence-based clinical practice can take place (Muir Gray 2004), and focuses on the needs of populations (e.g. should there be a national primary angioplasty service [Boyle 2006]), while EBP at the 'micro' level is concerned with individual decisions made for and with patients. Nurses have potential to influence at both macro and micro levels, as policy advisers working in government and with professional societies nationally and internationally, and in leading clinical teams. In the latter context, Thompson et al. (2000) studied the use of research information and decision-making by UK coronary care nurses. The largest number of decisions made by nurses was related to questions about the clinical effectiveness of treatments or interventions. Worryingly, guidelines and protocols were referred to only rarely (four times during 180h

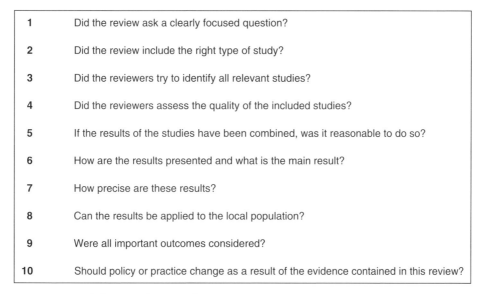

1	Did the review ask a clearly focused question?
2	Did the review include the right type of study?
3	Did the reviewers try to identify all relevant studies?
4	Did the reviewers assess the quality of the included studies?
5	If the results of the studies have been combined, was it reasonable to do so?
6	How are the results presented and what is the main result?
7	How precise are these results?
8	Can the results be applied to the local population?
9	Were all important outcomes considered?
10	Should policy or practice change as a result of the evidence contained in this review?

Figure 7.2 Ten questions to help you make sense of reviews.
Reproduced with permission from Public Health Resource Unit from Critical Appraisal Skills Program: Systematic Review Appraisal Tool

of observation). Coronary care nurses tended to draw on what Thompson et al. (2000) described as a 'personal memory bank' of past experience and intuition. The researchers suggested that, because more junior nurses felt that there was little time available to identify and assess the evidence base to assist with their decision-making, more effort should be focused on key or 'link' nurses, who could be sources of information for colleagues. In addition, the researchers also suggested that nurses need to develop skills in recognising problems and formulating clinical questions, and information (evidence) retrieval.

Several initiatives are underway to improve the translation of the evidence into practice to improved cardiovascular care. An example of this in England is the National Service Framework developed by the Department of Health which has brought about significant improvements through a range of strategies that included better-equipped ambulances and investment in staff, interventional facilities and procedures (Department of Health 2000, 2008). This was supported through a national programme targeted at service improvement which was led by a Heart Improvement Programme and included clinical networks and a cardiovascular diseases specialist library. A National Institute for Health and Clinical Excellence (NICE) was established in 1999 with special health authority status to promote the effective use of resources in England and Wales. NICE is an independent organisation that has developed robust methodologies for developing guidelines, and is thought to be the world's largest such programme (Chidgey et al. 2007). Other examples of practice improvement strategies include the CRUSADE quality improvement initiative in the United States (Blomkalns et al. 2007) and the National Institute of Clinical Studies (NICS) in Australia, which works to improve health care by helping to close important gaps between best available evidence and current clinical practice (NICS 2008).

Evaluating the impact of the evidence

A key component of EBP is evaluating the impact of the implementation of the best evidence and monitoring its sustainability. There are many different approaches to this evaluation; however, one of the common approaches is that of clinical audit. Clinical audit is a clinically led initiative which seeks to improve the quality and outcome of patient care (Burnett & Winyard 1998). It entails a systematic and critical look at health care practice. It is used to scrutinise the treatments and investigations that are undertaken, and the resources that are used. It is used to examine the outcomes of practice and to compare actual practice against expected practice. This is achieved through a structured peer review whereby clinicians examine their practices and compare the results against agreed standards. These agreed standards arise from best practice that has been identified through research.

The clinical audit acts as a cyclical process and entails:

- identifying a clinical problem
- determining the best practice
- practising evaluation
- comparing actual to the best practice
- making changes and improvements as required
- starting the cycle again if required

Some of the suggested benefits of clinical audit include the identification and promotion of good practice, improvement to service delivery, identification of how to better use resources and the improvement of outcomes for users of the service (Clouston et al. 2005). As a result of these benefits, clinical audit has become a common feature of health care, and staff at all levels are involved in the process.

Barriers to the evidence

There are many potential barriers to implementation of best evidence. Some have already been mentioned, such as the volume of literature, complexity of research reports research and poor research literacy skills. Another important barrier is that nurses, like all other health professionals, get comfortable in their routine practices (Grol & Grimshaw 2003). The implementation of new evidence threatens this comfort, and the security that accompanies routine practices. A lack of time to read the research literature is a barrier for some nurses. A study by Nagy et al. (2001) found that some nurses thought research was irrelevant, while Egerod & Hansen (2005) found that for Danish cardiac nurses unfamiliarity with English was a problem. However, factors relating to an health care organisation can also impact on EBP. For example, organisational support can be a barrier to the implementation of research evidence (Egerod & Hansen 2005), while a lack of coordinated implementation effort and negative attitudes can impede change (Ley 2001).

Conclusion

While there are many challenges to research implementation and practice improvement, the processes of EBP have been developed to help overcome the barriers. However, given the nature of research and health technologies, health care has become dynamic as treatments and support therapies continue to change and improve. Nurses, like other health workers, must accept that change is now a normal component of professional practice, and EBP can be used to ensure their practice is based firmly on the best available research evidence.

References

American College of Cardiology Foundation (ACCF) (2008). National Cardiovascular Data Registry, American College of Cardiology Foundation, United States of America. Retrieved online 12th February 2008 from http://www.accncdr.com/WebNCDR/Common/

Alexander, K.P., Newby, L.K., Bhapkar, M.V., et al. for the Symphony and 2nd Symphony Investigators (2006). International variation in invasive care of the elderly with acute coronary syndromes. *European Heart Journal*, **27**:1558–64.

Altman, D.G. (2002). Poor-quality medical research: what can journals do? *Journal of the American Medical Association*, **287**: 2765–7.

Antman, E.M., Lau, J., Kupeinick, B., Mosteller, F. & Chalmers, T.C. (1992). A comparison of results of meta-analyses of randomised controlled trials and recommendations of clinical experts. *Journal of the American Medical Association*, **268**:240–8.

Birkhead, J.S., Walker, L., Pearson, M., Weston, C., Cunningham, A.D. & Rickards, A.F. (2004). Improving care for patients with acute coronary syndromes: initial results from the national audit of myocardial infarction project (MINAP). *Heart*, **90**:1004–9.

Blomkalns, A.L., Roe, M.T., Peterson, E.D., Ohman, E.M., Fraulo, E.S. & Gibler, W.B. (2007). Guideline implementation research: exploring the gap between evidence and practice in the CRUSADE quality improvement initiative. *Academic Emergency Medicine*, **14**:949–54.

Booth, A. (1996). In search of the evidence: informing effective practice. *Journal of Clinical Effectiveness*, **1**:25–9.

Boyle, R.M. (2006). *Mending Hearts and Brains*. Department of Health, London.

Breen, A. & Feder, G. (1999). Where does the evidence come from? In: A. Hutchinson & R. Baker (eds), *Making Use of Guidelines in Clinical Practice*. Radcliffe Medical Press, Abingdon.

Burnett, A.C. & Winyard, G. (1998). Clinical audit at the heart of clinical effectiveness. *Journal of Qualitative Clinical Practice*, **18**:3–19.

Chidgey, J., Leng, G. & Lacey, T. (2007). Implementing NICE guidance. *Journal of the Royal Society of Medicine*, **100**:448–52.

Clouston, T.J., Westcott, L., Turner, A. & Palastanga, N. (2005). *Working in Health and Social Care: An Introduction for Allied Health Professional*. Elsevier, Amsterdam.

Counsell, C. (1997). Formulating questions and locating primary studies for inclusion in systematic reviews. *Annals of Internal Medicine*, **127**:380–7.

Department of Health (2000). *National Service Framework for Coronary Heart Disease*. Department of Health, London.

Department of Health (2008). *The Coronary Heart Disease National Service Framework: Building for the future – progress report for 2007*. Department of Health, London.

DiCenso, A., Cullum, N. & Ciliska, D. (1998). Implementing evidence-based nursing: some misconceptions. *Evidence-Based Nursing*, **1**:38–40.

Egerod, I. & Hansen, G.M. (2005). Evidence-based practice among Danish cardiac nurses: a national survey. *Journal of Advanced Nursing*, **51**:465–73.

Evans, D. (2003). Hierarchy of evidence: a framework for the ranking of evidence evaluating nursing interventions. *Journal of Clinical Nursing*, **12**:77–84.

Evans, D. & Kowanko, I. (2000). Literature reviews: evolution of a research methodology. *Australian Journal of Advanced Nursing*, **18**:31–6.

Fowkes, F.G.R. & Fulton, P.M. (1991) Critical appraisal of published research: introductory guidelines. *British Medical Journal*, **302**:1136–40.

Grol, R. & Grimshaw, J. (2003). From best evidence to best practice: effective implementation of change in patients' care. *The Lancet*, **362**:1225–30.

Guyatt, G., Cook, D. & Haynes, B. (2004). Evidence-based medicine has come a long way. *British Medical Journal*, **329**:990–1.

Hutchinson, A.M. & Johnson, L. (2004). Bridging the divide: a survey of nurses' opinions regarding barriers to and facilitators of, research utilisation in the practice setting, *Journal of Clinical Nursing*, **13**:304–15.

Ioannidis, J.P.A. (2005). Contradicted and initially stronger effects in highly cited clinical research. *Journal of the American Medical Association*, **294**:218–28.

Jones, T & Evans, D. (2000). Conducting a systematic review. *Australian Critical Care Nursing Journal*, **13**:66–71.

Kramer, J.M., Newby, L.K., Chang, W., et al. for the Symphony and 2nd Symphony Investigators (2003). International variation in the use of evidence-based medicines for acute coronary syndromes. *European Heart Journal*, **24**:2133–41.

Ley, S.J. (2001). Quality care outcomes in cardiac surgery: the role of evidence-based practice. *American Academy of Ambulatory Care Nursing Clinical Issues*, **12**:606–17.

Liebeskind, D.S., Kidwell, C.S., Sayre, J.W. & Saver, J.L. (2006). Evidence of publication bias in reporting acute stroke clinical trials. *Neurology*, **67**:973–9.

McCormack, B. (2006). Evidence-based practice and the potential for transformation. *Journal of Research in Nursing*, **11**:89–94.

Mills, J.L. (1993). Data torturing. *The New England Journal of Medicine*, **329**:1196–9.

Muir Gray, J.A. (2004). Evidence based policy making. *British Medical Journal*, **329**:988–9.

Nagy, S., Lumby, J., McKinley, S. & MacFarlane, C. (2001). Nurses' beliefs about the conditions that hinder or support evidence-based nursing. *International Journal of Nursing Practice*, **7**:314–21.

National Institute of Clinical Studies (NICS) (2008). National Institute of Clinical Studies (NICS), National Health and Medical Research Council, Australia. Retrieved online 14th February 2008 from http://www.nhmrc.gov.au/nics/asp/index.asp

National Health Service (NHS) (2008). Database of Uncertainties about the Effects of Treatments (DUETs), National Health Service, United Kingdom. Retrieved online 14th February 2008 from http://www.duets.nhs.uk/Uncertainties.asp

Newman, M., Papadopoulas, I. & Melifonwu, R. (2000). Developing organisational systems and culture to support evidence-based practice: the experience of the Evidence-Based Ward Project. *Evidence Based Nursing*, **3**:103–4.

Powell, J. & Clarke, A. (2002). The WWW of the World Wide Web: who, what and why. *Journal of Medical Internet Research*, **4**:e4.

PHRU (2008). Critical Appraisal Skills Program: systematic review appraisal tool, National Health Service. Retrieved online 14th February 2008 from http://www.phru.nhs.uk/Pages/PHD/resources.htm

Rosenberg, W. & Donald, A. (1995). Evidence based medicine: an approach to clinical problem solving. *British Medical Journal*, **310**:1122–6.

Sackett, D.L., Rosenberg, W.M., Muir Gray, J.A., Haynes, R.B. & Richardson, W.S. (1996). Evidence based medicine: what it is and what it isn't. *British Medical Journal*, **312**:71–2.

Thompson, C., McCaughan, D., Cullum, N., Sheldon, T. & Thompson, D. (2000). Nurses' use of research information in clinical decision making: a descriptive and analytical study – final report. NCC SDO, London.

Wilson, C.B. (2006). Adoption of new surgical technology. *British Medical Journal*, **332**:112–4.

Wilson, G., Walsh, T. & Kirby, M. (2007). Reflective practice and workplace learning: the experience of MSW students. *Reflective Practice*, **8**:1–15.

Useful Websites and Further Reading

United Kingdom

Cardiovascular Diseases Specialist Library: www.library.nhs.uk/cardiovascular

Heart Improvement Programme: www.heart.nhs.uk

National Institute for Health and Clinical Excellence (NICE): www.nice.org.uk

Database of Uncertainties about the Effects of Treatments (DUETS): www.duets.nhs.uk

Netting the evidence: http://www.shef.ac.uk/scharr/ir/netting/

The Cochrane Collaboration: http://www.cochrane.org/

Bandolier: http://www.jr2.ox.ac.uk/Bandolier/

Australia

National Institute for Clinical Studies: http://www.nhmrc.gov.au/nics/asp/index.asp

Australian Resource Centre for Healthcare Innovations: http://www.archi.net.au/index.phtml

Canada

Canadian Centres for Health Evidence: http://www.cche.net/

The Canadian Coordinating Office for Health Technology Assessment: http://www.cadth.ca/

United States of America

Agency of Health Care Policy and Research: http://www.ahcpr.gov/

National Guideline Clearinghouse: http://www.guidelines.gov/

8 Ethics of Research in Acute Cardiac Care

B.F. Williams & A.M. Kucia

Overview

Our understanding of the mechanisms of coronary artery disease has improved greatly over the last few decades, leading to the development of a number of new therapies. Some of these therapies have proved to be safe and effective, and some have not. We have to have a way of distinguishing therapies that are useful from those that are not, and given that we are using these therapies on humans, we also need to know which therapies are safe, and which may be harmful. Moreover, as resources are finite, we also need to look at cost efficacy of these new therapies. Researching new therapies is not cost-neutral. Pharmaceutical companies invest huge amounts of money in research and development of new therapies, and would like to see a return on this investment. Researchers and research teams invest a great deal of time and effort into trialling new therapies, and they would like to see this work recognised and rewarded, perhaps through publication. It is therefore imperative that determinations about the safety, efficacy and cost-effectiveness of a therapy are made in a fair and unbiased way. We rely upon well-designed scientific and clinical research to provide us with this information.

Scientific and clinical research is necessary for us to continue to make advances in knowledge about coronary artery disease and to develop better management strategies to improve outcomes for patients with this disease. This seems like a logical and straightforward assumption; however, there are a number of ethical issues to do with research, particularly where human subjects are involved. Acutely ill individuals, such as patients with acute coronary syndromes (ACS), are a vulnerable group when it comes to involvement in research, and this chapter will discuss some of the ethical issues that arise in using these patients as research subjects in clinical trials.

Learning objectives

After reading this chapter, you should be able to:

- Define an ethical dilemma.
- List the elements of informed consent.
- Discuss the reasons why patients with ACS may have difficulty giving an informed consent.
- Describe how nurses can advocate for patients who are invited to participate in clinical trials.
- Debate the value of research in ACS.

Evidence-based medicine and clinical trials

Significant advances in the treatment of ACS have been made over the past few decades, but ACS is still a major cause of morbidity and mortality in Western societies. As we are always looking to improve the human condition, the value of clinical trials to reduce mortality and morbidity due to cardiovascular disease should be indisputable. The goal is to progress the betterment of health by seeking and justifying new and better treatments, and making them available for public benefit. This is the underpinning concept of evidence-based practice.

Evidence-based medicine is defined as 'the use of the best available external clinical evidence in making treatment decisions for the care of individual patients' (Sackett et al. 1996). The best available evidence includes the findings of clinical trials, and the results of randomized clinical trials have become the scientific 'gold standard' for clinical evidence. It is considered unethical to introduce new therapies without verifying that they are better than, or at least equal to, existing ones.

Informed consent for trial participation

A crucial component of ethical research involving human subjects is to obtain the potential participant's voluntary and informed consent, allowing the person to consider the risk, potential benefits, and other aspects of the trial (Beecher 1966). The requirement for informed consent is founded in historical disciplines and social contexts. Legally, a doctor has a duty to inform patients and obtain their consent for treatment. Informed consent must be freely and autonomously given by people who understand the information that is presented to them. The elements of informed consent are presented in Box 8.1.

> ## Box 8.1   Elements of informed consent
>
> It is generally understood that discussion of the following aspects of a treatment or intervention should take place to allow the patient to be an informed participant in health care or research:
>
> - The nature of the decision/procedure
> - Reasonable alternatives to the proposed intervention
> - The relevant risks, benefits and uncertainties related to each alternative
> - Assessment of patient understanding
> - Voluntary acceptance of the intervention by the patient

There is evidence to suggest that acutely ill patients have some impairment in understanding, which creates doubt about their ability to give informed consent in the acute phase of their illness (Kucia & Horowitz 2000). However, it cannot be assumed that these patients are totally incapable of understanding proposed treatment and making choices. Seedhouse (1998) describes a basic concept of autonomy as being able to 'do' – to do something rather than nothing. The question then is, what information about a clinical trial should be offered to an acutely ill patient in a situation that requires a quick decision?

Presenting information and obtaining consent

Although regulations and guidelines require that patients are given a comprehensive information sheet and consent form prior to consenting to inclusion in a clinical trial, acutely ill patients are unlikely to have the ability to read and understand these lengthy, complex and difficult-to-understand documents in the required timeframe (Cassileth et al. 1980; Priestley et al. 1992; Grossman et al. 1994). It has been suggested that obtaining consent for trial participation from acutely ill patients is used to comply with perceived regulatory requirements rather than to truly inform the patient (Iserson & Mahowald 1992) and that patients often consider these forms to be for the protection of the physician rather than themselves (Cassileth et al. 1980; Boisaubin & Dresser 1987; Searight & Miller 1996).

A patient who is acutely ill may be vulnerable to persuasion to participate in a clinical trial due to the dependant nature of the doctor–patient relationship. Patients are largely dependant upon the treating doctor for information, including the potential risks and benefits of clinical trial participation. There is little or no control over the quality of information that is given verbally to patients: it is often unclear what verbal information has been given to the patient, and what has been omitted in soliciting their agreement to participate in a trial. A worrying trend is that the task of obtaining informed consent often falls to junior medical staff, who may themselves be ignorant of clinical trial details and the potential risks involved (Kerrigan et al. 1993). Information delivery may also play a part in modulating patient preferences: particular options may look more attractive than they otherwise would because of the manner in which information is delivered, particularly in terms of the risk:benefit ratio (Cocking & Oakley 1994). The order in which information is presented also plays a part. Consider the normal sequence in which information is given to patients: introducing oneself, explaining the medical problem to the patient, explaining the proposed treatment option/s, expected outcome and lastly potential risk. The later that information is presented in a conversation, the less likely it is to be absorbed by an acutely ill patient. Thus the patient is more likely to focus on the expected benefit, than the potential risks.

Difficulties in obtaining informed consent

It is often difficult for patients with limited medical knowledge to make decisions about their health when the situation is ideal; it is even more difficult for a critically ill patient make these decisions, especially as there is usually no time to consider or discuss the options (Schaeffer et al. 1996). Patients with ACS are often placed in this situation: they are under pressure to make urgent treatment decisions without in-depth medical knowledge (Ingelfinger 1972). There are those who suggest that presenting detailed information about treatments to an acutely ill patient can cause confusion (Ingelfinger 1972; Brewin 1982), increased anxiety (Simes et al. 1986) and that confronting

seriously ill patients with the possibility of adverse outcomes as a result of essential treatment can be needlessly cruel (Tobias & Souhami 1993). It has been suggested that often, a patient just wants reassurance that the situation is under control, and that a clear explanation of what treatment is going to be used, rather than a detailed explanation of potential unpleasant outcomes is all that is required (Tobias & Souhami 1993).

The thrombolytic trials raised a number of ethical issues, particularly regarding the difficulty of obtaining informed consent from acutely ill patients. This issue has not been resolved and is present in current studies of new therapies involving patients with ACS, particularly where there is high risk of complications such as bleeding. In early thrombolytic trials, an assumption was made that patients with an acute myocardial infarction (AMI) would not be able to give an informed consent due to the severity of their condition (Gruppo Italiano per lo Studio della Streptochinasi nell'Infarto Miocardio [GISSI] 1986; ISIS-2 Collaborative Group 1988; GISSI-2 1990). This assumption is supported by studies of patient consent in ACS that have found that few patients suffering AMI read the written information presented to them during the consent process for trial participation, and they remember little of the information given to them verbally (Kucia & Horowitz 2000; Yuval et al. 2000; Agård et al. 2001; Williams et al. 2003). Some physicians feel that too much information has to be given to prospective trial participants (Agård et al. 2004) and have suggested that it is 'time to adjust the informed consent process to the patient's capacity' (Agård et al. 2001).

The usual methods of obtaining informed consent for trial participation from patients during a clinical emergency are impractical and inadequate. However, if such research were to require lengthy and explicit consent from the potential participant, it would result in the exclusion of all acutely ill patients from clinical trials (Iserson & Mahowald 1992). It can be argued that excluding acutely ill patients as a group from involvement in research is unethical, as this group then would be denied the opportunity to benefit from potentially improved outcomes resulting from research. With this in mind, alternatives to the standard consent process have been explored for patients with a life-threatening illness, such as proxy consent, given by a person who considers themself morally responsible for the person unable to consent. Decisions of proxy consent should be made with only the interests of the individual person in mind, rather than the 'greater good' (Ashley & O'Rourke 1982), but proxy consent is subject to the same kind of impediments as obtaining informed consent from an acutely ill person: family members also suffer emotional shock and stress which interferes with their ability to assimilate information and to appreciate the inherent risks of research that may not be present in conventional therapy (Marson et al. 2000).

Deferred consent has been suggested as a method for obtaining consent from individuals or their proxies who are not able to consent at the time of enrolment into a trial, but who some time later may be competent to do so (Abramson et al. 1986).

The Declaration of Helsinki, an international code for ethical research, allows for research in individuals from whom it is not possible to obtain informed consent, but only if the physical/mental condition that prevents obtaining informed consent is a necessary characteristic of the research population. Consent to remain in the research should be obtained as soon as possible from the individual or a legally authorised proxy (World Medical Association 2000). Whether patients with ACS fit this latter criterion is arguable.

What is an ethical dilemma?

An ethical dilemma is said to exist where there is no clear 'right or wrong answer' to an issue. Seedhouse (1998) describes ethical analysis as being similar to looking at the tip of an iceberg and seeing the ethical problem, and then considering the broader ethical issues that lie underneath. What is right? What actions are in the best interests of your patient? In many cases, nurses are in the best position to be the patient's advocate. Awareness of ethical issues can enhance delivery of nursing care.

It is considered unethical to introduce new therapies without verifying that they are equal to, or better than, existing ones. Patients with ACS potentially have a lot to gain through new and improved therapies, but may also face substantial

risk. These patients may not be capable of fully understanding the information presented to them in the consent process, and therefore are not in a position to make an informed decision about accepting the risk in these trials. Moreover, as has previously been discussed, these acutely ill patients are a vulnerable group. There are potentially positive outcomes from to clinical trial involvement for the patient, but potentially negative ones too. For patients in your care, clinical trial involvement may result in ethical dilemma for you in how best to provide information to the patient to enable them to make an informed choice about trial participation, particularly if you feel the patient has been inadequately informed, misinformed or has felt pressured to agree to trial participation. On the contrary, nurses are in the best position to give ongoing support to trial participants by way of explanations of trial procedures and reassurance. Risks of side effects such as bleeding may be no greater than with standard clinical treatment. Participation in clinical trials may offer some advantages to patients as a result of more intense scrutiny and follow-up. Trial participants may have access to treatments that may not be readily available to non-trial patients. Mortality for many potentially lethal conditions is potentially lower for clinical trial participants, even after adjustment for prognostic factors such as age, gender, revascularisation and co-morbidity scores in clinical trial groups, including those in the placebo arm, than that in the general hospital population (Jha et al. 1996; Schmidt et al. 1999). Regardless of any of the perceived benefits above, patients must freely make their own decision whether or not to participate in a clinical trial, and the nurse should advocate for the patient, where necessary, to ensure that this happens. Furthermore, before a clinical trial can proceed it must be scrutinised and approved by an ethics committee.

Although most of the research discussed here refers to large clinical trials, smaller studies can also be ethically problematic. It should be remembered that any research with human subjects, even qualitative types of investigation that may seem more in line with quality assurance activities, may have the potential to cause psychological harm to the patient. All research studies involving patients should be submitted to the institution's ethics committee for consideration.

Genetic research

In the practice of evidence-based medicine, generalised evidence from clinical trials is applied to an individual patient. Consideration is not given to groups of patients who respond differently to the statistical mean. Genetic analysis of an individual's response to a specific drug opens the way for personalised medicines (Marshall 1998). Since the sequencing of the human genome, advances in technology now exist to better link genetic risk factors to phenotypic characteristics. Thus, genetic research is vital to the development of medications and therapies capable of saving lives, reducing morbidity and improving quality of life. Clinical trials now frequently include collection of blood samples from subjects for genetic analysis, usually as an optional sub-study attached to a trial of investigational drugs.

As with all human research it is important that participation in genetic research is voluntary and that refusal to participate has no effect on a patient's access to other treatments. Benefits for participants agreeing to blood sampling for genetic analysis are indirect. Genetic studies will help further understanding of health and disease, which may improve health care for future generations. Long-term benefits include identification of patients who may benefit from, or are at adverse risk from, a specific drug (Marshall 1998; Evans & Relling 1999).

Risks to participants are largely hypothetical, and pharmaceutical companies have gone to great lengths to anonymise samples so that it is impossible to link an individual's identity to a specific sample. Thus, immediate ethical issues may relate to the fact that once a DNA sample has been anonymised it is not possible for a person to withdraw from the genetic study. Other ethical issues to be considered are related to hypothetical risks such as the anonymisation process for the DNA sample might be faulty and a person's identity might remain linked to their sample or, erroneously, be linked to another person's sample leading, for example, to personal genetic discrimination in terms of employment or health/life insurance. Also there are fears that a person's DNA could be immortalised or used for cloning. In study protocols and informed consent documents, pharmaceutical companies provide assurances of the

ethical integrity of the proposed genetic study, and ethics committees and regulatory authorities have a responsibility to ensure that the ethical integrity is upheld.

Considering an offer for the unit to participate in a clinical trial

Cardiac units in large teaching hospitals often have a well-established research unit and close collaborative links with international research networks. To be able to enrol many tens of thousands of patients in multi-centre clinical trials with a large sample size, these networks have extended to include smaller community hospitals. The nursing staff in these units may be involved in the process of deciding whether or not it is feasible to conduct the trial in their unit. In order to make an informed decision, both the benefits and the resource implications for participation need to be considered.

Clinical trials provide an opportunity for staff to improve their knowledge of the clinical condition under investigation and provide first-hand experience with new medications and treatments. In most trials the investigational treatment and the control treatment are provided free of charge to both the unit and the trial participant. This alone can represent a large budgetary saving if a trial of an expensive pharmaceutical agent runs for a year or longer. In addition, to cover the costs incurred by the institution and the staff carrying out the trial procedures, most trials pay a set amount per patient recruited. Consideration needs to be given to whether the nursing staff can carry out the trial procedures as part of their clinical workload and whether a study coordinator is needed to supervise trial procedures and complete the trial documentation. Resource and payment issues for pharmacy and laboratory involvement in the trial also need to be considered.

It is important to review the eligibility criteria for the trial and compare these with the unit admission records to ensure that sufficient potentially eligible patients will be admitted during the period of the trial. A review of the trial medications and procedures may highlight issues that could pose cultural difficulties. For example, a trial using a medication of porcine or bovine origin such as heparin might raise religious difficulties for trial participants of Jewish, Islamic or Hindu origin. Some ethnic groups, for example New Zealand Maori, may raise concerns if biological samples are sent out of the country of origin for analysis in a central laboratory, and consultation with local ethnic groups might be required.

Ethical issues in marketing and pricing of new pharmaceutical agents

The majority of clinical trials of drugs and therapeutic devices are funded by industry. Drug and device development is lengthy and expensive, and consequently, the high cost of new products often results in inequity of access to these products, particularly in underdeveloped countries, and often amongst the population that has been used to test the product. It is not unusual for a patient to be involved in a clinical trial of a drug, which has been found to be effective in treating their condition, only to be denied ongoing access to the drug due to financial and/or marketing considerations (Angell 2000). The pharmaceutical industry has faced increasing scrutiny due to soaring costs of drugs (Angell 2000). A somewhat cynical suggestion is that whilst a percentage of newly marketed products actually do fill an unmet medical need, many are similar to currently marketed products and are cleverly promoted to highlight small advantages which have been demonstrated in industry-sponsored clinical trials that have been carefully designed to obtain these desired results (Langreth 1998). The development of new therapeutic products is expensive and many are never approved for use or find a niche on the market: thus, pharmaceutical companies need to recoup the costs involved in the research and development of new innovative products that meet a medical need (Rosner 1992) and are marketable.

Conclusion

In this chapter, we have touched upon a few common ethical issues that arise in research with ACS patients. It is likely that you will encounter one or more of these issues in your practice, and many others that have not been included in this discussion. In the study of ethics, we find that often there are no clearly defined right or wrong answers, but often, just different ways of looking at things. This often causes tension or disagreement between people or groups of people that can be difficult to resolve, particularly where there are potential advantages to some and disadvantages to others. Knowledge gained from research has the potential to offer benefits to large groups of people in the future, but may offer no benefit, or in fact actually harm those involved in the research. Altruism is not always the first concern in research, and this is why ethics committees are needed to protect the subjects of human research. Nurses may find themselves in a position of patient advocacy to ensure that the best interests of the patient are being observed, or at least that the patient is able to understand what clinical trial participation involves and freely consents to participation.

Learning activities

You are working on a coronary care unit that is involved in a number of clinical research studies. A new patient is admitted with a rare clotting disorder and a myocardial infarction. You need to take routine cardiac enzymes and clotting studies, and the patient has intravenous access for blood taking. The cardiologist tells you to take an extra 50 mL of blood for some laboratory tests that are not clinically indicated and are for research purposes only. Consider the ethical issues and what your actions would be.

You want to do a survey with patients admitted to your ward to see how many of them are able to identify their own cardiac risk factors on admission. You have decided you will do this with a questionnaire whilst they are in hospital. Do you need to get their consent if you are just asking them to fill in a questionnaire? What are the ethical issues involved?

References

Abramson, N.S., Meisel, A. & Safar, P. (1986). Deferred consent. A new approach for resuscitation research on comatose patients. *Journal of the American Medical Association*, **255**:2466–71.

Agård, A., Hermerén, G. & Herlitz, J. (2001). Patient's experiences of intervention trials on the treatment of myocardial infarction: is it time to adjust the informed consent procedure to the patient's capacity? *Heart*, **86**:6232–7.

Agård, A., Herlitz, J. & Hermerén, G. (2004). Obtaining informed consent from patients in the early phase of acute myocardial infarction: physicians' experiences and attitudes. *Heart*, **90**:208–10.

Angell, M. (2000). The pharmaceutical industry – to whom is it accountable? *New England Journal of Medicine*, **342**:1902–4.

Ashley, B.M. & O'Rourke, K.D. (1982). *Health Care Ethics – A Theological Analysis*, 2nd edn. Catholic Health Association of the United States, St. Louis.

Beecher, H.K. (1966). Ethics and clinical research. *New England Journal of Medicine*, **274**:1354–60.

Boisaubin, E.V. & Dresser, R. (1987). Informed consent in emergency care: illusion and reform. *Annals of Emergency Medicine*, **16**:62–7.

Brewin, T.B. (1982). Consent to randomized treatment. *The Lancet*, **2**:919–21.

Cassileth, B.R., Zupkis, R.V., Sutton-Smith, K. & March, V. (1980). Informed consent – why are its goals imperfectly realized? *New England Journal of Medicine*, **302**:896–900.

Cocking, D. & Oakley, J. (1994). Medical experimentation, informed consent and using people. *Bioethics*, **8**:293–311.

Evans, W.E. & Relling, M.V. (1999). Pharmacogenomics: translating functional genomics into rational therapeutics. *Science*, **286**:487.

Grossman, S.A., Piantadosi, S. & Covahey, C. (1994). Are informed consent forms that describe clinical oncology research protocols readable by most patients and their families? *Journal of Clinical Oncology*, **12**:2211–5.

Gruppo Italiano per lo Studio della Streptochinasi nell'Infarto Miocardio (GISSI) (1986). Effectiveness of intravenous thrombolytic treatment in acute myocardial infarction. *The Lancet*, **1**:397–402.

Gruppo Italiano per lo Studio della Sopravvivenza nell'Infarto Miocardio (GISSI-2) (1990). A factorial randomized trial of alteplase versus streptokinase and heparin versus no heparin among 12,490 patients with acute myocardial infarction. *The Lancet*, **336**:65–71.

Ingelfinger, F.J. (1972). Informed (but uneducated) consent. *New England Journal of Medicine*, **287**:465–6.

Iserson, K.V. & Mahowald, M.B. (1992). Acute care research: is it ethical? *Critical Care Medicine*, **20**:1032–7.

ISIS-2 Collaborative Group (1988). Randomised trial of intravenous streptokinase, oral aspirin, both, or neither among 17187 cases of suspected acute myocardial infarction: ISIS-2. *The Lancet*, **2**:349–60.

Jha, P., Doeboer, D., Sykora, K. & Naylor, C.D. (1996). Characteristics and mortality outcomes of thrombolysis trial participants and nonparticipants: a population based comparison. *Journal of the American College of Cardiology*, **27**:1335–42.

Kerrigan, D.D., Thevasagayam, R.S., Woods, T.O., et al. (1993). Who's afraid of informed consent? *British Medical Journal*, **306**:298–300.

Kucia, A.M. & Horowitz, J.D. (2000). Is informed consent to clinical trials an upside selective process? *American Heart Journal*, **140**:94–7.

Langreth, R. (1998). Drug marketing drives many clinical trials. *Wall Street Journal*. 16th November.

Marshall, A. (1998). Laying the foundations for personalized medicines. *Nature Biotechnology*, **16**(Suppl.):6–8.

Marson, S.A. & Allmark, P.J. for the Euricon Study Group (2000). Obtaining informed consent to neonatal randomised controlled trials: interviews with parents and clinicians in the Euricon study. *The Lancet*, **356**:2045–51.

Priestley, K.A., Campbell, C., Valentine, C.B., et al. (1992). Are patient consent forms for research protocols easy to read? *British Medical Journal*, **305**:1263–4.

Rosner, F. (1992). Ethical relationships between drug companies and the medical profession. *Chest*, **102**:266–9.

Sackett, D.L., Rosenberg, W.M., Gray, J.A.M., et al. (1996). Evidence based medicine: what it is and what it isn't. *British Medical Journal*, **312**:71–2.

Schaeffer, M.H., Krantz, D.S., Wichman, A., Masur, H. & Reed, E. (1996). The impact of disease severity on the informed consent process in clinical research. *American Journal of Medicine*, **100**:261–8.

Schmidt, B., Gillie, P., Caco, C., Roberts, J. & Roberts, R. (1999). Do sick newborn infants benefit from participation in a randomised clinical trial? *Journal of Pediatrics*, **134**:151–5.

Searight, H.R. & Miller, C.K. (1996). Remembering and interpreting informed consent: a qualitative study of drug trial participants. *Journal of the American Board of Family Practitioners*, **9**:14–22.

Seedhouse, D. (1998). *Ethics. The Heart of Health Care*, 2nd edn. John Wiley & Sons, Chichester, UK.

Simes, R.J., Tattersall, M.H.N. & Coates, A.S. (1986). Randomised comparison of procedures for obtaining informed consent in clinical trials of treatment for cancer. *British Medical Journal*, **293**:1065–8.

Tobias, J.S. & Souhami, R.L. (1993). Fully informed consent can be needlessly cruel. *British Medical Journal*, **307**:1199–200.

Williams, B.F., French, J.K. & White, H.D. for the HERO-2 consent substudy investigators (2003). Informed consent during the clinical emergency of acute myocardial infarction (HERO-2 consent substudy): a prospective observational study. *The Lancet*, **361**:918–22.

World Medical Association (2000). Ethical principles for medical research involving human subjects (Declaration of Helsinki), 6th edn. Edinburgh, Scotland. Retrieved online on 21st September 2007 from http://www.wma.net/e/policy/b3.htm

Yuval, R., Hanlon, D.A., Merdler, A., et al. (2000). Patient comprehension and reaction to participating in a double-blind randomized clinical trial (ISIS-4) in acute myocardial infarction. *Archives of Internal Medicine*, **160**:1142–6.

Useful Websites and Further Reading

American Association of Critical Care Nurses Ethics in Critical Care Nursing Research: http://www.aacn.org/AACN/research.nsf/0/daddec18fb7e925788256826007dec91?OpenDocument

Benatar, S.R. Singer, P.A. (2000). A new look at international research ethics. *British Medical Journal*, **321**:824–6. Available online at http://www.bmj.com/cgi/reprint/321/7264/824

International Council of Nurses Code of Ethics for Nurses: http://www.icn.ch/icncode.pdf

Medi-Smart Nursing Education Resources Nursing Legal Issues: http://medi-smart.com/ethics.htm

National Institutes of Health Bioethics Resources on the Web: http://bioethics.od.nih.gov/

Nursing Ethics.ca: http://www.nursingethics.ca/

Steinke, E.E. (2004). Research ethics, informed consent, and participant recruitment. *Clinical Nurse Specialist*, **18**:88–97.

The World Medical Association Ethics Unit: http://www.wma.net/e/ethicsunit/helsinki.htm

Tully, J., Ninis, N., Booy, R. & Viner, R. (2000). The new system of review by multicentre research ethics committees: prospective studies. *British Medical Journal*, **320**:1179–82. Available online http://www.bmj.com/cgi/reprint/320/7243/1179

University of Surrey's International Centre for Nursing Ethics: http://portal.surrey.ac.uk/portal/page?_pageid=731,131416&_dad=portal&_schema=PORTAL

9 Cardiovascular Assessment

A.M. Kucia & S.A. Unger

Overview

Assessment data is obtained from a patient's history, physical examination and diagnostic tests. This information is used to establish a clinical diagnosis, establish goals of care and evaluate outcomes. Assessment is undertaken by various members of the health care team, and synthesis of this information allows a comprehensive plan of care to be developed for the patient that takes into consideration immediate and long-term health care needs. The immediate assessment needs of a patient who presents with an acute cardiac condition will be somewhat different from those who present with a chronic or stable disease because rapid assessment and treatment can have a significant impact upon outcomes for those with an acute cardiac condition. This chapter outlines the components of assessment for a patient with an acute cardiac condition.

Learning objectives

After reading this chapter, you should be able to:

- Describe the components of the cardiovascular history.
- Explain the information required in the assessment of chest pain.
- Describe the steps of the cardiovascular physical examination.
- Explain the steps in cardiac auscultation and the origin of heart sounds and murmurs.
- Describe the aspects of cardiovascular examination that assess cardiac output and circulation.

Key concepts

Health history; precordial inspection; palpation; cardiac auscultation

Health history

The health history provides physiological and psychosocial information that guides the physical assessment, the selection of diagnostic tests and the choice of treatment options. A health history is obtained from the patient but may also contain information from secondary sources such as the patient's family. This will contain information about the symptoms that the patient is experiencing, any previous or related illness experiences and information about the patient's coping mechanisms, including the meanings that the patient places on the illness such as causation, impact on life and treatment options.

The history should focus on the following areas:

- Comprehensive history of the presenting problem
- Past health history
- Risk factors for cardiovascular disease (CVD)
- Medication history
- Social and personal factors that impact on cardiovascular health

Presenting problem

The patient is asked about the symptoms or problem that has prompted them to seek care. The nature of the problem will guide the nurse in asking further questions to explore the nature of the complaint. Ask the patient about other symptoms or problems that are associated with the chief complaint, such as chest pain, breathlessness, cough, nausea or vomiting, diaphoresis, swelling of feet or ankles, palpitations, dizziness/lightheadedness, nocturia and intermittent claudication.

Key point

When taking the patient's history, a differentiation needs to be made between dyspnoea (a subjective complaint of true difficulty in breathing) and breathlessness (a response that follows a sudden burst of activity such as running up flights of stairs). It should be established whether difficulty in breathing occurs only with exertion or at rest, and whether position is a factor in dyspnoea. If dyspnoea is present when the patient lies flat and is relieved by sitting or standing, it is known as orthopnoea. If the onset of breathing difficulties occur a couple of hours after sleep onset and the symptoms are relieved by sitting upright or getting out of bed, the condition is known as paroxysmal nocturnal dyspnoea (PND) (Morton & Tucker 2005).

Chest pain is one of the most common presenting complaints to emergency departments and general practice surgeries. Box 9.1 outlines some of the questions that may be asked to obtain information from a patient presenting with chest pain.

Box 9.1   Assessment of chest pain using the PQRST mnemonic

Using the PQRST mnemonic may help you to remember the questions that need to be asked in assessing a patient with chest pain.

P   Precipitating and palliative factors

Questions that will yield information about what changes the intensity of the pain include:

What were you doing when the pain started?

Was there anything that seemed to trigger or cause the pain?

Was it associated with anything in particular, such as exertion, stress or before, during or after meals?

Does anything relieve the pain?

Get the patient to sit up – note any grimacing or difficulty in moving and changing position. Ask the patient to take a deep breath in as quickly as they can – if it causes pain in the patient, you often will be able to see by the patient's expression or the patient will be unable to take a deep breath in. Ask the patient whether changing position or taking a deep breath made any difference to the pain.

Q   Quality

Ask the patient to describe how the pain feels. Try to avoid prompting the patient with descriptors of pain such as heavy, dull, sharp, tight, burning – they will often agree with whatever you are suggesting, even if you are suggesting conflicting things.

R   Region and radiation

Ask the patient where the pain is. Get the patient to point to the areas where pain is located.
Ask if the pain travels anywhere else, such as the arm, back, neck or jaw.

S   Severity

It is important to obtain a baseline assessment of the severity of pain. A pain-rating scale is often used where 0 is scored as no pain and 10 is the most severe pain ever experienced. This baseline can then be used to compare pain at time intervals to see whether it is improving or worsening, and whether therapy is having the desired effect.

Table 9.1	Risk factors for CVD.
Non-modifiable risks	Age
	Gender
	Family history of CVD
Modifiable risk factors	Hypertension
	Dyslipidaemia
	Overweight/obesity
	Diabetes/insulin resistance
	Renal disease
Behavioural risk factors	Tobacco smoking
	Physical inactivity
	Poor nutrition
	Excessive alcohol consumption
Psychosocial risk factors	Depression
	Stress
	Anxiety
	Social isolation

T   Time

Ask the patient questions that will establish pain onset such as:

When did the pain start?

Did it start suddenly or gradually?

Has the pain been continuous since it started or does it come and go?

Have you had this type of pain before and if so, how often has it occurred?

Associated features

Ask the patient about whether they have symptoms commonly associated with chest pain such as breathlessness, nausea or vomiting, diaphoresis or dizziness/lightheadedness.

- History of CVD
- History of peptic ulcer disease, gastro-oesophageal reflux or frequent ingestion of non-steroidal anti-inflammatory drugs/steroids
- Recent operations (such as cardiothoracic surgery)
- History of pulmonary embolus or long period of inactivity or immobility (such as long journey, recent operation or illness)
- Recent viral illness

Key point

Chest pain may result from a cardiovascular problem other than myocardial ischaemia. For example, pain that is made worse by lying down, moving or deep breathing may be caused by pericarditis. Pain that is retrosternal and accompanied by sudden shortness of breath and peripheral cyanosis may be caused by a pulmonary embolism (Morton & Tucker 2005).

Risk factors for CVD

Additionally, it is important to assess for the presence of cardiac risk factors or diseases that are associated with an increased risk of CVD. These are listed in Table 9.1 and discussed in detail in Chapters 5 and 6.

Medications

A comprehensive medication history should be obtained addressing the following elements:

- Identify prescribed medications currently taken including dosage, frequency, length of time taken, side effects and compliance.
- Identify over-the-counter medications taken regularly or recently and the reason for use.

Past health history

The past history usually includes information about childhood and adult illnesses, accidents and injuries, operations and interventions that may or may not be relevant to the current illness. The patient is also asked about current medications and known allergies.

Previous illnesses and operations

Previous illnesses and operations may provide important clues to the current condition or offer potential alternative diagnoses where the problem is not clearly cardiac in nature. These include:

- Identify any known allergies to medications.
- Identify any contraindications to medications that may be prescribed, such as aspirin or beta blockers in asthmatics, or streptokinase in patients in whom it has previously been administered.

Social and personal history

Social and personal factors that affect cardiovascular health should be included in the patient's history. These include factors such as:

- Family composition/significant other support
- Living conditions
- Daily routine and activities
- Occupation and employment
- Cultural/religious beliefs
- Coping patterns

It is important to know the person as well as the illness. These details will give some indication as to how the person will cope with illness, what supports are available to them, what services need to be offered or put into place to assist the patient through the illness and achieve optimal health, and involve the patient in formulating a plan of care that takes into account their individual needs and preferences.

Physical examination

A baseline physical examination is obtained and this will determine the requirement and timing of further assessment. Subsequent assessment can be compared with baseline to look for improvement or deterioration.

Learning activity

Visit St George's University London Clinical Skills Online available at http://www.elu.sgul.ac.uk/cso/video.php?skill=cvs for video clips of various examinations, including a cardiovascular examination.

General appearance

Information gathering about the patient starts from the first interaction and begins with first impressions from the patients appearance. These include things such as whether the patient appears well groomed or unkempt, and may have implications about the patient's ability or motivation to perform self-care activities. If obesity or cachexia is present, an observation is made about the patient's nutritional state. Facial expressions and body language are some of the first things that are noticed and may give an indication as to whether the patient appears anxious, distressed or in pain. Their affect and how they interact with the nurse will become evident when you introduce yourself and explain your intent in taking a history and examination. Observe if they make eye contact and respond appropriately to conversation. Other observations that can be made whilst taking a patient history are presence of pallor or cyanosis, diaphoresis, laboured breathing, coughing and vomiting.

Precordial inspection and palpation

With the patient supine and the head of the bed raised at a 45 degree angle, inspect the precordium for any visible pulsations, masses, scars, lesions, signs of trauma or previous surgery (such as median sternotomy). Locate the angle of Louis (sternal angle) also known as the notch of Louis (sternal notch), the raised notch where the manubrium and the body of the sternum are joined. This notch is at the level of the second rib and can, therefore, be used as a reference point for locating intercostal spaces.

Palpate the areas of the valves for any thrills (a palpable vibration felt as a result of turbulent blood flow). Palpate for any parasternal heaves (large movements best felt with the heel of the hand at the sternal border). Palpate for any epigastric pulsations. Aortic pulsations may be felt in the epigastrium, but an abnormally large pulsation may suggest pathology such as an abdominal aortic aneurysm.

Palpate the apex beat (also known as the 'point of maximal impulse') which is usually found in the fifth intercostal space and 1 cm medial to the

Box 9.2 Characteristics of the apex beat

S	Size	Is it larger than one intercostal space?
A	Amplitude	Is it strong or weak?
L	Location	Is it in the 5th intercostal space at the mid-clavicular line?
I	Impulse	Is it monophasic or biphasic?
D	Duration	Is it abnormally sustained?

mid-clavicular line. Characteristics of the apex beat can be described using the mnemonic in Box 9.2.

Key point

If the apex beat can be felt across a large area, feel for the most lateral and inferior position of pulsation. If the apex beat is located in the axilla, it would suggest cardiomegaly or mediastinal shift. The apex beat does not exactly correspond to the anatomical apex of the heart.

If you are having difficulty palpating the apex beat, keep the pads of your fingers in the position described earlier and ask the patient to roll on to their left side. It may not be possible to palpate the apex beat in obese patients or those with emphysema.

Learning activity

For short video clips on how to palpate the precordium, including palpation for thrills and heaves and the apex beat, visit the Arts and Science of Clinical Medicine webpage on Precordium Examination at http://www.radiationoncology.ca/ascm/Physical_Examination/ascm1/Precordial/index.htm

Jugular venous pressure

The jugular venous pressure (JVP) is an indirect measure of central venous pressure (CVP). The height of the level of blood in the right internal jugular vein (IJV) is an indication of right atrial pressure because there are no valves or obstructions

between the vein and the right atrium (Morton & Tucker 2005). The patient should be positioned in a semi-recumbent position at a 45 degree angle with the head turned slightly to the left. If possible have a tangential light source that shines obliquely from the left. Look for the surface markings of the right IJV that runs from the medial end of clavicle to the ear lobe. The JVP has a double waveform pulsation. Measure the level of the JVP by measuring the vertical distance between the sternal angle and the top of the JVP. This is usually less than 3–4 cm.

Key point

If you are having difficulty distinguishing the JVP from the carotid pulse, remember that the JVP has a double waveform pulsation (Figure 9.1). Time the jugular venous pulse waves by simultaneous palpation of the carotid arterial pulse. The *a* wave precedes the carotid arterial pulse, whereas the *v* wave closely follows the pulse.

Unlike the carotid pulse, the JVP pulse is not palpable, obliterated by pressure and decreases with inspiration. To confirm that the pulsation observed is caused by the JVP, apply firm pressure using the palm of the hand on the right upper quadrant and a transient increase in the JVP will be seen in normal patient's hepatojugular reflex.

Pulses

The arterial pulses should be palpated using the pads of the fingers. In a full cardiovascular examination, the carotid, brachial, radial, femoral, popliteal, posterior tibial and dorsalis pedis pulses should be palpated. In a targeted examination (such as in an acute admission), the radial pulse is the usual site for assessing the arterial pulse. Peripheral pulses are compared bilaterally for symmetry.

- The pulse is assessed for rate and rhythm. The normal pulse is regular and between 60 and 100 bpm.
- The strength of the pulse is assessed and this may be graded on a scale of 0–3 as described in Table 9.2.

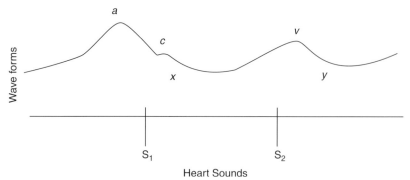

a wave is produced by right atrial contraction.
c wave represents tricuspid valve closure
x wave or x descent represents drop in pressure in the right atrium.
v wave represents passive right atrial filling late in systole or by ballooning of the
tricuspid valve during right venticular contraction.
y wave or descent represents drop in pressure in the right ventricle.

Figure 9.1   Jugular venous pulse wave form.

Table 9.2   Rating scale for strength of arterial pulses.

0	Absent
1	Weak, thready, easily obliterated
2	Normal
3	Strong, bounding, cannot be obliterated

- The character of the pulse is described. A pulse that alternates in strength with alternate beats is known as pulsus alternans and almost invariably is associated with severe left ventricular systolic dysfunction. A pulse that disappears during inspiration but reappears during expiration is known as pulsus paradoxus.

Key point

Pulsus paradoxus may be a normal finding. Changes in intrathoracic pressures during breathing are transmitted to the heart and great vessels, causing arterial blood pressure to fall with inspiration and rise with expiration. Increased venous return during inspiration causes right ventricle distension, and the interventricular septum bulges into the left ventricle (LV), thereby reducing its size. Increased pooling of blood in the expanded lungs decreases the return of blood to the LV, thereby decreasing stroke volume. Additionally, negative intrathoracic pressure during inspiration is transmitted to the aorta. Therefore, during inspiration the fall in the left ventricular stroke volume is reflected as a fall in the systolic blood pressure. The converse is true for expiration. During normal respiration, the changes in intrathoracic and blood pressure are minor, and the accepted upper limit for fall in systolic blood pressure with inspiration is 10 mmHg. Causes of pathologic pulsus paradoxus (fall in systolic blood pressure with inspiration >10 mmHg) include cardiac tamponade, pericardial effusion, constrictive pericarditis, restrictive cardiomyopathy, acute myocardial infarction, cardiogenic shock, pulmonary embolus, bronchial asthma, tension pneumothorax and extreme obesity (Khasnis & Lokhandwala 2002). To determine if pulsus paradoxus is a pathological finding, use a sphygmomanometer and allow the cuff to deflate until the pulse is heard only during expiration and note the corresponding pressure. Continue to deflate the cuff. The point at which the pressure is heard throughout the inspiratory and expiratory cycle is noted. The second systolic pressure reading is subtracted from the first; if the difference is >10 mmHg during normal respirations, it is considered pathological (Morton & Tucker 2005).

Peripheral vascular system

Skin temperature and colour

The skin temperature and colour (including the peripheries) should be noted. Colour should be uniform. Note any areas of cyanosis. Central cyanosis is generally distributed but best observed in the mucous membranes which appear dusky and bluish in colour. Central cyanosis is a sign of reduced oxygen concentration and is a late sign of hypoxia. Peripheral cyanosis, on the other hand, is localised in the extremities and protrusions (hands, feet, nose, ears and lips) and reflects impaired circulation (Morton & Tucker 2005).

Peripheral oedema

Observe the legs and feet for oedema. Although oedema can occur due to causes other than heart failure, this is a potential cause. Ask about the onset and of oedema development and duration, and whether it is relieved by elevation of the limbs.

Peripheral circulation

Look for any signs of thrombophlebitis, varicose veins, lesions and ulcers, and assess capillary filling time.

Blood pressure

The blood pressure should initially be taken on both arms and readings should not vary more than 10 mmHg between arms. In a full cardiovascular examination, blood pressure should be assessed in lying and standing positions, and readings should not vary by more than 5–15 mmHg with these position changes.

> **Key point**
>
> A blood pressure difference of ≥20 mmHg between the left and right arm may indicate aortic dissection, but significant inter-arm blood pressure differentials may be found in 20% of people without aortic dissection (Wiesenfarth 2007).
>
> A variation in blood pressure by 5–15 mmHg in the setting of dizziness or syncope may indicate postural (orthostatic) hypotension. To assess the patient for postural hypotension, the patient should lie for 10 min before the blood pressure and heart rate is obtained; then blood pressure and heart rate should be immediately assessed on arising and again after 2 min (Lance et al. 2000).

Blood pressure can be assessed using a number of non-invasive methods:

- Palpatory method: A systolic blood pressure reading can be obtained by palpating the brachial or radial artery and rapidly inflating the cuff to about 30 mmHg above the point where the pulse disappears. Slowly deflate the cuff and the point at which the pulse reappears is the approximate level of the systolic blood pressure. This method may be useful where a quick assessment of systolic pressure is needed.

> **Key point**
>
> Blood pressure should be assessed using appropriate equipment but as a rough guide (if equipment is not immediately available), if a radial pulse can be felt the systolic blood pressure is usually at least 80 mmHg (Hambly 2000).

- Auscultatory method: The auscultatory method requires a sphygmomanometer (mercury or aneroid) and stethoscope. The cuff should be appropriately sized as most inaccuracies result from the use of the wrong size of cuff: a narrow cuff wrapped round a fat arm will give an abnormally high reading and vice versa (Hambly 2000). The cuff bladder should be over the brachial artery with the lower edge of the cuff 2–3 cm above the antecubital fossa (Beevers et al. 2001).
- Automated devices: Automated blood pressure measurement devices are being increasingly used and although they are generally reasonably accurate, there are a number of situations where the device does not accurately represent the blood pressure reading. These devices tend to over-read at low blood pressures and under-read at very high blood pressures. The devices rely on a constant pulse volume, so are often inaccurate in the setting of an irregular pulse, such as atrial fibrillation. As with the manual auscultatory method, cuffs must be appropriately sized and applied.

Key point

Automated devices may have difficulty in 'reading' the blood pressure, and will continue to inflate and deflate which is likely to cause discomfort to the patient. This should be avoided especially when the patient has received thrombolytic, antiplatelet or anticoagulation therapy as substantial bruising can occur.

Learning activity

We use a number of devices in cardiovascular assessment. Understanding how these devices work may help us to ensure that we use them properly in order to get an appropriate result or reading. Obtaining a blood pressure is something that we take for granted, but manual and automated methods of obtaining blood pressure can be subject to operator error or equipment malfunction. Read the following articles for a better idea of how these devices work and the optimal way of using them to avoid inaccurate results:

  Beevers, G., Lip, G.Y.H. & O'Brien, E. (2001). ABC of hypertension. Blood pressure measurement Part II—conventional sphygmomanometry: technique of auscultatory blood pressure measurement. *British Medical Journal*, **322**(7293):1043–7. Available online at www.bmj.com
  Hambly, P. (2000). Measuring the blood pressure. Practical procedures, **11**(6):1. Available from http://www.nda.ox.ac.uk/wfsa/html/u11/u1106_01.htm

Cardiac auscultation

A good quality stethoscope with both a diaphragm and a bell is needed for cardiac auscultation. When using the diaphragm, it should be placed firmly on the chest wall to create a tight seal, and it is used to hear high-frequency sounds such as the first and second heart sounds (S_1, S_2), friction rubs, systolic murmurs and diastolic insufficiency murmurs. When using the bell, it should be placed lightly on the chest wall and is used to detect low-frequency sounds such as the third and

fourth heart sounds (S_3, S_4) and the diastolic murmurs of mitral and tricuspid stenosis (Morton & Tucker 2005). The physiology behind heart sounds is demonstrated in Table 9.3.

The patient should be positioned in a semi-recumbent position with the head of the bed elevated 30–45 degrees. Systematic auscultation of the precordium with the stethoscope diaphragm follows the following pattern:

- Right sternal border in the second intercostal space referred to as the aortic area.
- Left sternal border in the second intercostal space referred to as the pulmonic area.
- Left sternal border in the third intercostal space referred to as Erb's point where S_2 is best heard.
- Left sternal border in the fifth intercostal space referred to as the tricuspid area.
- Mid-clavicular line in the fifth intercostal space at the apex of the heart which may be referred to as the mitral area where S_1 is the loudest.
- This pattern is then repeated with the stethoscope bell. Figure 9.2 shows the positions in which to place the stethoscope.

In each of the positions auscultated, the normal heart sounds S_1 and S_2 should be identified. The intensity of the sound, respiratory variation and splitting should be noted. After S_1 and S_2 are identified, listen for the presence of any extra sounds, first in systole, then in diastole. Finally, each area is auscultated for the presence of murmurs and friction rubs (Morton & Tucker 2005).

Key point

To help hear abnormal sounds, the patient may be asked to roll partly onto the left side to help bring the LV closer to the chest wall (Morton & Tucker 2005).

Listen in the same area during inspiration and expiration to differentiate murmurs arising from the left or right side of the heart, as deep inspiration increases venous return to the right side of the heart and thus augments the intensity of right-sided murmurs while having little or no effect on murmurs arising from the left side of the heart (Skillings 2001).

Table 9.3   Heart sounds.

Sound	Cause
First heart sound (S_1)	This is a normal heart sound timed with closure of mitral and tricuspid valves at the beginning of ventricular systole. Mitral closure is responsible for most of the sound produced and so S_1 is best heard in the mitral area (apex). If the valves do not close at the same time, a 'split' S_1 sound may be heard. This may be physiological in a healthy individual or pathological (in conditions such as right bundle branch block). A split S_1 is best heard in the tricuspid area.
Second heart sound (S_2)	A normal heart sound produced by vibrations initiated by the closure of the aortic and pulmonic valves at the beginning of diastole best heard at Erb's Point. With inspiration, the pulmonic valve closes a bit later than the aortic valve, producing a split S_2 sound known as 'physiological splitting' which is best heard on inspiration with the stethoscope placed in the pulmonic area. The intensity of S_2 may be increased in the presence of aortic or pulmonic valvular stenosis or in pulmonary or systemic hypertension.
Third heart sound (S_3)	Low-frequency sound that occurs during the early, rapid-filling phase of ventricular diastole. May be a normal finding in children or young adults. In older adults, S_3 signifies a ventricular failure and is a sound caused by a non-compliant or failing ventricle that cannot distend to accept the rapid inflow of blood. The resulting turbulent flow causes vibration of the atrioventricular valvular structures or the ventricles themselves, producing a low-frequency sound. A left ventricular S_3 is best heard at the apex with the stethoscope bell. A right ventricular S_3 is heard best at the xiphoid or lower left sternal border and varies in intensity with respiration, becoming louder on inspiration (Gonce Morton & Tucker 2005).
Fourth heart sound (S_4)	An S_4, sometimes known as an atrial gallop, is a low-frequency sound heard late in diastole, just before S_1. The sound is produced by atrial contraction forcing blood into a non-compliant ventricle that is resistant to filling. Causes include systemic hypertension, acute myocardial ischaemia or infarction, cardiomyopathy and aortic stenosis (AS). S_4 is best heard with the bell of the stethoscope at the apex. Conditions affecting right ventricular compliance, such as pulmonary hypertension or pulmonic stenosis, may produce a right ventricular S_4 heard best at the lower left sternal border, becoming louder on inspiration (Gonce Morton & Tucker 2005).
Summation gallop	As ventricular diastole is shortened in rapid heart rates, if S_3 and S_4 are both present, they may fuse together and become audible as a single diastolic sound called a summation gallop. This sound is loudest at the apex and is heard best with the stethoscope bell while the patient lies turned slightly to the left side (Gonce Morton & Tucker 2005).
Heart murmurs	Sounds produced either by the forward flow of blood through a narrowed or constricted valve into a dilated vessel or chamber, or by the backward flow of blood through an incompetent valve or septal defect. The sound produced is described as blowing, harsh, rumbling or musical, and the intensity or loudness of a murmur is described using the following grading system.

- Grade I: faint and barely audible
- Grade II: soft
- Grade III: audible but not palpable
- Grade IV and V: associated with a palpable thrill
- Grade VI: is audible without a stethoscope

Systolic murmurs occur between S_1 and S_2.

- Stenosis of the aortic or pulmonic valve results in a mid-systolic ejection murmur. The quality of these murmurs is harsh and of medium pitch. AS is heard best in the aortic area and may radiate into the neck; pulmonic stenosis is heard best over the pulmonic area.
- Mitral or tricuspid valvular insufficiency (regurgitation) or a ventricular septal defect (VSD) produces systolic murmurs caused by the backward flow of blood from an area of higher pressure to an area of lower pressure, which are harsh and blowing in quality. The sound is described as holosystolic (the murmur begins immediately after S_1 and continues throughout systole up to S_2). Mitral regurgitation (MR) is best heard at the apex and radiating to the left axilla. Tricuspid regurgitation (TR) is best heard at the left sternal border and increases in intensity during inspiration. This murmur may radiate to the cardiac apex.

Table 9.3   *(cont'd)*

Sound	Cause
	• A VSD produces a harsh, blowing holosystolic sound caused by blood flowing from the left to the right ventricle through a defect in the septal wall during systole. This murmur is heard best from the fourth to sixth intercostal spaces on both sides of the sternum and is accompanied by a palpable thrill (Gonce Morton & Tucker 2005).
	Diastolic murmurs occur after S_2 and before the onset of the following S_1.
	• Aortic or pulmonary valvular insufficiency (regurgitation) produces a blowing diastolic murmur that begins immediately after S_2 and decreases in intensity as regurgitant flow decreases through diastole. These murmurs are described as early diastolic decrescendo murmurs. Aortic regurgitation (AR) is best heard in the aortic area and may radiate along the right sternal border to the apex. Pulmonic valve regurgitation is best heard in the pulmonic area.
	• Mitral or tricuspid stenosis produces a diastolic murmur. This murmur decreases in intensity from its onset and then increases again as ventricular filling increases because of atrial contraction; this is termed decrescendo–crescendo. Mitral stenosis (MS) is best heard at the apex with the patient turned slightly to the left side. Tricuspid stenosis increases in intensity with inspiration and is loudest in the fifth intercostal space along the left sternal border (Gonce Morton & Tucker 2005).
Friction rubs	A pericardial friction rub may be heard anywhere over the pericardium with the diaphragm of the stethoscope. The rub may be accentuated by having the patient lean forward and exhale and, unlike a pleural friction rub, does not vary in intensity with respiration (Gonce Morton & Tucker 2005).

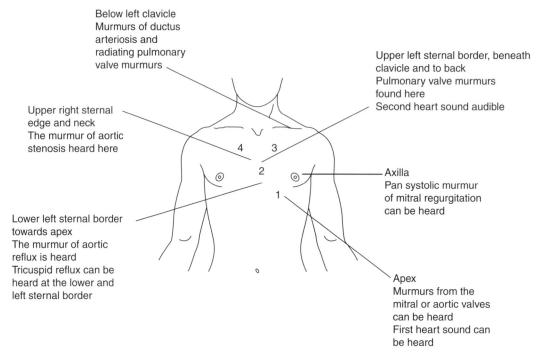

Below left clavicle
Murmurs of ductus arteriosis and radiating pulmonary valve murmurs

Upper left sternal border, beneath clavicle and to back
Pulmonary valve murmurs found here
Second heart sound audible

Upper right sternal edge and neck
The murmur of aortic stenosis heard here

Axilla
Pan systolic murmur of mitral regurgitation can be heard

Lower left sternal border towards apex
The murmur of aortic reflux is heard
Tricuspid reflux can be heard at the lower and left sternal border

Apex
Murmurs from the mitral or aortic valves can be heard
First heart sound can be heard

1 – Mitral regurgitation: apex, axilla
2 – Aortic regurgitation: lower left sternal border
3 – Pulmonary stenoses: upper left sternal border/clavicle
4 – Aortic stenoses: apex, upper right sternal border, neck

Figure 9.2   Sites for cardiac auscultation.
Source: From White (2002). Copyright Elsevier 2002.

Respiratory assessment

A respiratory assessment should be undertaken to detect any evidence of heart failure or other respiratory pathology.

Ask the patient about any symptoms of dyspnoea:

- Establish whether it occurs on exertion or at rest
- Establish whether the patient experiences orthopnoea – asking the patient how many pillows they use to sleep is often useful to establish whether orthopnoea is present
- Establish whether there is any evidence of PND

Ask the patient about any symptoms of cough or sputum production. Patients with heart failure may experience a dry irritating cough which may occur particularly at night (National Heart Foundation of Australia [NHFA] & Cardiac Society of Australia and New Zealand [CSANZ] 2006).

Observe the patient's pattern and cycle of breathing, including:

- The respiratory rate (in a healthy adult, inaudible respirations should occur between 12 and 20 times per minute)
- The duration of the inspiratory/expiratory cycle and any note if there is any difficulty in expelling air (expiration [E] should take around twice as long as inspiration [I], giving an I:E ratio of 1:2)

- Use of accessory muscles of respiration (sternocleidomastoid, spinal, neck and abdominal muscles)
- Intercostal retractions (visible indentations between the ribs as the intercostal muscles aid in breathing)
- Nasal flaring (intermittent outward movements of the nostrils)
- Pursed lip breathing (partial closure of the lips to allow air to be expired slowly) (Habel 2006)

Note the patient's posture, including whether the patient needs to sit upright and is unable to tolerate lying down. Auscultate the patient's posterior chest, beginning with the areas above the scapulae. Move downward in a stair-step fashion, comparing your findings from one side with those from the other side. Listen to the character of the breath sounds. Normal vesicular breath sounds are heard over most lung fields. See Table 9.4 for types and causes of abnormal (also known as adventitious) breath sounds.

Table 9.4 Abnormal breath sounds.

Type of breath sound	Nature of the sound	Potential causes
Crackles (rales)	Discontinuous breath sounds that sound like crinkling plastic wrap or can be simulated by rubbing strands of hair together between two fingers near one's ear. May be further described as: • Fine crackles are short high-pitched sounds • Coarse crackles are longer-lasting low-pitched sounds	Signify distension of fibrotic lung tissue or opening of collapsed alveoli most commonly with atelectasis and alveolar filling processes such as: • Pulmonary oedema • Interstitial lung disease (Merck & Co, Inc. 2005)
Rhonchi	Low-pitched respiratory sounds that can be heard during inspiration or expiration	Probably relate to variations in obstruction as airways distend with inhalation and occur in a variety of conditions including: • Chronic bronchitis (Merck & Co, Inc. 2005) • Pneumonia and infections of the lungs
Wheezes	Whistling, musical breath sounds that are worse during expiration than inspiration and are commonly associated with dyspnoea. May be audible without a stethoscope.	• Asthma or chronic obstructive pulmonary (airways) disease (COPD) • Acute allergic reaction
Stridor	High-pitched, predominantly inspiratory sound that can normally be heard without a stethoscope formed by extrathoracic upper airway obstruction.	It is a serious finding and often signifies a life-threatening upper airway obstruction (Merck & Co, Inc. 2005).
Decreased breath sounds	Poor air movement in airways	Usually caused by disease processes or mechanisms limiting airflow. May signify: • Bronchospasm • Pleural effusion • Pneumothorax • Asthma or COPD (Merck & Co, Inc. 2005)
Bronchial breath sounds	Louder, harsher and higher pitched than normal breath sounds	• Normal finding over trachea • May be caused by lung consolidation in conditions such as pneumonia (Merck & Co, Inc. 2005)
Bronchophony	Clear transmission of the patient's spoken voice through the chest wall	Results from alveolar consolidation such as in pneumonia (Merck & Co, Inc. 2005)
Egophony	Occurs when a patient says the letter 'e' and the examiner hears the letter 'a' on auscultation	Any condition that results in pulmonary consolidation such as pneumonia (Merck & Co, Inc. 2005)
Whispered pectoriloquy	Transmission of the patient's whispered voice through the chest wall at an increased volume	Pneumonia
Friction rubs	Grating or creaking sounds that fluctuate with the respiratory cycle	Sign of pleural inflammation associated with: • Pleurisy • Post thoracotomy • Empyema (Merck & Co, Inc. 2005)

Pulse oximetry is used to monitor the percentage of haemoglobin (Hb) which is saturated with oxygen. The pulse oximeter is a computerised device that detects the percentage of Hb saturated with oxygen via a probe that is attached to the patient's finger or ear lobe. The device has a visual display and an audible signal for each pulse beat and alarms that respond to a slow or fast pulse rate, or oxygen saturation below 90% as a fall in PaO_2 below this level represents serious hypoxia. Oxygen saturation should be above 95%, although patients with long-standing respiratory or congenital heart disease may have lower readings reflecting the underlying severity of the disease. It should be remembered that pulse oximeters give no information about the level of CO_2 and therefore have limitations in the assessment of patients developing respiratory failure due to CO_2 retention (Fearnley 1995).

Key point

When using devices in cardiovascular assessment, nurses should be aware of situations that may affect the accuracy or reliability of the device. A pulse oximeter may not give accurate readings in the following situations:

Reductions in peripheral pulsatile flow due to peripheral vasoconstriction (due to hypovolaemia, severe hypotension, cold, cardiac failure, some cardiac arrhythmias) or peripheral vascular disease may result in an inadequate signal for analysis. Venous congestion may result in low pulsatile readings. Inflation of a blood pressure cuff on the same limb or any circumstance that obstructs blood flow to the limb will result in inability of the device to obtain a reading.

If the probe is placed over nail varnish, falsely low readings may result. The units are not affected by dark skin or jaundice (Fearnley 1995).

Pulse oximetry cannot distinguish between different forms of Hb. Carboxy-haemoglobin (Hb combined with carbon monoxide) registers as 90% oxygenated Hb and 10% desaturated Hb – therefore the oximeter will overestimate the saturation and should not be used in carbon monoxide inhalation. The units should still be accurate in anaemia (Fearnley 1995).

Key point

As part of a respiratory assessment, look for signs of cyanosis, conscious level and mentation. An altered state of consciousness, anxiety, restlessness, confusion or other changes in mental status are important signs of potential respiratory problems.

Conclusion

Cardiovascular assessment is a systematic process that involves a thorough history and examination of the patient. In emergency situations, a targeted history and examination may be needed, and further information is obtained when the patient is stabilised. Many of the skills required to perform cardiovascular assessment need to be practiced, and so every opportunity should be taken to perfect the techniques required.

References

Beevers, G., Lip, G.Y.H. & O'Brien, E. (2001). ABC of hypertension. Blood pressure measurement Part II—Conventional sphygmomanometry: technique of auscultatory blood pressure measurement. *British Medical Journal*, **322**:1043–7.

Fearnley, S.J. (1995). Pulse oximetry. Practical procedures, 5:1. Retrieved online 25th July from http://www.nda.ox.ac.uk/wfsa/html/u05/u05_003.htm

Morton, P.G. & Tucker, T. (2005). Patient assessment: cardiovascular system. In: P. Gonce Morton (ed.), *Critical Care Nursing: A Holistic Approach*, 8th edn. Lippincott Williams & Wilkins, Philadelphia, pp. 211–91.

Habel, M. (2006). Respiratory assessment. RNCEUS. Retrieved online 25th July 2008 from http://www.rnceus.com/resp/respframe.html

Hambly, P. (2000). Measuring the blood pressure. Practical procedures, 11:1. Retrieved online 24th July 2008 from http://www.nda.ox.ac.uk/wfsa/html/u11/u1106_01.htm

Khasnis, A. & Lokhandwala, Y. (2002). Clinical signs in medicine: pulsus paradoxus. *Journal of Postgraduate Medicine*, **48**:46–49. Retrieved online 24th July 2008 from http://www.jpgmonline.com/text.asp?2002/48/1/46/153

Lance, R., Link, M., Padua, M, Clavell, L.E., Johnson, G & Knebel, A. (2000). Comparison of different methods of obtaining orthostatic vital signs. *Clinical Nursing Research*, **9**:479–91.

Merck & Co, Inc. (2005). Pulmonary disorders: Introduction. *The Merck Manuals Online Medical Library*. Retrieved online 25th July 2008 from http://www.merck.com/mmpe/sec05/ch045/ch045a.html

National Heart Foundation of Australia and the Cardiac Society of Australia and New Zealand (Chronic Heart Failure Guidelines Expert Writing Panel) (2006). Guidelines for the prevention, detection and management of chronic heart failure in Australia. Retrieved online 28th March 2009 from http://www.heartfoundation.org.au/SiteCollectionDocuments/CHF%202006%20Guidelines%20NHFA-CSANZ%20WEB.pdf

Skillings, J.E. (2001). Can I improve my skills in auscultation? *Medscape Nurses*. Retrieved online 25th July from http://www.medscape.com/viewarticle/412518

Wiesenfarth, J.M. (2007). Dissection, aortic. *eMedicine*. Retrieved online 24th July 2008 from http://www.emedicine.com/emerg/TOPIC28.HTM

White, M. (2002). The cardiovascular system. In: S. Cross & M. Rimmer (eds.), *Nurse Practitioner Manual of Skills*, 6th edn. Baillière Tindall, Edinburgh, pp. 116–34.

Useful Websites and Further Reading

Levine, B.S. (2005). History taking and physical examination In: S.L. Woods, E.S.S. Froelicher, S. Underhill Motzer & E.J. Bridges (eds), *Cardiac Nursing*, 5th edn. Lippincott Williams and Wilkins, Philadelphia, pp. 229–64.

St George's University London Clinical Skills Online: Available at http://www.elu.sgul.ac.uk/cso/video.php?skill=cvs

10 Electrocardiogram Interpretation

A.M. Kucia & C. Oldroyd

Overview

Electrocardiography has been used diagnostically for many years. It provides useful information about heart rate, rhythm, electrocardiographic intervals, electrical axis, bundle branch block (BBB) and hypertrophy. It is central to the diagnosis of myocardial ischaemia and infarction and is useful in detecting drug toxicity, electrolyte imbalance and hypothermia. The ability to interpret an electrocardiogram (ECG) is a useful skill for most nurses, and is a 'must have' skill for nurses working in a cardiac environment. ECG abnormalities can only be appreciated when one is familiar with the range of normal findings, which can be seen to vary markedly between individuals. The theoretical basis of electrocardiography and practical applications will be discussed in this chapter, including normal ECG parameters and causes of abnormal ECG findings.

Learning objectives

After reading this chapter, you should be able to:

- Describe the procedure for obtaining a 12-lead ECG.
- Identify the anatomical zones of the heart associated with the 12 ECG leads.

- Describe the ECG changes associated with acute myocardial ischaemia and evolving myocardial infarction (MI).
- Explain the term 'electrical axis' and calculate the electrical axis using Leads I and aVf.
- Identify the electrocardiographic features of left and right BBB, atrial and ventricular hypertrophy, and changes due to drug toxicity, electrolyte imbalance and hypothermia.

Key concepts

ST-segment changes; T-wave changes; bundle branch block; electrical axis; atrial and ventricular hypertrophy

Normal sequence of depolarisation and repolarisation

The normal sequence of myocardial depolarisation and repolarisation was discussed in Chapter 3. To recap, the heart has specialised conduction cells that are designed to rapidly transmit electrical activity through the heart. This electrical activity produces sequential characteristic waveforms on the 12-lead ECG. Under normal conditions, the sinoatrial (SA) node is the most rapidly depolarising tissue, and thus sets the heart rate. The electrical impulse then spreads via the internodal tracts throughout the left and right atria, and to the atrioventricular (AV) node. As the SA node is located at the superior right border of the heart, the direction of the impulse tends to be downward and to the left. The atrial walls have little muscle mass, thus the electrical activity produced by their depolarisation causes only a small deflection on the 12-lead ECG. This is known as the P wave (Figure 10.1). In the normal heart, the only pathway for the electrical impulse to travel from the atria to the ventricles is via the AV node. There is a short delay whilst the impulse is transmitted

through the AV node before travelling down the common bundle of His and the bundle branches. As these structures are small, their depolarisation is not seen on the surface of 12-lead ECG and this time interval is known electrocardiographically as the isoelectric PR interval. As the wave of depolarisation passes through the bundle branches, the septum begins to depolarise from left to right, and in a slightly downward direction. Septal depolarisation produces a characteristically small deflection (small negative deflection in Lead I and small positive deflection in V1). As the impulse spreads through the distal bundle branches and Purkinje fibres, the larger bulk of the ventricular myocardium depolarises from the septum to the

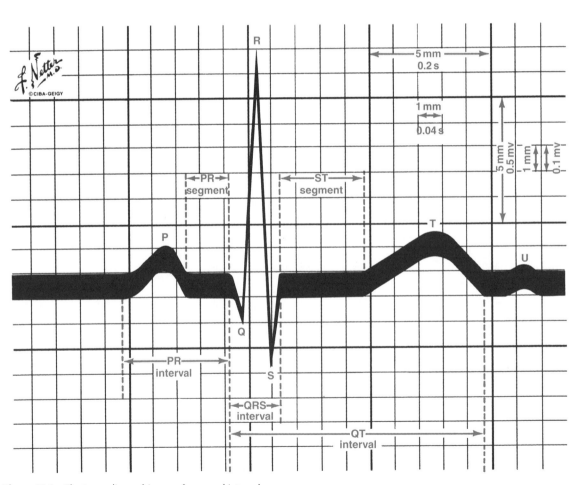

Figure 10.1   Electrocardiographic waveforms and intervals.
Source: From Scheidt (1986). Copyright Novartis A.G. Used with permission.

apex and then the left and right free ventricular walls. As depolarisation of the left and right ventricles is meant to happen simultaneously, the left bundle branch divides into anterior and posterior fascicles to enable the impulse to be transmitted quickly throughout the larger bulk of the left ventricular myocardium. Given that the left ventricle is about 10 mm thick, compared with 3 mm for the right ventricle, the left ventricle generates substantially greater electrical activity; thus, the QRS complex, which denotes ventricular depolarisation on the ECG, is largely a reflection of left ventricular electrical activity when conduction is normal. Following depolarisation of the ventricles, there is little activity until repolarisation begins. This appears on the 12-lead ECG as the isoelectric ST segment. Repolarisation of the ventricles begins from endocardium to epicardium and appears on the ECG as the T wave (Scheidt 1986). Figure 10.1 shows the elements of the ECG complex which represent one cardiac cycle (one heart beat).

Theoretical basis of electrocardiography

Electrical changes resulting from the depolarisation and repolarisation of myocardial cells are recorded using electrodes that are placed in specific positions on the limbs and chest wall. These electrical changes are then transcribed on to graph paper to produce a 12-lead ECG. Electrical activity is recorded on the ECG as a positive or negative deflection. Conventionally, if the electrical impulse is travelling towards the lead, the deflection from the isoelectric line (baseline) is upwards (positive). If the electrical impulse is travelling away from the lead, the deflection from the isoelectric line is downwards (negative). If the wave of depolarisation is at right angles to the lead, the deflection is equiphasic (Meek & Morris 2002). A biphasic deflection may be more positive or negative, depending upon its orientation in relation to the wave of depolarisation.

The 12 ECG leads all record the same electrical events within the heart at a given time, but each of the leads looks at a different view. The standard limb leads (II, III and aVF) are bipolar electrodes:

- Lead I records the electrical potential between the left arm (LA) electrode, which is designated

to be the positive pole in this lead, and the right arm (RA) electrode which is the negative pole in this lead.
- Lead II records the electrical potential between the left leg (LL), which is designated as the positive pole in this lead, and the RA electrode, which is the negative pole in this lead.
- Lead III records the electrical potential between the LL electrode, which is the positive pole in this lead, and the LA electrode, which is the negative pole in this lead (Scheidt 1986).

Where a fourth lead is attached to the right leg (RL), this is used as a ground electrode, and is not seen on the 12-lead ECG.

Learning activity

Think about the normal path of the cardiac conduction system from the SA node to the AV node and down the bundle branches. Which of the bipolar limb leads is likely to have the most positive deflection from the isoelectric line, and why?

Key point

You may hear the term 'Einthoven's triangle' used in relation to the standard limb Leads II, III and aVf. Einthoven was a Dutch doctor and physiologist who invented the first practical ECG in 1903 and received the Nobel Prize in Medicine for this work in 1924. The term refers to an imaginary inverted equilateral triangle described by Einthoven, which is centred on the chest, with the points being the standard leads on the arms and leg. Many of the conventions established by Einthoven provided the basis for modern electrocardiography, including the identification of PQRST waves.

Leads aVR, aVL and aVF are referred to as the 'augmented limb leads'. These leads measure the electric potential at one point with respect to zero potential. Zero potential means that no significant variation in electric potential is registered during contraction of the heart. It is obtained by comparing the electrical potential of one of the leads against the sum electrical potential of the other two leads. For example, in Lead aVF, the electric potential of the LL is compared to zero potential which is obtained by adding together the potential of Leads aVR and aVL. The positive pole of aVR is at the right arm, the positive pole of aVL is at the LA, and the positive pole of aVF is at the LL. Bipolar and augmented limb leads are frontal plane leads. If the three bipolar and three augmented limb leads are superimposed on a single diagram, they encompass a 360° circle (Figure 10.2). Conventionally, the positive pole of Lead I is taken as 0° and coordinates are measured at 30° intervals. This becomes important when determining the cardiac axis (Scheidt 1986).

The precordial leads (V1–V6) examine cardiac electrical activity in the horizontal plane (from sternum to vertebral column) (Figure 10.3).

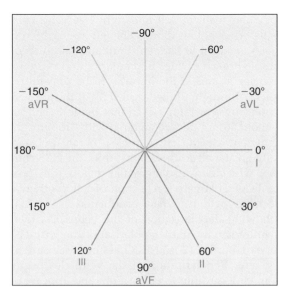

Figure 10.2   The hexaxial reference system.
Source: Reproduced from Meek and Morris (2002). With permission from BMJ Publishing Group Ltd.

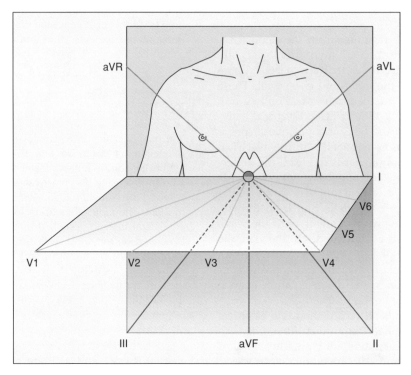

Figure 10.3   Vertical and horizontal perspective of the leads. The limb leads 'view' the heart in the vertical plane and the chest leads in the horizontal plane.
Source: Reproduced from Meek and Morris (2002). With permission from BMJ Publishing Group Ltd.

Determining the cardiac axis

The flow of electrical current through the heart is fairly uniform since it normally follows a well-defined conduction pathway. The cardiac axis represents the mean direction that the electrical impulse takes as it spreads through the myocardium, which is usually from 11 o'clock to 5 o'clock. There is a common misconception that the axis represents the anatomical position of the heart, but this is not the case. An axis deviation does not mean that the heart has moved to point in another direction. It merely represents an alteration in the general direction that the wave of depolarisation takes as it flows through the ventricles (Houghton & Gray 2003). The mean QRS axis represents the direction of electrical activity as seen from the frontal plane leads. Electrical activation is considered to occur from a point within the centre of a circle, and in addition to the radii representing the six limb leads, six further radii are produced. This is known as the hexaxial reference system (Figure 10.2). The axis is determined using this hexaxial reference system, with Lead I designated as 0°. An axis lying above this line is described as a negative number up to −180°, and an axis below as positive up to +180°. A normal axis lies between −30° and +90°. An axis greater than −30° is referred to as a left axis deviation (LAD), whereas an axis of greater than +90° is referred to as a right axis deviation (Meek & Morris 2002).

Axis determination is useful in the diagnosis of a variety of conditions including broad complex tachycardias, pre-excitation syndromes such as Wolff–Parkinson–White (WPW) syndrome, pulmonary embolism, conduction defects (hemiblocks) and congenital heart disease (Jowett & Thompson 2003). In some cases, an axis deviation

can be normal for an individual. Common causes of axis deviation are summarised in Table 10.1.

There are various ways of calculating the cardiac axis, some of which are more precise than others. In most cases, a rough approximation is sufficient to detect an abnormality which can then be referred on to a specialist for more accurate determination. One quick and easy method of determining the cardiac axis involves using Leads I and aVF. Referring back to the hexaxial reference system (Figure 10.2), the circle can be divided into quadrants (four equal parts) and labelled as normal (0 to +90°), left axis (0 to 90°), right axis (+90 to +180°) and extreme left or right (−90° to ±180°) also referred to colloquially as 'No man's land'. By looking at the directions of Leads I and aVF on the 12-lead ECG, it is possible to place the axis within one of the quadrants, thereby providing a rough indication at a glance as to whether the cardiac axis lies within normal limits.

If a more accurate estimate is required, it is necessary to examine all six limb leads. A positive deflection on an ECG indicates that the electrical current is moving towards that lead and a negative deflection indicates that the current is moving away from that lead; so if Lead I is the most positive limb lead, it can be assumed that the axis is bearing in that direction, which corresponds to 0° on the hexaxial reference system. A lead that lies at 90° (perpendicular to the current) will appear on the ECG as equiphasic, and this information can be used to as follows to determine the cardiac axis more precisely:

• Identify the most equiphasic limb lead. The axis lies at 90° to the right or left of this lead. If, for example, Lead II is considered to be the most equiphasic lead, it can be assumed that

Table 10.1 Common causes of axis deviation.

Left axis deviation (>−30º)	Right axis deviation (>+90º)	Extreme axis deviation (No man's land)
• Left anterior hemi-block • WPW syndrome with right-sided, accessory pathway • Inferior MI	• Right ventricular hypertrophy • WPW with left-sided, accessory pathway • Anterolateral MI • Dextrocardia • Left posterior hemi-block	• Ventricular tachycardia • ECG leads incorrectly applied

the axis is running perpendicular to this lead and lies at either $+150°$ or $-30°$.

- Looking back at the hexaxial diagram, identify which leads lie at 90° to the equiphasic lead and decide whether this lead is positive or negative on the ECG. If Lead II was identified as the most equiphasic, the lead lying at 90° is aVL. If aVL is positive on the ECG, then the axis lies at $-30°$, since the current must be travelling towards this electrode to produce a positive deflection. If aVL is negative, then the current must be moving away from the electrode and lies at $+150°$ (Meek & Morris 2002).

This more-precise estimate can be useful for nurses working in specialist areas such as coronary care units and cardiothoracic centres, but for the majority of nurses it is sufficient to simply be able to identify if the axis is normal or abnormal and understand the implications.

Determination of heart rate and electrocardiographic intervals

The horizontal axis on ECG paper represents time. The ECG is normally recorded on standard paper that travels at a speed of 25 mm/second (s), although this can be generally changed in most machines if required. The ECG paper is divided into large squares with darker lines, each of which is 5 mm wide and equates to 0.2 s. Each of these large squares has five smaller squares within it. These small squares are 1 mm wide and equivalent to 0.04 s (Figure 10.1).

The vertical axis on the ECG paper represents voltage amplitude. Electrical activity detected by the ECG machine is measured in millivolts. ECG machines are calibrated so that a signal with an amplitude of 1 mV moves the recording stylus vertically 1 cm; therefore 0.1 mV = 1 mm (one small square).

Key point

A number of conditions can influence the amplitude in ECG leads. Large myocardial mass, such as in ventricular hypertrophy, is likely to result in increased amplitude of the ECG waveform. If current flow is impeded through tissue, such as occurs with pericardial fluid build-up, pulmonary emphysema or obesity, the waveform amplitude is likely to be reduced (Meek & Morris 2002).

Heart rate

Most modern ECG machines and monitors record the ventricular heart rate on printouts. Some will also include printouts of other electrocardiographic intervals. There may be times when you want to calculate atrial rate which may be different to the ventricular rate. In regular rhythms, calculating heart rate (atrial or ventricular) is a simple process. One large box represents 0.2 s; thus there are five large boxes in a second. Count how many complexes are there in a second and multiply by 60. That will give you the heart rate. This method is not reliable for irregular heart rates. For irregular heart rates, it is suggested that the heart rate is calculated by counting the complexes that occur over 6 s (30 large boxes) and multiply by 10. Most ECG paper has markings in the top or bottom margin such as a vertical line or a dot that are spaced at 3-s intervals (every 15 large boxes). This gives an estimate of the heart rate but is not an accurate measure.

Heart rhythm

The normal heart rhythm is sinus rhythm. The rate should be between 60 and 100 beats per minute. A normal P wave should precede each QRS complex and the PR interval should be of normal duration. Refer to Table 10.2 for normal criteria for these waveforms and intervals. Diagnosis of arrhythmias is dealt with in more detail in Chapter 23.

Learning activity

Collect rhythm strips (regular and irregular heart rhythms) and practice calculating the heart rate.

Electrocardiographic waveforms and intervals

There are a number of standard electrocardiographic intervals that provide useful information about conduction (Table 10.2).

Table 10.2 Normal waveforms and electrocardiographic intervals.

Waveform/Interval	Significance	Normal interval
P wave	Represents atrial depolarisation. Measured from the first upward deflection from baseline to return to baseline.	Width <0.11 s (3 small squares)
PR interval	Represents the delay between conduction from atria to ventricles through the AV node. Measured from the end of the P wave to the beginning of the QRS complex.	Width 0.12–0.20 s (3–5 small squares)
QRS interval	Represents ventricular depolarisation. Measured from the first upward/downward deflection from baseline until return to baseline.	Width 0.06–0.10 s (1.5–2.5 small squares)
J point	The point at which the QRS complex ends and the ST segment begins.	The J point may deviate from the baseline due to: • early repolarisation • epicardial or endocardial ischaemia or injury • pericarditis • bundle branch block • ventricular hypertrophy • digitalis effect (Hurst 1998)
ST segment	Represents the time between ventricular depolarisation and ventricular repolarisation. Measured from the end of the QRS to the beginning of the T wave.	Width dependant upon heart rate.
T wave	Represents ventricular repolarisation. Measured from the first upward/downward deflection to return to baseline.	
QT interval	Measured from the first upward/downward deflection of the QRS complex to return of the T wave to baseline.	Width markedly affected by heart rate (HR). The corrected QT (QTc) is commonly calculated using Bazett's formula and should be between 0.3 and 0.44s.
U wave	Thought to represent afterdepolarisations which interrupt or follow repolarisation and are more prominent at slower heart rates	

Learning activity

We refer to ventricular depolarisation as the QRS complex on the ECG, but is there always an identifiable Q wave, R wave and S wave in every complex? Obtain a 12-lead ECG and look at the QRS complexes. In some leads, you will see that the first deflection from the isoelectric line is upwards; in others it is downwards. If the first deflection is downward from the isoelectric line, it is known as a Q wave. If the next deflection upwards crosses above the isoelectric line before returning to baseline, then that deflection is known as an R wave. If the next deflection downwards crosses the isoelectric line before returning to baseline, it is known as an S wave. If the first deflection is upwards, it is an R wave. There is no Q wave in that complex. If the next deflection downwards crosses the isoelectric line before returning to baseline, it is known as an S wave. Some complexes may just have a Q wave before the stylus returns to baseline or an R wave. Go through the 12-lead ECG that you have obtained and identify the waveforms in all of the 12 leads.

Chamber enlargement

The ECG is examined for evidence of atrial enlargement by examining the amplitude (height), duration and contour of the P wave. In right atrial enlargement (RAE) or hypertrophy, the P wave is characteristically tall and peaked, and this can be best seen in Leads II, III and aVF. Criterion for RAE is P wave amplitude ≥2.5 mm (Scheidt 1986). RAE is usually caused by pressure or volume overload in the RA, commonly associated with primary hypertension and conditions resulting in pulmonary hypertension.

Left atrial enlargement (LAE) or hypertrophy is associated with (1) a wide P wave ≥0.11 s in duration; (2) a notch in the top of the P wave with the two peaks being ≥0.04 s apart in any lead and (3) a negative deflection in the terminal end of the P wave in V1 ≥1 mm deep and ≥1 mm wide. LAE is commonly the result of mitral valve insufficiency or stenosis. It is often associated with an increased workload in filling the left ventricle and is commonly associated with left ventricular hypertrophy (LVH) resulting from systemic hypertension, aortic valvular disease, hypertrophic cardiomyopathy and other conditions that reduce left ventricular compliance (Scheidt 1986).

The ECG is then examined for evidence of ventricular enlargement by examining the amplitude of components of the QRS complex. Right ventricular hypertrophy (RVH) is characterised by (1) R wave in V1 ≥7 mm that exceeds the S wave depth in V1; (2) right axis deviation; (3) relatively taller R waves in the right precordial leads and relatively deeper S waves in the left precordial leads than normally seen. RVH may be due to abnormalities of the pulmonary valve (uncommon in adults), congenital lesions such as atrial or ventricular septal defect, tricuspid regurgitation, or by primary hypertension and conditions resulting in pulmonary hypertension (Scheidt 1986).

Key point

A tall R wave in V1 can result from posterior infarction or counterclockwise rotation of the heart. In contrast to these conditions, RVH is associated with right axis deviation and inverted T waves in V1 (and sometimes in V2 and V3) (Scheidt 1986).

A number of methods have been proposed for ECG diagnosis of LVH, with varying degrees of sensitivity and specificity. The Cornell voltage criteria (Casale et al. 1987) provide a relatively simple ECG diagnostic criterion for LVH and are based upon echocardiographic correlative studies designed to detect a left ventricular mass index >132 g/m^2 in men and >109 g/m^2 in women. The voltage criteria are as follows:

- For men: S in V3 + R in aVL >2.8 mV (28 mm)
- For women: S in V3 + R in aVL >2.0 mV (20 mm)

Conditions resulting in LVH include systemic arterial hypertension, aortic stenosis or insufficiency, and other conditions resulting in volume or pressure overload of the left ventricle (Scheidt 1986).

Bundle branch block

Bundle branch block can occur in either the right or left bundle branches. Ventricular depolarisation is abnormal in complete right or left BBB as conduction is not facilitated across specialised conduction fibres within the His–Purkinje system, and the impulse has to travel to various parts of the myocardium via the myocardial cells, resulting in a widened QRS.

Right bundle branch block (RBBB) is characterised by a widened QRS and has the following diagnostic criteria:

- The heart rhythm must be supraventricular in origin.
- The QRS duration must be ≥0.12 s (three small squares).
- There should be a terminal R wave in Lead V1 (usually has an RSR' pattern).
- There should be a slurred S wave in Leads I and V6.

In RBBB, the T wave generally is deflected in the opposite direction of the QRS complex. This is known as appropriate T-wave discordance with BBB (Figure 10.4). A T wave that deflects in the same direction of the QRS complex may suggest ischaemia or MI. RBBB generally is due to degenerative conduction system disease and ischaemic heart disease in the anterior septum (Scheidt 1986).

Right bundle branch block

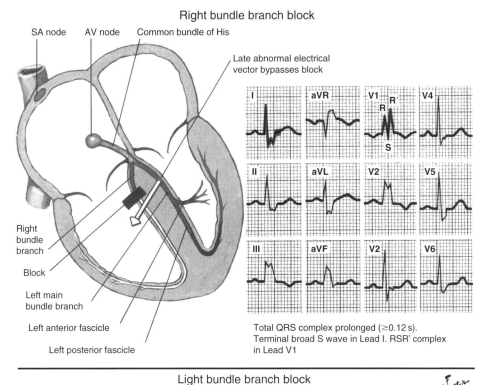

Total QRS complex prolonged (≥0.12 s).
Terminal broad S wave in Lead I. RSR' complex
in Lead V1

Light bundle branch block

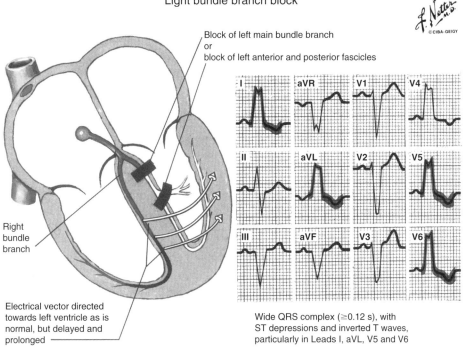

Wide QRS complex (≥0.12 s), with
ST depressions and inverted T waves,
particularly in Leads I, aVL, V5 and V6

Figure 10.4 Right and left bundle branch block.
Source: From Scheidt (1986). Copyright Novartis A.G. Used with permission.

Key point

In some cases, the QRS has an RSR' pattern in V1 and is just above the normal duration of the QRS (<0.10 s), but under the RBBB criteria of ⩾0.12 s duration. The ECG is sometimes interpreted as having an 'incomplete' or 'borderline' RBBB, but this does not necessarily reflect the anatomical abnormality; rather it is a description of the ECG. This type of abnormality may also be referred to as intraventricular conduction delay or right ventricular conduction delay (Scheidt 1986).

In left bundle branch block (LBBB), the ventricle cannot be depolarised normally from the left bundle; so depolarisation must proceed down the right bundle, across the intraventricular septum to the left ventricle. As the wave of depolarisation has a right to left orientation (as is the case in normal depolarisation), the QRS complex, though wide, has the same general directional orientation as a normally conducted complex on the 12-lead ECG. A number of variations in shape can be seen in the QRS complex in LBBB and the complex is usually notched. The following criteria should be used to diagnose LBBB on the ECG:

- The heart rhythm must be supraventricular in origin.
- The QRS duration must be ⩾1.2 s (three small squares).
- There should be a QS or RS complex in Lead V1.
- There should be a monophasic R wave in Leads I and V6.

The LBBB generally indicates widespread myocardial disease due to degenerative conduction disease, ischaemic heart disease and conditions that produce LVH, but in some people, it can develop in the absence of any apparent heart disease (Scheidt 1986). As with RBBB, the T wave generally is deflected in the opposite direction of the QRS complex.

Key point

You may see in some publications that lowercase and capital letters are used to describe QRS components, depending on the relative size of each wave. For example, an Rs complex would be positively deflected, while an rS complex would be negatively deflected. If both complexes were labelled RS, it would be impossible to appreciate this distinction without viewing the actual ECG.

The left bundle branch divides into the left anterior fascicle and the left posterior fascicle. A block in the left anterior fascicle is known as left anterior fascicular block (LAFB) or left anterior hemi-block (LAHB). In LAFB, the heart must be depolarised from areas other than the normal conduction pathway. In hemi-blocks, the spread of depolarisation is not greatly delayed and thus the duration of the QRS complex is within normal limits and generally, is of normal shape, without the characteristic notching found in complete LBBB. However, the axis is shifted to the left, and diagnosis of LAFB is made on LAD. LAFB is commonly caused by degenerative conduction disease or ischaemic heart disease. Unless it occurs in the setting of acute MI (AMI), it is usually benign and only rarely is a precursor of complete LBBB in the short term (Scheidt 1986).

Like LAFB, left posterior fascicular block (LPFB) or left posterior hemi-block (LPHB) does not result in a prolonged QRS, but in this case, the electrical axis is shifted to the right. It is more difficult to recognise than LAFB as the axis, although orientated towards the right, often remains within normal limits. LPHB is uncommon and rarely diagnosed on a routine ECG. The causes and prognostic significance of LPHB are similar to that of LAHB.

Key point

As the RBBB has one fascicle and the LBBB has two fascicles, there are three pathways through the ventricles for AV conduction. This gives rise to the notion of trifascicular conduction. A block in conduction in two fascicles is often referred to as "bifascicular block" and in clinical practice usually involves an LAFB plus RBBB; a blockage in three is referred to as "trifascicular block" and in clinical practice usually involves LAFB plus RBBB plus first degree AV block. Bifascicular and trifascicular blocks are common ECG findings. Some patients with these findings develop severe AV conduction abnormalities whilst others develop no further problems (Scheidt 1986).

Learning activity

Locate an ECG with a paced rhythm. In what ways does this resemble a BBB pattern and why? How might the type of pacemaker and lead placement change the QRS configuration?

ECG changes related to myocardial ischaemia and infarction

The 12-lead ECG is the single-most important source of data in assessment of patients with a potential acute coronary syndrome (unstable angina pectoris or MI). Acute myocardial ischaemia or infarction causes characteristic changes in the ST segment and T wave that are related to repolarisation abnormalities. Progressive development of Q waves or loss of R waves in infarct-related leads can often be detected as an MI evolves.

Sub-endocardial ischaemia

Myocardial ischaemia usually occurs first in the sub-endocardial region as these deeper myocardial layers are farthest from the blood supply and have greater intramural tension and need for oxygen. Repolarisation normally proceeds in an epicardial-to-endocardial direction, and delayed recovery in the sub-endocardial region due to ischaemia does not reverse the direction of repolarisation but merely lengthens it. Thus, sub-endocardial ischaemia prolongs local recovery time, resulting in a prolonged QT interval and/or increased amplitude of the T wave in the electrodes overlying the ischaemic region on the 12-lead ECG. In the setting of severe ischaemia, injury to the myocardial cells results, and is manifested on the ECG by ST-segment depression (American Heart Association [AHA] 2007).

Sub-epicardial or transmural ischaemia

Transmural ischaemia refers to sub-epicardial ischaemia which has a more visible effect on recovery of sub-epicardial cells compared with sub-endocardial cells. Recovery is more delayed in the sub-epicardial layers than in sub-endocardial muscle fibres. Repolarisation is endocardial-to-epicardial, resulting in inversion of the T waves in leads overlying the ischaemic regions. In the setting of severe ischaemia, injury to the myocardial cells results, and is manifested on the ECG by ST-segment elevation (AHA 2007).

Myocardial infarction

Myocardial infarction refers to necrosis (death) of myocardial cells. The left ventricle is the predominant site for MI, but the right ventricle can also be involved. The process of MI involves various stages of ischaemia. There is usually a central area of necrosis that is generally surrounded by an area of injury, which in turn is surrounded by an area of ischaemia. MI can be classed as:

- ST-elevation MI (STEMI)
- Non-ST elevation MI (non-STEMI)

depending upon the presence or absence of ST elevation in the presence of elevated cardiac enzymes. MI may also be referred to as:

- Q wave acute MI (QAMI), which is diagnosed by the presence of pathological Q waves and may (but not always) be associated with *transmural infarction*.
- Non-Q wave acute MI (NQAMI), which is diagnosed in the presence of ST depression and T-wave abnormalities (AHA 2007).

Key point

The distinction between ischaemia and necrosis is whether or not the phenomenon is reversible. Transient reversible ischaemia appears on the ECG as T wave changes, and sometimes ST-segment changes, that can be reversed without producing permanent damage or serum enzyme elevation. Elevation of serum enzymes is expected in infarction. In the absence of enzyme elevation, ST and T-wave abnormalities are interpreted as due to injury or ischaemia rather than infarction (AHA 2007).

The ST segment

The ST segment may become depressed or elevated during episodes of myocardial ischaemia or infarction. Taken in context with a patient history and examination, ST-segment elevation is usually the product of intense transmural ischaemia indicating MI. ST-segment elevation represents the most severe condition in the acute coronary syndrome spectrum and carries the poorest prognosis (Hasdai et al. 2002). Prompt management with pharmacological or percutaneous reperfusion is critical. The GUSTO ECG criteria are commonly used to identify ST-segment elevation MI:

- $\geqslant 0.1\,mV$ (one small square in height) of ST-segment elevation in two or more limb leads; or
- $\geqslant 0.2\,mV$ (two small squares in height) of ST-segment elevation in two or more contiguous precordial leads (GUSTO Investigators 1993).

Another cause of ST elevation is pericarditis. A thorough history of the features of associated chest pain must be obtained to differentiate between pericarditis and MI. Pericarditis is usually a generalised pathophysiological process; thus the ST elevation associated with pericarditis is often widespread on the ECG, involving more than one area of the heart. Another ECG characteristic that may differentiate pericarditis from AMI is PR interval depression in the setting of diffuse ST-segment elevation (Marinella 1998).

Persistent ST elevation can occur in the presence of ventricular aneurysm following an MI. This is generally associated with Q waves in the infarct-related leads.

A normal variant known as early repolarisation (sometimes called high take-off) can be seen in asymptomatic people without significant coronary disease. This phenomenon can be seen across most of the population but is common in young male athletes. Early repolarisation is best seen in the precordial leads. ST segments in these leads appear elevated, upwards and concave and are often associated with peaked and slightly asymmetrical T waves with notch and slur on the R wave. The other accompanying features are a shorter and depressed PR interval, abrupt transition, counterclockwise rotation, presence of U waves and sinus bradycardia (Mehta et al. 1999).

ST depression may be described as 'upsloping', 'horizontal' or 'downsloping' (Figure 10.5), with downsloping ST depression being the most specific for myocardial ischaemia, and upsloping the least. Other causes of ST depression include RVH and LVH, RBBB and LBBB, and some drugs.

Non-specific ST depression is a common ECG finding and implies that the cause of the abnormality is not known, and that the ST segment change is minor. For ST-segment depression to be termed 'non-specific', the T-wave vector should be normal. If the T-wave vector is abnormal in the absence of other known causes of ST depression, it is suggestive of ischaemia. Significant ST depression has been defined as:

- deviation from the J point of $\geqslant 1\,mm$ (two small vertically ruled boxes)
- deviation of $\geqslant 1\,mm$ from 0.06 to 0.08 s after the J point (Scheidt 1986)

Key point

You will note in some studies of ST-segment depression, significant ST depression is defined as $\geqslant 0.5\,mm$ (one small square). Although this may be a more sensitive criteria for detecting ST-segment depression, in everyday clinical practice there is a lot of variability in ECG interpretation in terms of ST-segment amplitude; thus, setting the measurement criteria at this lower level may reduce diagnostic specificity.

Transient ST-segment depression with inverted T waves is usually a sign of reversible ischaemia affecting the sub-endocardial layers of myocardium (Scheidt 1986) and can occur as a result of acute reduction in coronary flow, or as a result of an acute increase in coronary demand, such as occurs with tachycardia (Sclarovsky 1999).

Downsloping ST-segment depression in the precordial leads, particularly in Leads V4 and V5 (Figure 10.5), are often due to extensive ischaemia as a result of stenosis of the left main coronary artery and/or triple vessel disease, and may produce life-threatening haemodynamic disturbance, both systolic and diastolic (Sclarovsky et al. 1986a). This type of ST depression needs urgent investigation.

Types of ST-segment depressions

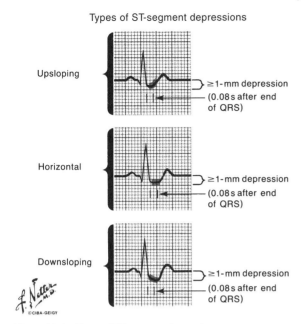

Upsloping
≥1-mm depression
(0.08 s after end
of QRS)

Horizontal
≥1-mm depression
(0.08 s after end
of QRS)

Downsloping
≥1-mm depression
(0.08 s after end
of QRS)

Figure 10.5 Types of ST-segment depression.
Source: From Scheidt (1986). Copyright Novartis A.G. Used with permission.

ST depression has been shown in several studies to be associated with poor outcomes (Anderson et al. 1996; Patel et al. 1996; Cannon et al. 1997; Boersma et al. 2000), and therefore should not be dismissed without further investigation in the absence of an obvious cause, such as tachycardia.

T-wave abnormalities

The T wave represents repolarisation of the ventricles. The wave of repolarisation moves predominantly from epicardium to endocardium (Hurst 1998). T-wave abnormalities often accompany abnormalities of the ST segment, but in some instances, occur in isolation. Although T-wave abnormalities are often associated with acute coronary syndromes, there are a number of other reasons why they may occur (Table 10.3) (Sclarovsky et al. 1986b).

Q waves

Pathological Q waves (initial downward deflection of ≥40 ms in duration in any lead except III and aVR) are the most characteristic ECG finding of transmural MI of the left ventricle. Q waves in

V2 through V6 are considered abnormal if greater than 25% of R-wave amplitude. Q waves appear when the infarcted muscle is electrically inert and forces from other areas of the myocardium (such as the opposite wall) are reflected on the ECG. These forces may be represented by a vector directed away from the site of infarction and thus are seen as a negative wave (Q wave) by electrodes overlying the infarcted region (AHA 2007).

Site of infarction

Twelve-lead ECG leads that best detect changes in anatomically described locations of the myocardium according to the AHA (2007) are classified in Table 10.4.

Incremental ECG leads

Right ventricular leads

In the case of inferior infarction where right ventricular involvement is suspected, ST-segment elevation ≥1 mm in Lead V4r, a lead placed in the right midclavicular line and 5th intercostal space, has been shown to be highly predictive of right ventricular infarction. Right ventricular involvement in inferior infarction is a strong, independent predictor of major complications and in-hospital mortality (Zahender et al. 1993).

Posterior leads

Infarction of the anatomically labelled posterior surface of the left ventricle is not associated with conventional changes in standard ECG leads. ST-segment elevation in Leads V7–V9 placed from the posterior axillary line to the paraspinal line identifies patients with a larger inferior MI because of concomitant posterolateral involvement who have an increased risk of re-infarction, heart failure or death compared to those without ST-segment elevation in Leads V7–V9 (Matetzky et al. 1998).

Learning activity

The Internet has a range of websites devoted to ECG interpretation and activities. Take some time to surf the Internet and see what is available and useful.

Table 10.3 T wave abnormalities.

T wave abnormality	Cause
'Flattened' T waves	• Considered to be a non-specific abnormality with a number of potential causes such as ischaemia, cardiac scar, evolving infarction and electrolyte abnormality (Scheidt 1986)
Tall peaked T wave ('hyperacute' T wave)	• First ECG sign of a sudden narrowing or obstruction of an epicardial artery – caused by potassium leak through damaged membranes in the area of the infarct (Chesebro et al. 1991) • Hyperkalaemia (Scheidt 1986)
Inverted T waves Deep symmetrical T-wave inversion	• Normal finding in Lead III, aVR and V1 • Normal finding in V1–V3 for infants and children, and may persist into adolescence and young adulthood (Scheidt 1986) • No obvious cause, particularly in women • Chronic pericarditis, ventricular hypertrophy, intraventricular conduction defects • Hyperventilation • Mitral valve prolapse • Ventricular pre-excitation • Myocarditis • Electrolyte imbalance • Cardio-active drugs (AHA 2007) • Myocardial ischaemia • MI • Cerebral disease such as sub-arachnoid haemorrhage (Scheidt 1986)
Biphasic T waves	• Myocardial ischaemia • Evolution of AMI (Scheidt 1986)
Pseudonormalisation of T waves	• Where the T wave has become inverted following an ischaemic event, a recurrent ischaemic event may result in the T wave first becoming biphasic and then returning to what appears to be a normal configuration, which may then be followed by ST-segment elevation

Table 10.4 Anatomical region of the heart and associated ECG lead/s.

Anatomical region of the heart	ECG Lead
Inferior (or diaphragmatic) wall	II, II and aVF
Septal	V1 and V2
Anteroseptal	V1, V2, Vf3 and sometimes V4
Anterior	V3, V4 and sometimes V2
Apical	V3, V4 or both
Lateral	I, aVL, V5 and V6
Extensive anterior	I, aVL and V1 through V6
Posterior	V1 and V2[a]

[a]Posterior wall infarction does not produce Q-wave abnormalities in conventional leads and is diagnosed in the presence of tall R waves in V1 and V2.

Obtaining a 12-lead ECG

Equipment preparation

A 12-lead ECG may be obtained using an ECG machine (that is usually located on a mobile trolley) or from a bedside monitor that has 12-lead capability.

- Check that the equipment has no broken cables/wires and no damage to the housing.
- Inspect the cables/wires for cleanliness. They should be cleaned between uses.
- If the machine requires an external power source, plug the machine into a grounded alternating current wall outlet. If battery operated, ensure that the machine has been charged.

- Ensure that the machine has the appropriate cable/lead configuration attached.
- Ensure that there are sufficient consumables to undertake the procedure (ECG paper, 10 adhesive electrodes).
- Turn the machine on and ensure it is functional.
- Turn the ECG machine on and input patient information details if that is the unit practice (name, age, date and any other relevant details).
- Check that paper speed is set at 25 mm/s; sensitivity is set at 1 or 10 mm/s and baseline at centre.

Patient preparation

Information and consent

Although having an ECG is not a new procedure for many patients, others may be unaware of what is involved, and the appearance of the ECG machine may be frightening.

- Explain to the patient that an ECG is not an invasive test and should not cause pain, although removal of adhesive electrodes can cause some discomfort.
- In most settings, an ECG will only require a verbal consent from the patient, but as with any procedure, this should be obtained prior to the procedure, after explaining the reason for obtaining the ECG and what is involved.

Positioning

If you want to get a good ECG trace on the first attempt, ensure that the patient is comfortable. If the patient is not comfortable, you will find that they will hold themselves rigidly or wriggle to try and get comfortable, resulting in muscle tremor and a poor ECG tracing. Lying completely flat is uncomfortable for many patients, particularly those with heart failure.

- Position the patient in a supine position, but lift the head of the bed slightly (around 15°). Ensure that the pillow is comfortably placed and not causing the patient to 'hunch' their shoulders or neck forward. For patients with heart failure and other acute respiratory conditions, the ECG will have to be taken in a position tolerated by the patient.

- Ensure that the patient's extremities are not in contact with bedrails or footboards. This may result in reduced quality of the ECG tracing.

Patient privacy

The procedure for obtaining a 12-lead ECG involves uncovering and exposing parts of the patient's body that are not normally exposed publicly. This may cause some embarrassment and anxiety for the patient, particularly if there is a likelihood of being observed by others who are not involved in the procedure of obtaining an ECG.

- Ensure that privacy is maintained and that unwelcome visitors during the procedure are discouraged.
- Demonstrate consideration of the patient's dignity by not exposing any more of the patient than needed to complete the ECG procedure.
- Cover the patient where possible during the procedure. Keeping them covered as much as possible and maintaining warmth will also prevent shivering which could result in a poor ECG tracing.

Skin preparation

Taking time to prepare the patient's skin for electrode adhesion will save time in the long run and contribute to obtaining a quality ECG trace.

- Ask the patient to remove jewellery from any area that may impede electrode placement.
- If the patient is diaphoretic, has excess oils or any material on the skin that may result in poor attachment of the electrodes, clean the skin with a cloth and warm water (soap can be used if it does not irritate the patient's skin) and dry thoroughly.
- If the patient has excess body hair, remove the hair in the areas where electrodes will be placed, taking care not to cause any abrasions (with clippers if available, rather than shaving devices). Explain the rationale prior to removing body hair and get the patient's verbal permission to proceed. Excess body hair will result in poor attachment of the electrodes and a poor ECG trace. Furthermore, removal of the electrodes after the procedure will also result in a painful removal of the attached body hair.

Attaching the electrodes

Correct lead placement is an important aspect of obtaining a 12-lead ECG, particularly when sequential ECGs are expected to be performed.

Limb leads

Limb leads (using extremities) should be placed on the fleshy, lower aspects of the limbs, taking care to avoid bony prominences and muscle mass.

Key point

Electrocardiograms recorded with torso placement of the extremity electrodes cannot be considered equivalent to standard ECGs and thus should not be used interchangeably with standard ECGs for serial comparison (Kligfield et al. 2007).

Precordial leads

The 'angle of Louis', also known as the 'sternal notch', is the point where the clavicle joins the sternum. Run you finger from the top of the sternum and over the bony prominence of the sternal notch. Directly under this notch and to the side, you will palpate the second intercostal space. Slide your finger over the third and fourth ribs until you palpate the fourth intercostal space. Chest lead placement is as follows.

Lead V1 is placed in the fourth intercostal space to the right of the sternum.
Lead V2 is placed in the fourth intercostal space to the left of the sternum.
Lead V3 is placed directly between Leads V2 and V4.
Lead V4 is placed in the fifth intercostal space in the midclavicular line.
Lead V5 is placed horizontally with V4 in the anterior axillary line.
Lead V6 is placed horizontally with V4 and V5 in the midaxillary line.

- Precordial electrodes should be placed under the breast in women as breast tissue may impede conduction.
- If using pre-gelled electrodes, remove the backing and attach them firmly.
- Attach the lead wires to the electrodes.

Obtain the ECG

Ask the patient to relax and refrain from movement whilst obtaining the ECG. Obtain the 12-lead ECG by pressing the appropriate acquisition selector.

Check the quality of the ECG

The ECG quality should be reviewed prior to disconnecting the patient.

- The ECG should have a straight baseline. If there is a wandering baseline, check that the leads are connected properly. Request that the patient does not move during the procedure and repeat the ECG.
- The ECG should have clearly defined waveforms and intervals. If there is artefact, this may be due to electrical interference or skeletal muscle tremor. Unplug or move any unnecessary electrical equipment away from the patient. Ensure that the patient is warm (reduce potential for shivering). Repeat the ECG.

Interpret the ECG

The ECG should be interpreted by someone with the knowledge and skills to do so. In the case of a patient who is symptomatic, if the nurse/technician performing the ECG does not have ECG interpretation skills, a senior nurse or doctor who is able to interpret the ECG should be promptly notified to do so. If no further ECG is required, the equipment should be disconnected and the patient made comfortable. The ECG leads should be cleaned prior to re-use on another patient.

Documentation

Interpretation of the ECG should be documented in the patients case notes or file. If the ECG is part of an assessment for chest pain, the level of pain at the time the ECG is obtained (according to a pain scale) and should be documented on the ECG and in the case notes/file.

Conclusion

The 12-lead ECG has for some years been used in cardiac assessment. Nurses working in a cardiac environment require advanced skills in ECG interpretation to recognise abnormalities that may indicate rhythm disturbance, ischaemia and infarction and other conditions with associated ECG abnormalities.

References

American Heart Association (AHA) (2007). Myocardial injury, ischaemia and infarction. Retrieved online 6th November 2007 from http://www.americanheart.org/presenter.jhtml?identifier=251

Anderson, K., Eriksson, S.V. & Dellborg, M. (1996). Non-invasive risk stratification within 48 hours of hospital admission in patients with unstable coronary disease. *European Heart Journal*, **18**:780–8.

Boersma, E., Pieper, K.S., Steyerberg, E.W., et al. (2000). Predictors of outcome in patients with acute coronary syndromes without persistent ST-segment elevation. *Circulation*, **101**:2557–67.

Cannon, C.P., McCabe, C.H., Stone, P.H., et al. (1997). The electrocardiogram predicts one-year outcome of patients with unstable angina and non-Q-wave myocardial infarction: results of the TIMI III Registry ECG Ancillary Study: Thrombolysis in Myocardial Ischaemia. *Journal of the American College of Cardiology*, **30**:133–40.

Casale, P.N., Deveroux, R.B., Alonso, D.R., Campo, E. & Kligfield, P. (1987). Improved sex-specific criteria of left ventricular hypertrophy for clinical and computer interpretation of electrocardiograms: validation with autopsy findings. *Circulation*, **75**:565–72.

Chesebro, J.H., Zolhelyi, P. & Fuster, V. (1991). Pathogenesis of thrombosis in unstable angina. *American Journal of Cardiology*, **68**:B2–10.

Hasdai, D., Behar, S., Wallentin, L., et al. (2002). A prospective survey of the characteristics, treatments and outcomes of patients with acute coronary syndromes in Europe and the Mediterranean basin: The Euro Heart Survey of Acute Coronary Syndromes (Euro Heart Survey ACS). *European Heart Journal*, **23**:1190–201. Retrieved online 5th November 2007, doi:10.1053/euhj.2002.3193, available online at http://www.idealibrary.com

Houghton, A.R. & Gray, D. (2003). *Making Sense of the ECG: A Hands-On Guide*, 2nd edn. Hodder Arnold, London.

Hurst, J.W. (1998). Naming of the waves in the ECG, with a brief account of their genesis. *Circulation*, 98:1937–42.

Jowett, N.I. & Thompson, D.R. (2003). *Comprehensive Coronary Care*, 3rd edn. Bailliere Tindall, London.

Kligfield, P., Gettes, L.S., Bailey, J.J., et al. (2007). Recommendations for the standardization and interpretation of the electrocardiogram. Part I: the electrocardiogram and its technology. A scientific statement from the American Heart Association Electrocardiography and Arrhythmias Committee, Council on Clinical Cardiology; the American College of Cardiology Foundation; and the Heart Rhythm Society. *Circulation*, **115**:1306–24.

Marinella, M.A. (1998). Electrocardiographic manifestations and differential diagnosis of acute pericarditis. *American Family Physician*, **57**:699–704. Retrieved online 5th November 2007 from http://www.aafp.org/afp/980215ap/marinell.html

Matetzky, S., Freimark, D. & Chouraqui, P. (1998). Significance of ST segment elevations in posterior chest leads (V7 to V9) in patients with acute inferior myocardial infarction: application for thrombolytic therapy. *Journal of the American College of Cardiology*, **31**:506–11.

Meek, S. & Morris, F. (2002). ABC of clinical electrocardiography: Introduction I – Leads, rate, rhythm, and cardiac axis. *British Medical Journal*, **324**:415–8.

Mehta, M., Jain, A.C. & Mehta, A. (1999). Early repolarization. *Clinical Cardiology*, **22**:59–65.

Patel, D.J., Holdright, D.R., Knight, C.J., et al. (1996). Early continuous ST segment monitoring in unstable angina: prognostic value additional to the clinical characteristics and the admission electrocardiogram. *Heart*, **75**:222–8.

Sclarovsky, S., Davidson, E., Strasberg, B., et al. (1986a). Unstable angina pectoris evolving to acute myocardial infarction: significance of ECG changes during chest pain. *American Heart Journal*, **112**:462.

Sclarovsky, S., Davidson, E., Strasberg, B., et al. (1986b). Unstable angina: the significance of ST segment elevation or depression in patients without evidence of increased myocardial oxygen demand. *American Heart Journal*, **112**:463–7.

Sclarovsky, S. (ed.) (1999). *Electrocardiography of Acute Myocardial Ischaemic Syndromes*. Martin Dunitz Ltd., London.

Scheidt, S. (1986). *Basic Electrocardiography*. Ciba-Geigy Pharmaceuticals, New Jersey.

The Global Use of Strategies to Open Occluded Coronary Arteries in Acute Coronary Syndromes (GUSTO) Investigators (1993). An international randomized trial comparing 4 thrombolytic strategies for acute myocardial infarction. *New England Journal of Medicine*, **329**:673–82.

Zahender, M., Kasper, W., Kauder, E., et al. (1993). Right ventricular infarction as an independent predictor of prognosis after acute inferior myocardial infarction. *New England Journal of Medicine*, **328**:981–8.

Useful Websites and Further Reading

Edhouse, J., Thakur, R.K. & Khalil, J.M. (2002). ABC of clinical electrocardiography: conditions affecting the left side of the heart. *British Medical Journal*, **324**:1264–7. Available online at http://www.bmj.com/cgi/reprint/324/7348/1264

Goodacre, S. & Mcleod, K. (2002). ABC of clinical electrocardiography: paediatric electrocardiography. *British Medical Journal*, **324**:1382–5. Available online at http://www.bmj.com/cgi/reprint/324/7350/1382

Harrigan, R.A. & Jones, K. (2002). ABC of clinical electrocardiography: conditions affecting the right side of the heart. *British Medical Journal*, **324**:1201–4. Available online at http://www.bmj.com/cgi/reprint/324/7347/1201

Kligfield, P., Gettes, L.S., Bailey, J.J., et al. (2007). Recommendations for the standardization and interpretation of the electrocardiogram. Part I: the electrocardiogram and its technology. A scientific statement from the American Heart Association Electrocardiography and Arrhythmias Committee, Council on Clinical Cardiology; the American College of Cardiology Foundation; and the Heart Rhythm Society. *Circulation*, **115**:1306–24.

Meek, S. & Morris, F. (2002). ABC of clinical electrocardiography: Introduction I – Leads, rate, rhythm, and cardiac axis. *British Medical Journal*, **324**:415–8. Available online at http://www.bmj.com/cgi/reprint/324/7334/415

Meek, S. & Morris, F. (2002). ABC of clinical electrocardiography: Introduction II – Basic Terminology. *British Medical Journal*, **324**:470–3. Available online at http://www.bmj.com/cgi/reprint/324/7335/470

Slovis, C. & Jenkins, R. (2002). ABC of clinical electrocardiography: conditions not primarily affecting the heart. *British Medical Journal*, **324**:1320–3. Available online at http://www.bmj.com/cgi/reprint/324/7349/1320

M2H Nursing. EKG 12-lead placement activity. Available at http://www.m2hnursing.com/ecg_demo/12lead.php

Patient UK. ECG: a methodological approach. Available at http://www.patient.co.uk/showdoc/40000508/

The Alan E. Lindsay ECG Learning Center in Cyberspace. Available at http://library.med.utah.edu/kw/ecg/index.html

Wikipedia (2007). Electrocardiogram. Available at http://en.wikipedia.org/wiki/ECG

11 Cardiac Monitoring

A.M. Kucia & C. Oldroyd

Overview

Continuous electrocardiographic (ECG) monitoring has evolved over the past four decades from simple single-lead channels that tracked heart rate and basic rhythm to more advanced systems that can detect complex arrhythmias, myocardial ischaemia and abnormalities of components of the ECG cycle, such as the QT interval. ECG monitoring may be initiated for a variety of reasons and in a number of settings. The choice of the monitoring system will depend upon the clinical indication for monitoring the patient, the types of monitoring system available, the available evidence-based guidelines and institutional policies and practices. When ECG monitoring is initiated, the nurse has a responsibility to ensure that it is maintained, continuously observed and that any abnormalities detected are appropriately acted upon. Thus, nurses who are caring for patients with ECG monitoring should have appropriate skills to undertake these aspects of management. In a practical sense, there is a lot more to ECG monitoring than interpreting information and acting upon it. Nurses who are responsible for the delivery of care to patients with continuous ECG monitoring should be aware of specific issues related to electrical safety for patients and staff, the dignity and comfort of patients and the maintenance of skin integrity. This chapter will address a range of issues related to care of the monitored patient.

Learning objectives

After reading this chapter, you should be able to:

- Describe the types of ECG monitoring systems currently available and the indications for their use.
- List the indications for undertaking ECG monitoring.
- Describe the types of settings where cardiac monitoring may be used.
- Discuss the elements of equipment and patient preparation for ECG monitoring.
- Discuss nursing responsibilities in the delivery of care to patients with cardiac monitoring.

Key concepts

Arrhythmia monitoring; ischaemia monitoring; monitoring systems; electrical safety; telemetry

ECG monitoring systems and lead formats

The basic elements of ECG monitoring systems include a display screen, an amplifier to amplify the signal voltage, and leads and electrodes for connection to the patient. Basic ECG monitoring systems also have a small computer which allows two or three lines of the display to be retained in its memory which can be frozen and examined and also to provide a non-fading view of the last few seconds of the ECG recording. There is usually also a display of the average heart rate over the last few seconds (Brown 2000). Hardwire monitors are usually located at the bedside and transmit information to a central monitor where it can be printed, stored and analysed. Contemporary monitoring systems have become quite sophisticated and are capable of monitoring and displaying multiple leads simultaneously, advanced arrhythmia and ischaemia detection and calculation of ECG intervals. Many cardioscopes are used in conjunction with defibrillator, pacemaker and diathermy apparatus; thus, the circuits must be capable of withstanding relatively high voltages without damage and with almost instant recovery of the correct display (Brown 2000).

Key point

The modern ECG monitoring system display bears very little resemblance to the original cathode ray oscilloscopes. Monitoring systems have become increasingly complex and, in addition to arrhythmia monitoring and detection, are designed to monitor, collect and process data for a number of other clinical parameters. Most basic ECG monitors now come with additional software and equipment to monitor non-invasive blood pressure, SpO_2, respirations, invasive haemodynamics and temperature and allow acquisition and printout of a 12-lead ECG from the bedside. Most systems also offer 12-lead ST-segment analysis. Several other options can be added in areas such as intensive care, neonatal intensive care, paediatrics and anaesthetics.

Despite the advanced technology that is now available in cardiac monitoring systems, it is still necessary for experienced health care professionals to evaluate the information obtained from ECG

monitoring, including the detection of false alarms, and to make decisions on a course of action in response to the information obtained. The type of monitoring selected for use in a given clinical situation should be selected by health professionals who have expertise in the management of conditions in which ECG monitoring is indicated.

Three-electrode monitoring systems

Conventional cardiac monitoring using a 3 or 4 electrode configuration is the simplest and most common form of cardiac monitoring. The ECG leads normally monitored using this configuration are the modified limb leads I, II and III. Lead II is the usual choice for monitoring since it normally provides the best amplitude for both the P waves and the QRS complexes; however, leads I or III can be used if they provide a better signal (Sheppard & Wright 2000). The term 'modified' used in this context refers to the fact that the electrodes used for continuous ECG monitoring are placed on the torso rather than on the limb extremities, which is the traditional placement in electrocardiography. This is done to reduce artefact due to movement and to allow the monitored patient to freely move their limbs. The normal format of electrode placement is for the right arm (RA) electrode to be placed in the infraclavicular fossa close to the right shoulder; the left arm (LA) electrode to be placed in the infraclavicular fossa close to the left arm and the left leg (LL) electrode usually placed on the abdomen or lower left chest wall. If a fourth electrode (RL) is present, this is a ground or reference electrode and can be placed anywhere, but is usually placed on the right side of the abdomen (see Figure 11.1) (Drew et al. 2004). Electrode positions can be changed if circumstances (such as trauma or surgery) dictate. This system can also be used to monitor a modified chest lead (MCL) such as MCL1. As the name suggests, this lead provides a substitute for V1, which is reported to be the best lead position for recognising bundle branch block (Drew et al. 2004).

Caution must be exercised in interpreting broad complex tachycardias from a single lead as this may be due to differing QRS morphology in some patients (Drew & Scheinmann 1995). Most health care professionals who work in an acute environment, both in and out of hospital, are familiar with the 3-electrode monitoring configuration. This configuration is most frequently used for arrhythmia detection in short-term or emergency situations, and it is also the configuration most commonly found with defibrillators and portable monitors. The goal of this type of monitoring is to track heart rate, sense R waves for synchronised cardioversion and detect ventricular fibrillation, but is not adequate for sophisticated arrhythmia interpretation or ischaemia detection (Drew et al. 2004).

In emergency situations, alternatives to the three cable system may be available with the use of self-adhesive electrodes becoming the most favoured system in relation to defibrillation. Applied to the patient in the conventional defibrillator paddle positions, this system not only provides cardiac monitoring but also allows hands-free defibrillation if required.

Five-electrode monitoring systems

In 5-electrode monitoring systems, in addition to the electrodes previously described, a fifth electrode is used that can be placed in any of the precordial chest lead positions, although V1 is the most common. Unlike MCL1, this system provides a true recording of V1, but it is not possible to record more than one chest lead at a time. It is helpful in determining the origin of broad complex rhythms, but is not sensitive enough for use in monitoring for myocardial ischaemia (Bush et al. 1991). The anatomical placement of the RA, LA, RL, LL and V electrodes are the same as described in the Mason–Likar configuration described in Figure 11.1. Typically, cardiac monitors used with this electrode configuration have a 2-channel ECG display, so that a limb lead and a V lead can be visualised simultaneously (Drew et al. 2004).

Twelve-lead (10 electrode) monitoring systems

Continuous 12-lead ST-segment monitoring utilises 10 electrodes that are attached in a configuration similar to that of the standard ECG. In order to avoid artefact due to movement and for patient comfort, the limb leads are placed in the Mason–Likar configuration (Figure 11.1), with the RA electrode placed at the right infraclavicular fossa medial to the border of the deltoid muscle; the LA electrode placed in a corresponding position on the left; the LL electrode placed at the left iliac fossa and the RL electrode usually placed at the right iliac fossa, although it can be placed in any position. When making serial comparisons between ECGs, it is important to note that an ECG taken in a Mason–Likar configuration will differ from a standard 12-lead ECG with limb electrodes at the limb extremities, in that the limb lead QRS complexes may vary somewhat in amplitude and axis between the two configurations (Drew et al. 2004).

The standard 12-lead ECG has for some years been used to detect episodes of myocardial ischaemia and infarction, but has limitations. As standard ECGs are taken only at periodic intervals, transient episodes of ischaemia may go undetected, resulting in lost diagnostic and therapeutic opportunities (Kucia et al. 2002). 12-lead ST-segment monitoring with continuous 12-lead ECG

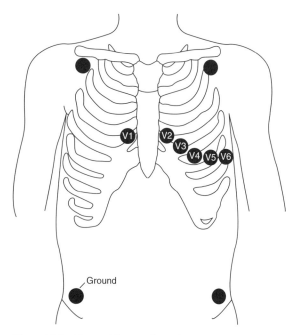

Figure 11.1   Mason–Likar configuration.
Source: Reprinted from Sejersten et al. (2006). Copyright 2006, with permission from Elsevier.

or vectorcardiography has been shown to be useful for detecting ischaemia during and after percutaneous coronary intervention (Krucoff 1988; Dellborg et al. 1991) and identifying successful reperfusion after thrombolytic treatment in patients with ST-elevation myocardial infarction (Krucoff et al. 1993; Dellborg et al. 1995; Shah et al. 2000). A number of studies have demonstrated the usefulness of continuous 12-lead ECG monitoring in risk stratification of patients with chest pain and a non-diagnostic ECG (Holmvang et al. 1999; Jernberg et al. 1999) particularly when used as an adjunct to troponin measurement (Jernberg et al. 1999, 2000a; Norgaard et al. 1999); and in a number of large international clinical trials it has been utilised as a strategy to identify responders to antithrombotic treatment (Klootwijk et al. 1998; Goodman et al. 2000; Jernberg et al. 2000b).

The new generation of cardiac monitoring systems generally has ST-segment monitoring and analysis software, but it is underutilized. Despite the accumulation of evidence that continuous ischaemia monitoring is useful in a number of settings, it does not appear to have been universally embraced by clinicians (Kucia 2007). Reasons for not using this extremely valuable technology are reported to be poor physician support, high number of false alarms and lack of education about how to use the technology and how to respond to alarms (Patton & Funk 2001).

Derived 12-lead ECG monitoring systems

Continuous 12-lead ECG monitoring can be conducted using eight electrodes in the Frank vectorcardiographic lead configuration with three channels of information (X, Y and Z leads), with vectorcardiographically derived information translated into a 12-lead ECG format that clinicians are familiar with. As the Frank system includes an electrode on the patient's back and one in the right axilla, it has been suggested that it may be a more sensitive configuration for detecting injury to the posterior wall of the heart and the right ventricle, but has limited practicability in continuous ECG monitoring as the patient must lie on two electrodes when supine which is uncomfortable and may cause a noisy signal (Drew et al. 2004). Similarly, the EASI 12-lead ECG uses five electrodes

to record three channels of ECG information which again is translated into a 12-lead ECG format that clinicians find familiar. As with the Mason–Likar modified lead configuration, clinicians must exercise caution when comparing these derived or modified configurations with other configurations, such as the standard ECG configuration with limb electrodes placed at limb extremities (Drew et al. 1999).

Telemetry monitoring systems

Telemetry literally means 'the measurement or recording of signals at a distance' and in the context of ECG monitoring, telemetry is used for the radio transmission of ECG signals to remove the need for connecting wires to the patient (Brown 2000). Telemetry systems may use the simple 3-electrode system described above for arrhythmia monitoring only; or they may take the form of more complex systems that are also capable of ischaemia monitoring and have adjuncts such as non-invasive blood pressure monitoring and pulse oximetry.

The telemetry transmitter is a small box which is attached to the patient by leads and electrodes (Figure 11.2). The transmitter sends a signal to a central monitoring system. This system is useful in that it allows the patient to mobilise within an area that is equipped to pick up the signal. This may be within a specific ward area, such as the coronary care unit (CCU), or in other wards that are equipped to receive the signal and transmit it to a central monitor in the CCU. One of the problems with this remote transmission, is that the responsibility for the maintenance of continued monitoring seems to fall somewhere between the nurses in a remote ward and those in the CCU. The patient often becomes disconnected from the monitoring system, either accidentally such as when an electrode becomes dislodged, or purposefully such as when the unit is removed for the patient to have a shower.

Another form of 'disconnection' from the monitoring system is when the patient wanders beyond the area where the signal can be picked up, or the patient may be sent to other departments for tests or procedures. This has ethical and medico-legal implications, and the line of responsibility for

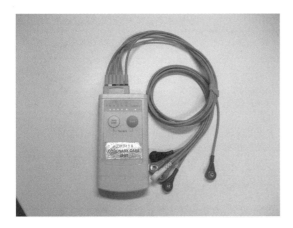

Figure 11.2   Telemetry monitor.

ensuring that monitoring remains intact should be described in institutional policy. Other problems that occur are that nurses in remote areas caring for the patient are not informed of the occurrence of arrhythmias and they may not get noted or documented. This may result in the assumption that the patient is not at increased risk of an arrhythmia when in fact this is not the case. Moreover, when a potentially lethal arrhythmia occurs, it may be difficult to locate patients if they are not at their bed space or have not informed the staff caring for them of their whereabouts. The telemetry receiver is an expensive piece of equipment, and can be easily lost if there is not a system in place for recording where it is being used and when it is returned. The demand for telemetry receivers is usually greater than the supply, so as previously mentioned, institutional guidelines for when telemetry monitoring should be instituted and when it should be removed should be in place. Evidence suggests that telemetry monitoring is often used inappropriately (Curry et al. 2003) and this has substantial workload impact on nurses working in the CCU, particularly with regard to remote telemetry monitoring.

Ambulatory ECG (Holter monitoring)

The Holter monitor is a battery-powered recording device which is strapped over a patient's shoulder or around his or her waist to detect car-

diac arrhythmias. The Holter monitor normally has 5–7 ECG electrodes which record heart rhythm and provide a 24-h record of the heart's electrical activity. Interpretation of a Holter monitor test is retrospective, often done on an outpatient basis and cannot be viewed in real time.

Indications for arrhythmia monitoring

Continuous ECG monitoring is commonly used in selected acute care settings such as intensive care units, CCUs, high dependency units, emergency departments, operating theatres and post-anaesthesia recovery rooms. The decision to undertake ECG monitoring in a patient will be influenced by local policies and guidelines and availability of monitored beds and equipment. According to Drew and colleagues (2004), there are a number of indications for ECG monitoring in the adult patient, as outlined in Table 11. 1.

Other illnesses that are not specifically cardiac conditions but may require ECG monitoring include trauma, sepsis, acute respiratory failure, acute pulmonary embolus, major surgery, renal failure, electrolyte disturbance and ingestion of toxic substances. Although there are some suggested time intervals for continuation of ECG monitoring indicated in each of the clinical situations above, there are no definitive rules as to when cardiac monitoring should be discontinued. Given that resources such as monitored beds and portable telemetry units are often in short supply, discontinuation of cardiac monitoring can often pose some difficulties and may have medico-legal and ethical implications, particularly where monitoring must be discontinued on one patient to enable it to be used on another who appears to be in more need at a given time. Institutional guidelines can be a helpful support in making these decisions.

Nursing considerations in the care of the patient with ECG monitoring

There are a number of practical aspects to be considered when caring for the patient with ECG monitoring and these are represented in Table 11.2.

Table 11.1   Indications for arrhythmia monitoring in adults.

Indication	Timeframe
Resuscitation from cardiac arrest	Until the cause of the arrest is detected and treated
Suspected/known acute coronary syndromes	Presentation until acute coronary syndrome is ruled out; ischaemia is resolved or for at least 24 h after acute myocardial infarction
Cardiac surgery	Minimum of 48–72 h following cardiac surgery; or until discharge if there is a risk of atrial fibrillation
Newly diagnosed left main disease (or equivalent) requiring urgent bypass surgery	Diagnosis until 24–72 h following cardiac surgery or until discharge if there is a risk of atrial fibrillation
Non-urgent percutaneous intervention with complications such as vessel dissection, abrupt closure or no reflow	Minimum of 24 h
Temporary transvenous or transcutaneous pacing or permanent pacemaker lead implantation where the patient is pacemaker dependant	Until the cause of bradyarrhythmia is corrected or permanent pacemaker function is established
Severe bradyarrhythmias and/or advanced AV block including Mobitz Type II, complete heart block or new-onset bundle branch block in the setting of myocardial infarction (particularly anterior myocardial infarction)	Until the cause of bradyarrhythmia is corrected or definitive therapy (such as permanent pacing) is instituted
Re-entrant tachyarrhythmias such as Wolff–Parkinson–White (WPW) with rapid anterograde conduction	Until a definitive therapy is established or a successful ablation procedure is undertaken
Ventricular arrhythmias such as ventricular tachycardia, ventricular fibrillation, Torsades de Pointes, or potential for ventricular arrhythmias due to prolonged QT syndrome	Until the cause of the arrhythmia is corrected or a definitive therapy, such as implantation of a cardioverter defibrillator, has been established
Intra-aortic balloon counterpulsation (IABP)	Until IABP therapy is ceased (no further need to track rhythm for IABP function) and the patient is haemodynamically stable
Acute heart failure/pulmonary oedema	Until the signs and symptoms of heart failure are resolved; therapies that may contribute to arrhythmias (positive inotropic drugs) are discontinued; causative mechanisms such as ischaemia or tachyarrhythmias such as atrial fibrillation are resolved or controlled
Anaesthesia or conscious sedation	Until the patient is properly awake and alert
Haemodynamic instability whatever the course	Until the cause of haemodynamic instability is corrected and the patient is clinically stable

Learning activities

Observe the trace in Figure 11.3. What are the likely causes of the poor trace and how may this be rectified?

You are working on a general medical ward and you have two patients who are on telemetry monitoring. The cardiac rhythm is transmitted directly to the CCU monitor and you have no visual display of the cardiac rhythm in the medical ward. What are your responsibilities in caring for these patients?

Table 11.2   Nursing considerations in the care of the patient with ECG monitoring.

Assemble the equipment that you will require

Monitor/transmitter	When using electrical equipment, such as a cardiac monitor, nurses should ensure that it has had a safety check as per the manufacturer's recommendations (usually annual). Nurses should be trained in the use of such equipment. Cables and leads should be intact and not frayed.
	Patients who have cardiac monitoring in place are often attached to other electrical devices such as infusion pumps, and have breaks in the skin for intravenous cannulation, which put them at increased risk of electrical shock. For this reason, cardiac monitoring areas should be cardiac protected according to national standards.
	If a telemetry transmitter is to be used, it will require fresh batteries appropriately inserted. A telemetry pouch or pocket will be needed to hold the device.
Disposable electrodes	Standard adhesive electrodes are usually the least costly option and for this reason most institutions would prefer that these are used in the first instance.
	For the diaphoretic patient, there are diaphoretic electrodes that are more expensive than the standard electrode, but they will not have to be replaced as often as on a diaphoretic patient and thus are likely to be more cost-effective in this situation.
	A number of patients are sensitive to the adhesive and/or the gel in electrodes and hypoallergenic electrodes may be required.
	The electrodes should be adhered in a way that ensures that there are no air bubbles beneath the electrode. It must be ensured that all backing material is removed from the electrode – any residual backing can cause irritation to the patient.
	Correct placement of the electrodes is required to ensure a tracing that can be correctly interpreted. Cables are usually colour coded, but it is important to realise that there may be international differences in the colour code.

Patient preparation

Patient education	The application of a cardiac monitor can cause anxiety in patients and their families, especially when there are irregularities with the cardiac trace (which may in fact be due to artefact) or when the heart rate changes. A little time spent in reassuring patients and families about the function of the monitor and letting them know that irregularities in rate and rhythm will trigger alarms in the central monitor that will alert nurses if there are any problems with heart rhythm of may allay their fears.
	When a patient is placed on telemetry, he or she needs to be educated about the area that they can mobilise within; to inform the nurse if an electrode becomes detached and not to shower or bath with the unit attached.
Skin preparation	Gauze swabs or a cloth to clean the skin may be required, particularly in diaphoretic patients. The skin should be clean and dry prior to attachment of the adhesive electrodes.
	If the patient has chest hair, it may need to be clipped. Shaving with a razor is not advised as it often results in grazing or small cuts which increases the risk of infection. If electrodes are placed directly over excess chest hair, impedance is increased, resulting in a poor trace and the electrode lifts, pulling at the chest hair, resulting in patient discomfort and a poor trace, electrodes have to be repeatedly replaced, resulting in discomfort to the patient each time the electrode is removed, increased cost in terms of electrode usage and the time taken to replace them frequently, and periods where the patient may be unmonitored due to 'loose lead'. A little time taken to attach electrodes properly when initiating monitoring will save time and resources and make the patient more comfortable.
	Regular checks of the skin are needed to detect allergy or irritation to the electrodes. Electrodes should be replaced if they roll up, lift or become soiled or wet. When monitoring is discontinued, the electrodes and any residual adhesive should be removed. Patients are often unaware that electrodes are still attached (particularly underneath a woman's breast).

Table 11.2 (cont'd)

Comfort and dignity	Exposure of the torso for the purpose of attaching electrodes is often embarrassing for the patient. Privacy must be ensured and the patient is covered as much as possible. It is often not practical for the patient to wear his or her own clothing when attached to cardiac monitoring and other devices such as infusion pumps. Hospital gowns can be less than discreet in covering the patient. When attaching electrodes and leads, it should be borne in mind how this will impact on the patient's clothing cover; do not attach the leads over the top of a gown as this will make the gown sag at the top and lift at the bottom, exposing the patient. The leads should be looped so that there is no tension on them. Tension may cause them to become disconnected or cause discomfort to the patient.
Hygiene needs	The patient with cardiac monitoring in place will need advice on how best to meet hygiene needs. The electrodes should not come into contact with water, and the patient may need some assistance in attending to hygiene.
Management of monitoring	
Obtain a good-quality trace on the cardiac monitor.	It must be ensured that the rhythm displayed on the monitor can be clearly seen and is free of artefact.
Obtain a rhythm strip, diagnose the rhythm and document	If any artefact is present, the cause must be rectified. It may be that an electrode has become detached or has poor contact with the skin. The electrode may be placed over the skeletal muscle or the patient's movement may result in artefact. Alternately, there may be electrical interference from another piece of electrical equipment such as an infusion pump or an electric bed.
Ensure that appropriate alarm limits are set.	Most systems will impose generic alarm settings, but this may need to be altered according to a patient's rhythm and condition. For example, a patient may normally be bradycardic due to beta blocker use: thus, the low rate alarm may need to be set lower to prevent continuous bradycardia alarms.
Ensure appropriate supervision.	It must be ensured that the monitored patient is under the direct care of a nurse who has had training in arrhythmia interpretation and management of arrhythmias.

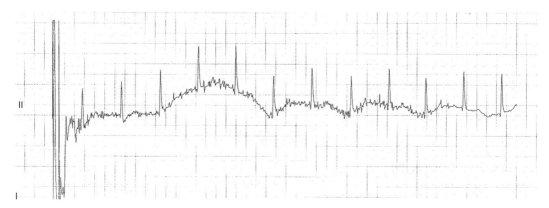

Figure 11.3 Cardiac trace with artefact.

References

Bush, H.S., Ferguson, J.J. III, Angelini, P. & Willerson, J.T. (1991). Twelve-lead electrocardiograph evaluation of ischaemia during percutaneous transluminal coronary angioplasty and its correlation with acute reocclusion. *American Heart Journal*, **121**:1591–9.

Brown, M.C. (2000). ECG monitor – Medical Equipment Dictionary. Retrieved online 26th August 2007 from http://www.medequipdict.com/

Curry, P.J, Hansen, P.W., Russell, M.W., et al. (2003). The use and effectiveness of electrocardiographic telemetry monitoring in a community hospital general care setting. *Anesthesia & Analgesia*, **97**:1483–7.

Dellborg, M., Emanuelsson, H., Riha, M. & Swedberg, K. (1991). Dynamic QRS-complex and ST-segment monitoring by continuous vectorcardiography during coronary angioplasty. *Coronary Artery Disease*, **2**:43–52.

Dellborg, M., Steg, P.G., Simoons, M., et al. (1995). Vectorcardiographic monitoring to assess early vessel patency after reperfusion therapy for acute myocardial infarction. *European Heart Journal*, **16**:21–9.

Drew, B.J. & Scheinman, M.M. (1995). ECG criteria to distinguish between aberrantly conducted supraventricular tachycardia and ventricular tachycardia: practical aspects for the immediate care setting. *Pacing Clinical Electrophysiology*, **18**:2194–208.

Drew, B.J. & Krucoff, M.W. for the ST-Segment Monitoring Practice Guideline International Working Group (1999). Multilead ST-segment monitoring in patients with acute coronary syndromes: a consensus statement for health professionals. *American Journal of Critical Care*, **8**:372–88.

Drew, B.J., Califf, R.M., Funk, M., et al. (2004). Practice standards for electrocardiographic monitoring in hospital settings: an American Heart Association Scientific Statement from the Councils on Cardiovascular Nursing, Clinical Cardiology, and Cardiovascular Disease in the young: endorsed by the International Society of Computerized Electrocardiology and the American Association of Critical-Care Nurses. *Circulation*, **110**:2721–46.

Goodman, S.G., Barr, A., Sobtchouk, A., et al. for the Canadian ESSENCE ST segment monitoring substudy (2000). Low molecular weight heparin decreases rebound ischemia in unstable angina or non-Q-wave myocardial infarction: the Canadian ESSENCE ST segment monitoring substudy. *Journal of the American College of Cardiology*, **36**:1507–13.

Holmvang, L., Andersen, K., Dellborg, M., et al. (1999). Relative contributions of a single admission 12-lead electrocardiogram and early 24-hour continuous electrocardiographic monitoring for early risk stratification in patients with unstable coronary artery disease. *American Journal of Cardiology*, **83**:667–74.

Jernberg, T., Lindahl, B. & Wallentin, L. (1999). ST-segment monitoring with continuous 12-lead ECG improves early risk stratification in patients with chest pain and ECG non-diagnostic of acute myocardial infarction. *Journal of the American College of Cardiology*, **34**:1413–9.

Jernberg, T., Lindahl, B. & Wallentin, L. (2000a). Combination of continuous 12-lead ECG and troponin T: a valuable tool for risk stratification during the first 6 hours in patients with chest pain and a non-diagnostic ECG. *European Heart Journal*, **21**:1464–72.

Jernberg, T., Abrahamsson, P., Lindahl, B., et al. (2000b). Continuous multi-lead ST-monitoring identifies patients with unstable coronary artery disease who benefit from long-term antithrombotic treatment. FRISC II-substudy. *European Heart Journal*, **21**(Suppl.):518.

Klootwijk, P., Meij, S., Melkert, R., Lenderink, T. & Simoons, M.L. (1998). Reduction of recurrent ischemia with abciximab during continuous ECG-ischemia monitoring in patients with unstable angina refractory to standard treatment (CAPTURE). *Circulation*, **98**:1358–64.

Kucia, A.M., Stewart, S. & Zeitz, C.J. (2002). Continuous ST-segment monitoring: a non-intensive method of assessing myocardial perfusion in acute myocardial infarction. *European Journal of Cardiovascular Nursing*, **1**:41–3.

Kucia, A.M. (2007). Continuous 12-lead electrocardiographic monitoring for ischaemia: does it still have a place in the new millennium? Cardiovascular Specialist Diseases Library. Retrieved online 27th August 2007 from http://www.library.nhs.uk/cardiovascular/Page.aspx?pagename=ED23

Krucoff M. (1988). Identification of high-risk patients with silent myocardial ischemia after percutaneous transluminal coronary angioplasty by multilead monitoring. *American Journal of Cardiology*, **61**:29F–34F.

Krucoff, M.W., Croll, M.A., Pope, J.E., et al. for the TAMI Study Group (1993). Continuous 12-Lead ST-segment recovery analysis in the TAMI 7 study: performance of a non-invasive method for real-time detection of failed myocardial reperfusion. *Circulation*, **88**:437–46.

Norgaard, B.L., Andersen, K., Dellborg, M., et al. (1999). Admission risk assessment by cardiac troponin T in unstable coronary artery disease. *Journal of the American College of Cardiology*, **33**:1519–27.

Patton, J.A. & Funk, M. (2001). Survey of use of ST-segment monitoring in patients with acute coronary syndromes. *American Journal of Critical Care*, **10**:23–4.

Sejersten, M., Pahlm, O., Pettersson, J., et al. (2006). Comparison of EASI-derived 12-lead electrocardiograms versus paramedic-acquired 12-lead electrocardiograms using Mason-Likar limb lead configuration in patients with chest pain. *Journal of Electrocardiography*, **39**:13–21.

Shah, A., Wagner, G.S., Granger, C.G., et al. (2000). Prognostic implications of TIMI flow grade in the infarct related artery compared with continuous 12-lead ST-segment resolution analysis. *Journal of the American College of Cardiology*, **35**:666–72.

Sheppard, M. & Wright, M. (2000). *Principles and Practices of High Dependency Nursing*, Balliere Tindall, London.

Useful Websites and Further Reading

Drew, B.J., Califf, R.M., Funk, M., et al. (2004). Practice standards for electrographic monitoring in hospital settings: an American Heart Association scientific statement from The Councils on Cardiovascular Nursing, Clinical Cardiology, and Cardiovascular Disease in the young: endorsed by the International Society of Computerized Electrocardiology and the American Association of Critical Care Nurses. *Circulation*, **110**:2721–46. Available online at http://circ.ahajournals.org/cgi/content/full/110/17/2721

Wipro GE Healthcare (2007). Monitoring systems online CE/CME courses. Retrieved online 28th August 2007 from http://www.gehealthcare.com/inen/education/ceonline/ healthstream_ms.html

12 Laboratory Tests

D. Barrett, L. Jesuthasan & A.M. Kucia

Overview

Whenever you care for a patient with an acute cardiac condition, one of the initial elements of the assessment is a full set of serum laboratory (blood) tests. A great deal of useful information about physiological and biochemical states can be derived from blood tests, and they can help in the identification of the presence or progress of certain disease states. Blood tests are also useful in determining the mineral content of the blood and can be used to assess organ function and the therapeutic efficacy of some medications. In this chapter, standard laboratory investigations, such as urea and electrolytes, full blood count and clotting screens, will be explored. Laboratory investigations that are specific to patients presenting with an acute coronary syndrome (ACS) or acute heart failure will also be covered in detail, including exploration of which investigations need to be done, and most importantly, why they need to be done.

Learning objectives

By the end of this chapter, you will be able to:

- Discuss the reasons for performing standard blood tests in patients with suspected ACSs or heart failure.

- Recognise the diagnostic importance of specific biochemical markers in patients with ACSs.
- Describe the significance of natriuretic peptide measurement in patients with heart failure.
- Discuss some of the limitations of laboratory tests.
- Discuss nursing considerations in obtaining a serum laboratory sample.

Key concepts

Serum testing; haematological examination; coagulation studies; screening; therapeutic monitoring

Generic laboratory tests

Most patients who come under your care will have a range of fairly standard laboratory investigations. These will include tests for electrolytes (E), such as sodium (Na^+) and potassium (K^+), urea (U) and creatinine (CR), clotting times, full blood count, blood glucose and lipid screen. For patients with suspected acute cardiac conditions, these tests are vitally important for three reasons: (1) they will help you and your colleagues to rule out other possible causes of the symptoms; (2) they will give you information that will help to tailor your management of cardiac problems and (3) they give you a valuable baseline against which you can track any changes.

Electrolytes

Serum electrolytes (E) are obtained via a venous blood sample and are electrically charged elements found in blood and body tissues in the form of dissolved salts. They are important in maintaining fluid balance and stabilising the body's pH level. The main electrolytes in the body are:

* Sodium (Na^+) which is found mainly in the plasma and interstitial fluid.
* Potassium (K^+) which is found mainly in the cells but also in smaller amounts in the plasma and interstitial fluid. Abnormalities in K^+ levels can cause life-threatening arrhythmias, so it is important to keep K^+ within normal parameters.
* Chloride (Cl^-) which shifts in and out of cells to maintain electrical neutrality. Levels of Cl^- are often related to levels of Na^+.
* Bicarbonate which helps to maintain a stable pH level (acid–base balance) through excretion and reabsorption via the kidneys.

Other components that are often measured in a serum electrolyte screen are shown in Table 12.1.

Key point

In terms of the electrolytes, K^+ and magnesium ($Mg2^+$) are often viewed as the most significant in cardiac patients. Any patient with suspected ACS or acute heart failure is at risk of cardiac arrhythmias. This susceptibility to arrhythmias will be more pronounced if the serum K^+ and/or $Mg2^+$ levels are abnormal. Abnormalities in the levels of these electrolytes are not unusual. Drugs such as loop diuretics, for example, furosemide, may cause abnormally low levels of K^+ (hypokalaemia) and $Mg2^+$ (hypomagnesaemia). Conversely, conditions such as renal failure may lead to abnormally high levels of K^+ (hyperkalaemia) and $Mg2^+$ (hypermagnesaemia). These conditions can potentially result in fatal arrhythmias and must be identified and treated as quickly as possible.

Table 12.1 Components and normal value of a serum electrolytes screen.

Component	Reference range
Sodium	135–145 mmol/L
Potassium	3.8–4.9 mmol/L
Chloride	95–110 mmol/L
Bicarbonate	24–32 mmol/L
Calcium	10–2.55 mmol/L
Magnesium	0.8–1.0 mmol/L
Phosphate	0.70–1.50 mmol/L
Serum osmolality	280–300 mmol/kg water

Renal function

Together with electrolytes, measurement of CR, blood urea nitrogen (BUN) and estimated glomerular filtration rate (eGFR) and CR clearance will give useful information about renal function. This is important, as impaired renal function is closely associated with an increased risk of mortality in patients with cardiac disorders (National Heart Foundation of Australia and Cardiac Society of Australia and New Zealand 2006).

* Creatinine is a waste product of creatine phosphate metabolism in muscles. CR is produced at a relatively constant rate and excreted almost exclusively by the kidneys, so serum levels of CR are a good measure of renal function.
* Blood urea nitrogen is an indicator of the level of Urea (U) in the blood. Urea is formed as a waste product of protein metabolism and is released into the bloodstream and transported to the kidneys where it is filtered and excreted. A rise in urea levels can often indicate renal failure.

Measurement of an accurate GFR is complex, but the eGFR gives a reasonable estimate. CR clearance tests evaluate the amount of blood filtered in 24 h and include the measurement of CR in a blood sample taken just before or after collection of a 24-hour urine sample. Normal reference ranges for CR, urea, eGFR and CR clearance are shown in Table 12.2.

Key point

Radio-opaque contrast may impair renal function. Furthermore, the dose of some pharmacological agents (such as enoxaparin) may have to be reduced in those with impaired renal function.

Table 12.2   Renal function tests and normal reference ranges.

Test/component	Reference range
Creatinine	0.05–0.12 mmol/L
Urea	3.0–8.0 mmol/L
eGFR	>60 mL/min

Glucose measurement

Glucose is the main source of energy for the body and needs to be maintained at a certain level for normal cellular function. Insulin, a hormone produced by the pancreas, is needed to transport glucose into the cells and to stimulate glycogen synthesis. Amounts of glucose and insulin must be balanced to prevent hyperglycaemia or hypoglycaemia, both of which can be acutely life threatening if severe. Chronically high blood glucose levels, such as occurs in uncontrolled diabetes, can cause progressive damage to the heart, blood vessels and kidneys.

Key point

For patients with ACS, glucose level on admission to the hospital is a significant predictor of 1-year mortality (Capes et al. 2000). In the short term, any diabetic patient, or one with significantly raised blood glucose after a myocardial infarction (MI), will need aggressive glycaemic management to normalise blood glucose levels (Davies & Lawrence 2002) and will require frequent testing to guide insulin administration.

Up to 50% of patients with type 2 diabetes are undiagnosed (Ryden et al. 2007), and given that diabetes is a strong risk factor for cardiovascular disease, cardiac patients should be screened for diabetes, ideally using a fasting glucose test. Initial blood glucose measurement in a patient with suspected cardiac problems may be by serum laboratory testing or by a capillary sample using a point-of-care (bedside) device. Samples taken in an acute presentation are often non-fasting samples. When screening for glucose intolerance or diabetes, it is recommended that the patient fasts for at least 8 h prior to a laboratory blood sample being taken. The patient then drinks a liquid containing a specified amount of glucose and subsequent blood samples are taken at specified intervals for comparison.

Lipid profiles

Dyslipidaemia is a major risk factor for cardiovascular disease. Screening for dyslipidaemia involves obtaining a lipid profile through a venous blood sample in acute settings, but can be obtained using a point-of-care device and a capillary (finger prick) sample. The point-of-care device method is usually used during community screenings. The lipid profile includes:

- Total cholesterol.
- High-density lipid (HDL) cholesterol which has a role in the removal and disposal of excess cholesterol.
- Low-density lipid (LDL) cholesterol which is harmful in excess as it deposits excess cholesterol in the walls of the blood vessel and contributes to atherosclerosis.
- Triglycerides are the body's storage form of fat and are found mainly in the adipose tissue. Some triglycerides circulate in the blood to provide fuel for muscles to work and the levels are highest after eating a meal; thus, triglyceride testing should be done on fasting samples.
- Total cholesterol/HDL ratio which is a calculated value that reflects a risk score based on lipid profile results, age, gender and other risk factors.

Target lipid profiles for people with cardiovascular disease are discussed in Chapter 5.

Key point

Triglycerides increase and cholesterol levels decrease in inflammatory states such as ACSs. Lipid profiles are generally reliable within the first 24 h of an ACS. Testing should be done in this timeframe, but follow-up testing is required.

Complete blood examination

The complete blood examination (CBE), also called complete blood count or picture (CBC or CBP) or full blood examination or count (FBE or FBC), is a basic screening test and one of the most frequently ordered blood tests. Parameters measured in the CBE are shown in Table 12.3. It is a useful test in patients with a known or potential acute cardiac problem such as ACS or heart failure. Anaemia, detected by measuring haemoglobin levels, can be a precipitant of myocardial ischaemia and/or heart failure. Infection, such as pneumonia, or inflammatory processes, such as endocarditis, may have similar presentations to ACSs or heart failure, but elevated levels of white blood cells may assist diagnosis. A CBE also gives information about platelet levels, important in the therapeutic monitoring of antiplatelet and anticoagulation therapy.

Table 12.3 Complete blood examination.

Component	Reference range
Red blood cell (RBC)	M: 4.5–6.5 × 10^{12}/L F: 3.8–5.8 × 10^{12}/L
Haemoglobin (Hb)	M: 130–180 g/L F: 115–165 g/L
Haematocrit (Hct) – the percentage of RBCs in the plasma	M: 40–50% (0.40–0.54 L/L) F: 37–47% (0.37–0.47 L/L)
RBC indices	
Mean corpuscular volume (MCV)	80–100 fL
Mean corpuscular Hb	27–32 pg
Mean corpuscular Hb concentration (MCHC)	300–350 g/L
White blood cells	
White cell count (WCC)	4.0–11.0 × 10^9/L
Differential count[a]	
Neutrophils	2.0–7.5 × 10^9/L
Lymphocytes	1.5–4.0 × 10^9/L
Monocytes	0.2–0.8 × 10^9/L
Eosinophils	0.04–0.4 × 10^9/L
Basophils	<0.1 × 10^9/L
Platelets	
Platelet count	150–400 × 10^9/L

M, male; F, female.
[a]The proportion of each of the five types of white cells in a WCC sample is known as a differential count. The differential is usually needed to make a diagnosis in the setting of an abnormal WCC.

Clotting screen

Acute coronary syndrome is usually a disease process that involves the formation of an unstable plaque in the coronary arteries, with the tendency for blood clot formation. Treatment regimens normally include the use of drugs that interfere with normal clotting mechanisms; thus, careful monitoring of clotting function is essential. The main measurements are:

- Activated partial thromboplastin time (aPTT) which is used in the setting of abnormal bleeding, thrombosis and in therapeutic monitoring of anticoagulation with unfractionated heparin. A baseline aPTT should be obtained. Therapeutic targets are normally maintained by adjusting the levels of intravenous heparin according to aPTT results using a weight-based nomogram. The range of normal aPTT values often differs between laboratories.
- The International normalised ratio (INR) which is used to test clotting in patients who are receiving oral anticoagulation with warfarin.
- Activated coagulation time (ACT) which is used in the setting of high dose of anticoagulant therapy, such as measuring when clotting has recovered sufficiently to remove an arterial sheath following cardiac intervention. ACT is usually performed using a point-of-care device and is useful when a rapid result is needed to guide treatment.

Biochemical markers

There are two main types of biochemical markers that you need to consider for cardiac patients. Firstly, there are those that detect damage to the heart muscle – sometimes referred to as biochemical markers of myocardial necrosis (Morrow et al. 2007). These tend to be utilised whenever an ACS is suspected. The second type is those markers used in heart failure, known as the cardiac natriuretic peptides.

Markers of myocardial necrosis

When a cardiac cell dies (becomes necrotic), the cell membrane becomes disrupted, allowing the contents of the cell to leak into the bloodstream (Naik et al. 2007). A number of these substances are found only in the cardiac muscle and are therefore useful in detecting damage to the heart caused by MI.

Creatine kinase (CK) is an enzyme found within muscle cells throughout the body, including the heart. CK will be released in response to skeletal muscle damage or trauma in any part of the body. To make testing more accurate, one specific type of CK that is located mainly in the heart, known as CK-MB, is often utilised. However, even CK-MB can be found in parts of the body outside the heart, and may be elevated by non-cardiac causes (Naik et al. 2007).

Key point

CK elevation above serum reference range can be seen at 4–8 h, but levels peak at 12–24 h. If no further necrosis occurs, levels generally return to normal in 3–4 days. CK levels are usually taken on admission with serial CK levels taken thereafter. Some institutions will obtain CK levels 4 hourly, others repeat at 8–12 h and then daily for 24–72 h.

Of the commonly used markers of myocardial necrosis, the cardiac forms of the proteins troponin I (cTnI) and troponin T (cTnT) are the most sensitive. Following an MI, levels of cTnI and cTnT will begin to rise after 3–4 h of the occurrence of damage and may stay elevated for up to 2 weeks (Bassand et al. 2007). In patients presenting with chest pain that may be due to myocardial ischaemia, troponin levels should be tested on admission, and another sample is required 6–12 h later, since there can be a delay in troponin rise in some patients. Since the development of troponin testing, there has been much discussion about the level at which a rise becomes clinically significant. Generally speaking, any rise in levels of troponin within the bloodstream is suggestive of myocardial damage, though the exact level that is considered significant will vary between countries and clinicians. Though precise guidelines may vary slightly from place to place, there is no doubt that an increase in troponin levels is associated with an increased risk of death following an ACS. All

patients with a suspected ACS – with or without ST-segment elevation – should have their troponin levels tested to confirm or refute a diagnosis of acute MI and to inform the risk stratification process (Aroney et al. 2006).

It should be recognised that conditions other than those related to coronary artery disease can damage myocardial cells and can therefore prompt a rise in troponin levels. Chronic or acute heart failure may cause troponin elevation, as may disorders such as myocarditis (Bassand et al. 2007). Troponin testing should therefore be considered as just one part of your assessment of patients with acute cardiac disorders: results should be evaluated in partnership with the clinical history, physical examination and ECG findings to reach a definitive diagnosis.

Key point

Because both cTnT and cTnI are present in the bloodstream for several days (long half life), they are not useful for detecting reinfarction. However, if the patient with MI has delayed seeking medical attention, cTnT and cTnI are still detectable when other markers of infarction have returned to normal (Newby 2005).

Cardiac natriuretic peptides

Cardiac natriuretic peptides are hormones that are produced in response to increased pressures within the heart. Atrial natriuretic peptide (ANP), as the name suggests, is secreted predominantly from atrial cells, as a response to atrial walls being stretched. B-type natriuretic peptide (BNP) secretion is stimulated by stretching or tension of the myocardial wall, notably that of the left ventricle (Panteghini 2004). In relation to ACSs, raised BNP levels in a patient may be a useful indicator of long-term prognosis, but are of little value in the initial diagnosis.

The primary use of BNP in the clinical setting remains the diagnosis of heart failure in the community or acute settings. For patients who attend an emergency department with shortness of breath, BNP levels may assist in differentiating between cardiac and non-cardiac causes (Bassand et al. 2007). Measurement of BNP levels is extremely effective at helping clinicians rule out ventricular dysfunction; any patient with a negative BNP (<100 pg/mL) is very unlikely to have heart failure (Bettencourt 2005). A raised BNP does not necessarily mean that a patient does have heart failure, since elevated BNP levels are also seen in conditions with expanded fluid volume unrelated to cardiac failure. However, further cardiac investigations are recommended for anybody with a raised BNP to discover the specific cause.

C-reactive protein

C-reactive protein (CRP) is an inflammatory marker produced by the liver, and the levels in the bloodstream can rise in response to any inflammatory process that occurs in the body. Elevated CRP, measured by high-sensitive CRP (hsCRP) assays, has been associated with a high rate of adverse events. However, CRP lacks specificity and does not really serve any useful purpose in the initial diagnosis of ACS or acute heart failure, apart from diagnosis of coexisting infection or inflammation (Bassand et al. 2007).

Conclusion

For patients suffering from an acute cardiac condition, a number of laboratory investigations are required. Some basic laboratory investigations such as CBE, CR, urea and electrolytes and blood glucose are necessary to exclude any underlying pathology and guide therapy. Specific markers such as markers of myocardial damage or necrosis (troponin and CK) and BNP may assist in the diagnosis and management of relevant conditions. It is important to remember that laboratory tests only form a part of the clinical assessment in addition to history, physical examination and other investigations. Like any investigation, laboratory tests have their strengths and weaknesses, and results should always be considered in the context of other aspects of patient history and assessment.

Learning activity

You are working in an emergency department and a patient presents with an acute ST-segment elevation MI following 1 h of chest pain. What blood tests would you take on presentation and why? If the diagnosis is clear, is there any value in obtaining a troponin sample?

References

Aroney, C, Aylward, P, Kelly, A.-M., et al. for the Acute Coronary Syndrome Guidelines Working Group (2006). Guidelines for the management of acute coronary syndromes 2006. *Medical Journal of Australia*, **184**(Suppl.):S1–30. Available online from http://www.mja.com.au/public/issues/184_08_170406/suppl_170406_fm.pdf

Bassand, J., Hamm, C., Ardissino, D., et al. (2007). Guidelines for the diagnosis and treatment of non-ST-segment elevation acute coronary syndromes. *European Heart Journal*, **28**:1598–660. Available online from http://eurheartj.oxfordjournals.org/cgi/content/full/28/ 13/1598

Bettencourt, P. (2005) Clinical usefulness of B-type natriuretic peptide measurement: present and future perspectives. *Heart*, **91**:1489–94.

Capes, S.E., Hunt, D., Malmberg, K. & Gerstein, H.C. (2000). Stress hyperglycaemia and increased risk of death after myocardial infarction in patients with and without diabetes: a systematic overview. *The Lancet*, **355**:773–8.

Davies, M. & Lawrence, I. (2002) DIGAMI (Diabetes Mellitus, Insulin Glucose Infusion in Acute Myocardial Infarction): theory and practice. *Diabetes, Obesity and Metabolism*, **4**:289–95.

Morrow, D., Cannon, C., Jesse, R., et al. (2007). National Academy of Clinical Biochemistry Laboratory Medicine Practice Guidelines: clinical characteristics and utilization of biochemical markers in acute coronary syndromes. *Clinical Chemistry*, **53**:552–74.

Naik, H., Sabatine, M. & Lilly, L. (2007). Acute Coronary Syndromes. In: L. Lilly (ed.), *Pathophysiology of Heart Disease*, 4th edn. Lippincott, Williams and Wilkins, Philadelphia, pp. 168–96.

National Heart Foundation of Australia and Cardiac Society of Australia and New Zealand (2006). Guidelines for the management of acute coronary syndromes. *Medical Journal of Australia*, **184**:S1–30.

Newby, L.K. (2005). The role of troponin in risk stratification. In: E.J. Topol (ed.), *Acute Coronary Syndromes*, 3rd edn. Marcel Dekker, New York.

Panteghini, M. (2004). Role and importance of biochemical markers in clinical cardiology. *European Heart Journal*, **25**:1187–96.

Ryden, L., Standl, E., Bartnik, M., et al. (2007). European Society of Cardiology (ESC) and European Association for the Study of Diabetes (EASD) Guidelines on diabetes, pre-diabetes, and cardiovascular diseases: full text. *European Heart Journal*, **9**(Suppl. C):C3–74.

Useful Websites and Further Reading

Antman, E.M., Anbe, D.T., Armstrong, P.W., et al. for the American College of Cardiology/American Heart Association Task Force on Practice Guidelines (Committee to Revise the 1999 Guidelines for the Management of Patients with Acute Myocardial Infarction) (2004). ACC/AHA guidelines for the management of patients with ST-elevation myocardial infarction, American College of Cardiology. Retrieved online 9th February 2006 from http://www.acc.org/clinical/guidelines/stemi/Guideline1/index.h

Aroney, C., Aylward, P., Kelly, A.-M., et al. for the Acute Coronary Syndrome Guidelines Working Group (2006). Guidelines for the management of acute coronary syndromes 2006. *Medical Journal of Australia*, **184**(Suppl.):S1–30. Available online from http://www.mja.com.au/public/issues/184_08_170406/suppl_170406_fm.pdf

Fox, K., Birkhead, J., Wilcox, R., Knoght, C. & Barth, J. (2004). British Cardiac Society Working Group on the definition of myocardial infarction. *Heart*, **90**:603–9.

Higgins, C. (2007). *Understanding Laboratory Investigations for Nurses and Health Professionals*, 2nd edn. Blackwell Publishing, Oxford.

Morrow, D., Cannon, C., Jesse, R., et al. (2007). National Academy of Clinical Biochemistry Laboratory Medicine Practice Guidelines: clinical characteristics and utilization of biochemical markers in acute coronary syndromes. *Clinical Chemistry*, **53**:552–74.

Nieminem, M.S., Bohm, M., Cowie, M.R., et al. for the Task Force on Acute Heart Failure of the European Society of Cardiology (2005). Executive summary of the guidelines on the diagnosis and treatment of acute heart failure. *European Heart Journal*, **26**:384–416. Available online from www.escardio.org

13 Diagnostic Procedures

L. Belz, K. Mishra, S.A. Unger & A.M. Kucia

Overview

The diagnosis of acute cardiac conditions requires a multimodal approach that involves a thorough patient history and physical examination, laboratory tests and diagnostic procedures. There are a number of diagnostic procedures that can be utilised for assessing cardiac anatomy and physiology and pathophysiological conditions. As our scientific world advances, great progress has occurred in computer technology and imaging, enhancing our ability to diagnose heart disease. This chapter provides an overview of the basic concepts of diagnostic cardiac procedures, as well as the clinical indications for each procedure, and the role of the nurse in caring for clients undergoing diagnostic procedures.

Learning objectives

After reading this chapter, you should be able to:

- Describe diagnostic procedures available for the assessment of heart disease, the situations in which they may be utilised and the limitations of each of them.
- Discuss the preparation and management of the patient undergoing coronary angiography, and identify potential complications of coronary angiography.
- List the four echocardiographic modalities and recognise the imaging planes used in echocardiography to identify heart anatomy.
- Discuss methods of exercise tolerance (stress) testing and the preparation and care of the patient undergoing each mode of testing.
- Explain the purpose, process, risks and alternatives of each of the diagnostic procedures discussed to a patient/client.

Key concepts

Diagnostic imaging; radiological examination; exercise tolerance testing; myocardial perfusion imaging

Chest X-ray

A simple chest X-ray (CXR), also called a chest film, is often the first imaging done of the heart, and is the most commonly performed imaging procedure that looks at the cardiac and mediastinal contours, along with pulmonary vascular markings. CXRs are usually performed by a radiographer or radiology technologist and ultimately reported by a radiologist, though they may be viewed and interpreted by nursing and medical staff prior to a formal report being recorded. Increasingly, radiological imaging results are available via intranets in many organisations. The CXR is useful in obtaining a diagnosis and is generally readily available in most health care settings and relatively inexpensive. A CXR is generally a safe procedure, with radiation exposure during a routine CXR estimated to be about one-fifth of the annual exposure one normally gets from natural sources such as the sun (American Heart Association (AHA) 2008). It does not, however, image the interior chambers of the heart or arteries.

Penetration of X-ray through the body is inversely proportional to tissue density. The chest has four levels of density: gas or air, water, fat and bone. X-ray beams pass easily through air-filled tissue such as the lung and appear black on the film. Dense matter such as bone is more difficult for the X-ray beam to penetrate and therefore appears white or opaque. For CXRs to be interpreted, the degrees of blackness, or density, on the film are examined and compared to previous films.

A CXR can be obtained from the standard postero-anterior (PA) position, anterior–posterior (AP) position (which is the position used by portable X-ray machines) and lateral (left or right) positions. The PA position is preferred as the X-ray beam travels from the posterior to the anterior of the chest and puts the heart closer to the film allowing the cardiac outline to be seen more clearly (Huseby & Ledoux 2005). A portable CXR can be taken when a patient is acutely unwell and is unable to be transported to the radiology department; however, it is important to note that the quality of the chest film will be inferior due to the probable difficulty in positioning the patient.

Interpretation of the CXR

Review of the X-ray takes place in a systematic pattern known as the directed search method. Soft tissues, bones and diaphragm are examined first, then the lungs are examined from apex to base, followed by the outline of the heart and aorta (Huseby & Ledoux 2005). Apart from evaluating anatomical structures in the chest and assisting in identification of conditions such as cardiomegaly, dissection or dilatation of the aorta, pericardial effusions and calcification of the heart valves or pericardium, the CXR is useful in evaluating placement of devices such as pacemakers, defibrillators, invasive catheters and chest tubes.

Cardiomegaly

Cardiomegaly can be detected by assessing the cardiothoracic ratio (CTR) which is the widest diameter of the heart compared to the widest internal diameter of the ribcage. The widest diameter of the heart should be no more than 50% of the widest internal diameter of the ribcage. Some common conditions where the CTR is abnormal but the heart is normal are AP CXR, obesity, pregnancy or ascites.

Key point

X-rays are subject to divergence and reflection, which makes structures more distant from the film appear magnified and less distinctly outlined (Huseby & Ledoux 2005). When a CXR is taken on a portable X-ray machine in the AP position, the heart is distant from the film and may make the heart appear to be enlarged when, in fact, it is normal. The heart appears larger in expiration than inspiration; thus, individuals who are pregnant, obese or have ascites may not be able to take a full inspiration which makes the heart look bigger than what it actually is (Herring 2007).

Left ventricular failure

There are several radiological signs associated with left ventricular (LV) failure. Pulmonary venous congestion occurs initially in the upper zones (referred to as upper lobe diversion or congestion), which appears on the CXR as increased density of the interstitial markings of the lung fields. As pulmonary venous congestion continues to increase (usually above 20 mmHg), fluid may be visible in the horizontal interlobar fissures. Kerley B lines – very specific patterns on the X-ray film that identify the presence of interstitial oedema – are short, horizontal lines that are perpendicular to the lateral aspects of the lung in the costophrenic angles, may be evident. When pulmonary venous pressures elevate above 25 mmHg, frank pulmonary oedema becomes evident (Davies et al. 2000). Fluid accumulates in the alveoli, which gives a bilateral fluffy appearance on the CXR. The fluffy appearance is often referred to as 'bats wings' or a 'butterfly effect' as it spreads out from the hilar region (Reading 2002). Additionally, pleural effusions may occur, usually bilaterally, but if unilateral, more often occurring on the right side.

Learning activity

Several online courses are available that give a basic introduction to the principles of CXR interpretation and is a good way to develop and practice your skills in CXR interpretation.

Using the link http://nps.freeservers.com/chestxra.htm takes the reader to an online course in a self-programmed format whereby one can review chest films with accompanying case histories and answers, by which nurses can correlate their knowledge of pathophysiology and cardiopulmonary physical assessment (theory and skills) with findings demonstrable on a CXR.

Another useful website by William Herring is available at http://www.learningradiology.com/medstudents/medstudtoc.htm

Key point

The Cardiac Society Australia and New Zealand Acute Coronary Syndrome Guidelines Working Group (Aroney et al. 2006) state that in the setting of acute coronary syndromes (ACS), a CXR is useful for assessing cardiac size, evidence of heart failure and other abnormalities (grade D recommendation), but should not delay reperfusion treatment where indicated. In the setting of unstable angina or non-ST-elevation acute coronary syndrome (NSTEACS), unless the patient has had a previous myocardial infarction (MI) the heart size should be normal (Topol 2007). Transient pulmonary oedema may occur with global ischaemia and is suggestive of the possibility of a left main coronary artery stenosis (Topol 2007).

In preparing a patient for CXR, nurses should ask the patient to remove metal objects such as necklaces and also ensure that the patient is not pregnant. If a patient with suspected or known ACS needs to be transported to another area or department for a CXR, consideration should be given to ensuring safe transport with a suitably qualified nurse, and monitoring defibrillation and resuscitation equipment.

Cardiac catheterisation (angiogram)

Cardiac catheterisation (coronary angiography or angiogram) is the most definitive procedure and indeed the 'gold standard' for diagnosis of most cardiac conditions. It determines the presence, location and severity of coronary artery disease and, with newer techniques, provides direct measurement of coronary flow reserve to evaluate the significance of coronary lesions (Deelstra & Jacobsen 2005). Coronary angiography also enables the measurement of haemodynamics, including intracardiac pressure measurements, and measurements of oxygen saturation and cardiac output (Olade & Safi 2006). When combined with LV angiography, it provides an assessment of global and regional LV function (ACC/AHA 2007). Cardiac catheterisation is also used in the evaluation of congenital or valvular heart disease (Deelstra & Jacobsen 2005). Despite the diagnostic usefulness of coronary angiography, it has some limitations. Coronary angiography produces a silhouette of the coronary artery and does not provide details about the vessel wall or identify vulnerable plaque (Kern et al. 2006). Indications for cardiac catheterisation are shown in Table 13.1.

Once the domain of major tertiary referral hospitals, many regional hospitals are now establishing their own catheter laboratories to provide their

Table 13.1   Indications for coronary angiography.

Known or suspected coronary artery disease	• Identification of the extent and severity of coronary artery disease and evaluation of LV function • Assessment of the severity of valvular or myocardial disorders such as aortic stenosis and/or insufficiency, mitral stenosis and/or insufficiency, and various cardiomyopathies to determine the need for surgical correction • Collection of data to confirm and complement non-invasive studies • Determination of the presence of coronary artery disease in patients with chest pain of uncertain origin • Identified as high risk following non-invasive testing • Successful resuscitation from sudden cardiac death
Unstable coronary syndromes	• Identified as being at intermediate or high risk of adverse outcomes • Angina refractory to adequate medical therapy or recurrent symptoms following stabilisation with medical therapy • Suspected variant (Prinzmetal's) angina (Scanlon et al. 1999)
Post-revascularisation ischaemia	• Suspected abrupt closure or suspected in-stent thrombosis • Recurrent angina within 9 months of revascularisation (Scanlon et al. 1999)
Initial management of NSTEACS	• There is some evidence to suggest that an early invasive strategy in patients with NSTEACS leads to a long-term reduction in death and MI, particularly in high-risk groups (Fox et al. 2005)
Initial management of ST-elevation acute coronary syndrome (STEACS)	• PTCA is the preferred option for management of acute MI where it can be offered within 90 min of presentation and performed by a skilled operator with appropriate backup facilities • Following failed thrombolysis (rescue PTCA)
During hospital admission with an ACS	• Spontaneous myocardial ischaemia provoked by minimal exertion during recovery phase of MI • Prior to definitive therapy for post-MI mechanical complications • Persistent haemodynamic instability (Scanlon et al. 1999)

patient population with an accessible diagnostic service, particularly now that percutaneous transluminal coronary angioplasty (PTCA) is the preferred method of reperfusion in patients with acute MI (Keeley et al. 2003) if available in a timely manner by an experienced operator.

Patient preparation

There are a number of activities to be undertaken to prepare patients for cardiac catheterisation. As with all invasive procedures, the patient should be informed about the purpose, benefits and risks of the procedure and any diagnostic alternatives. A written consent should be obtained. In the setting of an acute cardiac condition, a targeted history, including documentation of any allergies and current medications, is completed. Physical examination should include the usual

admission baseline observations. A temperature >37.5°C should be reported to the cardiologist performing the angioplasty prior to the procedure. As part of the preparation for coronary angiogram, the nurse should check and document the status of the peripheral pedal pulses, presence or absence, colour, warmth, movement and sensation of the lower limbs distal to the proposed puncture site. A complete blood count, blood chemistries, CXR and electrocardiogram (ECG) should be obtained prior to the procedure. An activated partial thromboplastin time (aPTT) should be obtained for patients with heparin infusions. Patients with diabetes need to have blood glucose levels checked, particularly when they are fasting. Instructions for fasting pre-procedure vary. Most institutional policies mandate that patients fast from food and fluid for 6–8h pre-procedure. Water and clear fluids are allowed up to 2h prior to the procedure in many places. In an emergency, it is not possible to fast the patient, and an antiemetic may be ordered prior to the procedure. Premedication with a mild sedative is common, and some operators administer diphenhydramine or a narcotic (Olade & Safi 2006), but the patient, unless a child, is generally not anaesthetised during an angiogram procedure. If conscious sedation is ordered, the nurse should be familiar with the institutional policy for caring patients with conscious sedation. Consideration of a smaller dose of sedation should be given for elderly patients and those with impaired renal function.

For a femoral approach, the patient requires a bilateral groin shave. The patient can undertake to perform the shave themselves if they are able, but the nurse should check that it has been done appropriately prior to the procedure.

Safety

The risk of a major complication during diagnostic cardiac catheterisation is <1–2%. The risk of procedure-related MI is <0.03%; stroke around 0.06% and death approximately 0.08% (Olade & Safi 2006). There are relatively few contraindications for coronary angiography that cannot be corrected prior to the procedure. Patients with insulin-dependent diabetes mellitus, renal insufficiency, peripheral vascular disease, contrast allergy or long-term anticoagulation use are at a higher risk of procedure-related complications, but appropriate therapies can generally minimise these risks (Olade & Safi 2006). Adequate hydration before and after the procedure will reduce the risk of worsening renal function as a result of contrast-induced nephropathy. There is some evidence to suggest that treatment with intravenous or oral *N*-acetylcysteine, an antioxidant, in addition to good hydration, may be useful in preventing contrast-induced nephropathy in patients with pre-existing renal impairment (Duong et al. 2004). Individuals with a history of allergy to iodine-containing substances such as contrast medium or seafood should receive non-ionic contrast and pre-treatment with steroids and an antihistamine (diphenhydramine) and to diminish the likelihood of an allergic reaction to contrast (Olade & Safi 2006).

> **Key point**
>
> Patients with ACS who are receiving antiplatelet therapy and/or anticoagulants have an increased risk of bleeding, as do patients undergoing cardiac catheterisation following thrombolytic therapy (rescue angioplasty). In the GUSTO study (GUSTO Angiographic Investigators 1993), 6% of patients who had angiography within 24 h of thrombolysis had major bleeds requiring blood transfusion and 1.4% required vascular repair.

In addition to relative contraindications already mentioned, others include severe uncontrolled hypertension, ventricular arrhythmias, acute stroke, severe anaemia, active gastrointestinal bleeding, uncompensated congestive failure (patient cannot lie flat), unexplained febrile illness and/or untreated active infection, electrolyte abnormalities (such as hypokalaemia) and severe coagulopathy (Olade & Safi 2006). The risk to benefit ratio of cardiac catheterisation should be assessed for patients with relative contraindications to the procedure, but in an emergency situation, there may be little choice other than to proceed with cardiac catheterisation.

> **Key point**
>
> Cardiac catheterisation involves radiation exposure for staff and patients. The dose of radiation is minimised for the patient by placing lead shielding (in the form of blankets or pads) over certain body parts and by minimising time of fluoroscopy. Staff working in the cardiac catheterisation laboratory wear lead jackets or aprons and have radiation badges to cumulatively monitor their exposure to radiation. Radiographic/fluoroscopic systems may be equipped with movable lead shields that can be placed between staff members and the source of radiation during the procedure. Catheterisation laboratories have a warning sign or light that indicates fluoroscopic activity and staff that are not protected by lead should not enter the laboratory at this time.

Peri-procedural considerations

Cardiac catheterisation is performed using a percutaneous (through the skin) approach from the femoral, radial, brachial or axillary artery. If catheter access to the right side of the heart or pulmonary arteries is required, right heart catheterisation can be performed from the femoral, internal jugular or subclavian veins using percutaneous access methods (Olade & Safi 2006). Cardiac catheterisation can be approached from the upper or lower extremities, and the various approaches with relative advantages and disadvantages are shown in Table 13.2. Access from the upper extremity is preferred in the presence of significant iliac or femoral artery stenosis, prior to bypass grafting of these vessels or in severe obesity, where location of landmarks is difficult (Olade & Safi 2006).

Once the catheter is in place, several diagnostic techniques may be used. The tip of the catheter can be placed into various parts of the heart to measure the pressure within the chambers, (intracardiac pressure). The catheter can be advanced into the coronary arteries and a contrast medium injected into the left and right coronary arteries (coronary angiography). With the use of fluoroscopy (a special type of X-ray), the interventionalist can tell where any blockages in the coronary arteries are located as the dye moves through the arteries. A small sample of heart tissue can be obtained during the procedure, to be examined later under the microscope for abnormalities (myocardial biopsy). The procedure takes approximately 20–30 min and is performed under local anaesthesia, but will take longer if the operator proceeds to PTCA.

Table 13.2   Benefit and risks associated with approach and technique for coronary catheterisation.

Approach/Technique	Benefits and risks
Brachial approach (Sones method)	Usually percutaneous using a 5F or 6F sheath in the brachial artery. Surgical exposure of the brachial artery is still used by some operators.
Radial approach	Access from the radial artery is increasing in popularity. Standard catheters may be used from the radial approach, and several new shapes have been developed to facilitate easy cannulation of the coronary arteries. Patients can mobilise soon after the procedure and there is less risk of bleeding and vascular complications. Disadvantages are that the radial approach involves a longer learning curve for the operator and occasionally severe arterial spasm occurs, which impairs manipulation of the catheter. Performing an Allen test before the procedure is necessary to ensure continuity of the arterial arch in the hand should the radial artery occlude during or after the procedure (Olade & Safi 2006).
Axillary approach	The advantage of this approach is that it avoids the potential for injury to the median nerve and provides a better platform for compression of the artery against the humerus to obtain haemostasis (Olade & Safi 2006).
Femoral approach (Judkins technique)	The femoral approach is widely used for ease and safety. Access to the femoral artery must be properly placed as vascular complications are increased if the arterial puncture is made either above or below the common femoral artery. The main disadvantage of this technique is the need for an extended period of bed rest (between 2 and 6h) after completion of the procedure. Advances in the development of active vascular closure devices (VCDs) mean that closure can be performed immediately at the end of the procedure, regardless of anticoagulation status and time to haemostasis which is generally <5 min with Angio-Seal, Perclose and staple/clip-mediated VCD (Sanborn et al. 1993; Baim et al. 2000; Nasu et al. 2003; Hermiller et al. 2006) compared with 15–30 min with standard 6F manual compression (Dauerman et al. 2007). This results in a substantially shortened period of bed rest, but complication rates with these closure devices are similar to conventional manual compression (Olade & Safi 2006).

Apart from the major risks of cardiac catheterisation already mentioned, intraprocedural complications are listed below.

- Transient hypotension may occur due to administration of large volumes of ionic contrast agents, particularly if ventricular filling pressures are low.
- Acute pulmonary oedema may develop due to the osmotic pressure of the contrast agents and fluid administration during the procedure, particularly in people with impaired LV function, which may require aborting the procedure.
- Chest pain/myocardial ischaemia may occur in patients sensitive to the vasodilatory effects of the contrast medium.
- Minor arrhythmias and conduction disturbances may occur but do not usually need treatment.
- Ventricular tachycardia and/or fibrillation occur in approximately 0.4% of patients, usually as a result of catheter manipulations or the injection of contrast directly into a coronary artery or bypass graft.
- Bradycardia and hypotension is common following right coronary artery injection of high-osmolar agents or during the administration of local anaesthesia in the groin.
- The incidence of infection is low as cardiac catheterisation is a sterile procedure, but the brachial approach has a 10-fold higher infection risk compared with the femoral approach (0.62% vs 0.06%) (Olade & Safi 2006). To minimise infection risk, the laboratory should be cleaned between procedures and staff that are not required for the procedure should not enter the laboratory.
- Allergic (anaphylactic) reactions to iodinated contrast agents occur in approximately 1% of patients with symptoms such as sneezing, urticaria, angioedema, bronchospasm and profound hypotension. Severe reactions may require intravenous dilute adrenalin.

Key point

Latex-induced allergic reactions are being recognised more frequently that are usually localised, but systemic reactions may occur.

Post-procedural care

Immediate assessment should take place when the patient returns from the cardiac investigation unit. This will include level of pain, ECG, vital signs, oxygenation level, urine output, cardiac and respiratory assessment. Particular attention must be paid to the arterial puncture site for any evidence of outward bleeding or haematoma formation. Neurovascular assessment of the lower extremities including colour, warmth, sensitivity, movement, pulses and capillary return should be conducted on the affected limb and the other limb for comparison. Pain or change in sensation at the puncture site or of the affected limb should be assessed. These observations continue at 15–30 min intervals until the sheath is removed, and for 2h following sheath removal (or according to unit policy).

The patient may have the arterial and venous (if used) sheaths removed soon after the procedure or may return to the ward with the sheaths in situ. Often, this depends upon the clotting time which is generally assessed by measuring the activated clotting time (ACT) as patients are often given large doses of heparin during the procedure, and the clotting time will need to be below a certain level to decrease the risk of bleeding when the sheath is removed. For patients who have had a femoral arterial puncture and have a sheath in situ should be placed on bed rest with the head of the bed elevated no higher than 30 degrees. Immediately following removal of the sheath, the patient must lie flat until haemostasis is achieved. The patient should be reminded to limit movement in the bed and to keep the affected limb straight. Advise the patient to apply pressure to the puncture site whilst coughing, sneezing or urinating and to notify nursing staff if any ooze, swelling or feeling of warmth or wetness at the puncture site occurs. Patients become incapable of maintaining self-care as a result of having to be supine for 2–4h (and sometimes longer if the sheath is not removed immediately following the procedure or if the patient is on high-dose anticoagulation or bleeding complications occur). The goal of nursing intervention is to move a patient towards responsible self-care by reducing discomfort due to prolonged bed rest.

Post-procedural complication

It is not uncommon for patients to experience a vasovagal reaction, characterised by hypotension and bradycardia with symptoms of yawning, nausea and sweating, during or soon after sheath removal. This is precipitated by the application of pressure to obtain femoral artery haemostasis and can be aggravated by fasting from fluids for a number of hours prior to the procedure or poor oral fluid intake due to maintaining a supine position for patients with sheaths in situ for a prolonged period of time. The management for vasovagal reaction is intravenous fluids and atropine if required.

Bleeding is the most common vascular complication following coronary angiography using a femoral approach. If the patient starts to bleed outwardly or a haematoma starts to form, pressure should be applied on the femoral artery above the puncture site until haemostasis is achieved.

Key point

When pressure is applied to stop bleeding, the pulse distal to the puncture site must be occluded for no more than 2–5 min. Thereafter, the pressure must be lessened until return of the distal pulse is felt (Deelstra & Jacobsen 2005).

Changes to neurovascular observations and ability to palpate pulses should be reported immediately as it may represent serious arterial occlusion which is a vascular emergency. The patient may experience pain, numbness or tingling if this occurs (Deelstra & Jacobsen 2005).

The patient should be encouraged to commence oral fluids to aid contrast dye removal from the kidneys. A light diet may be given. Maintain the patient on hourly fluid intake and output.

Retroperitoneal bleeding results from a high needle puncture above the inguinal ligament, where blood can enter the retroperitoneum. Typically, the patient complains of abdominal or back pain without any obvious haematoma formation in the groin, and severe back or loin pain after cardiac catheterisation should alert the clinician to this possibility. Retroperitoneal bleed can result in severe blood loss in the absence of pain. Unexplained hypotension and a decreasing haematocrit level should alert the nurse to the possibility of retroperitoneal haematoma formation. A diagnostic abdominal ultrasound or computerised tomography (CT) scan should be performed if there is suspicion of retroperitoneal bleed (Wong et al. 2006). Another potential source of bleeding is through the development of a pseudoaneurysm, which can develop if a connection persists between a haematoma and the arterial lumen. It presents as a pulsatile mass, sometimes with a systolic bruit, and requires a duplex ultrasound for confirmation of the diagnosis. Pseudoaneurysms may be managed conservatively using prolonged compression or thrombin injection in selected patients, but surgical correction is necessary for large pseudoaneurysms with a wide connection to the parent artery (Wong et al. 2006).

An arteriovenous fistula may occur if bleeding from the arterial puncture tracks into the adjacent venous puncture. These are usually small and resolve spontaneously, but surgical repair may be required to fix enlarging fistulae (Wong et al. 2006).

Key point

The Position and Mobilisation Post-Angiography Study (PAMPAS) was one of the largest, prospective, randomised controlled trials that looked at early mobilisation post-angiography.

Evidence suggests early mobilisation can be commenced if there is no bleeding from puncture site and anticoagulation has not been recommended within 2.5 h and that it is as safe as sitting up at 4 h and mobilising at 4.5 h (Pollard et al. 2003).

Echocardiography

Echocardiography is a diagnostic procedure that uses ultrasound to examine the heart and provide anatomical and haemodynamic information. In recent times, it has become one of the most commonly used, cost-effective, portable and widely available tools in diagnosis of heart problems. There are no known risks associated with this diagnostic test and an uncomplicated case may be completed within 30–45 min.

Transthoracic echocardiography

Transthoracic echo (TTE) is an ultrasound of different frequencies that are transmitted from a transducer (probe) which is placed on the patient's anterior chest wall in a number of standard positions (echo windows) to obtain different views or axes of the heart. 'Axes' refer to the plane in which the ultrasound beam travels through the heart (Kaddoura 2002).

Three modes of echo are commonly used.

1   Two-dimensional (2D) or 'cross sectional' echo gives a real-time image of the heart, chambers and blood vessels.
2   Motion or M-mode produces a graph representing changes in movement (such as valves opening and closing, or ventricular wall movement. Measurement of the size and thickness of cardiac chambers can also be made.
3   Doppler echo uses the reflection of ultrasound by moving red blood cells and provides haemodynamic information. It can be used to measure the severity of valvular stenosis or

regurgitation, and detect intracardiac shunts such as ventricular and atrial septal defects (Kaddoura 2002). Commonly used Doppler techniques are (1) spectral Doppler, which is a combination of continuous wave Doppler and pulsed wave Doppler which together allow a geographical representation of velocity against time; and (2) colour flow mapping, which is an automated 2D version of pulse wave Doppler that calculates blood velocity and direction at multiple points. Velocities and directions of flow are colour encoded, with blood flow away from the transducer coded blue and blood flow towards the transducer coded red (known as the BART convention: Blue Away Red Towards; Kaddoura 2002).

The patient usually lies in the left lateral position during the procedure which assists in obtaining quality images because the heart falls forward and the lungs are out of view and the patient's left arm is positioned above the head to aid in the separation of the ribs.

Transoesophageal echocardiography

Examining the heart with a transducer in the oesophagus is called a transoesophageal echocardiography (TOE). The procedure is similar to that of an endoscopy and the benefit is that it allows examination of the heart without the barriers of the lungs, chest wall and ribs that obscure the image with TTE. The TOE enables high-resolution imaging of posterior structures of the heart, in particular the aorta, the left atrium (including the left atrial appendage) and the mitral valve. Disadvantages are that it is invasive, uncomfortable for the patient and not without risk, including oesophageal trauma, risks associated with intravenous sedation and aspiration of stomach contents into lungs. The patient should be fasted for at least 4 h prior to the procedure; and oxygen, suction and continuous ECG monitoring should be available. A short acting sedative is generally used, and a local anaesthetic is sprayed directly on the patient's pharynx. The patient is placed in the left lateral position during the procedure with the neck fully flexed to allow easy insertion of the transducer. Post-procedure, the patient will be drowsy and have a numb throat. Nursing care involves airway protection. The patient should not eat or drink for at least 1 h in case of aspiration.

Other echocardiography techniques

Stress echocardiography is a useful technique in diagnosing ischaemia and is discussed in more detail in the section on stress testing. Contrast studies (bubble studies) are useful in detection of atrial or ventricular septal defects of patent foramen ovale. 3D echo provides 3D representations of the structure and function of heart chambers which avoids geographical assumptions. The main roles of 3D echo are infarct size estimation, evaluation of distorted ventricles and serial LV volume measurements in people with valvular regurgitation (Kaddoura 2002). There are a number of indications for echocardiography in both acute and chronic cardiac disorders. Indications for echocardiography in acute cardiac conditions are listed in Table 13.3.

Learning activity

Understanding echocardiography is a skill that takes a lot of practice and exposure to the various methods and modes. Reviewing pictures taken from the different echocardiographic windows and in different axis can help. The Atlas of Echocardiography at Yale University has a comprehensive library of normal and abnormal echocardiographic pictures at http://www.med.yale.edu/intmed/cardio/echo_atlas/contents/index.html

Stress testing

Exercise tolerance (stress) test

The exercise tolerance test (ETT) also known as the exercise stress test (EST) is a commonly used cardiac assessment technique used to assess the cardiac response to exercise routinely in patients

Table 13.3   Indications for echocardiography in acute cardiac care.

Indication	Clinical features
Chest pain	• suspected acute myocardial ischaemia when baseline ECG and laboratory markers are non-diagnostic (if the echo can be obtained during pain or within a few minutes of pain resolution) • suspected aortic dissection • severe haemodynamic instability • clinical evidence of valvular, pericardial or primary myocardial disease • left bundle branch block (LBBB) or paced rhythm
Risk stratification	• identify areas of reversible ischaemia and myocardial viability using stress echo
Assessment of mechanical function following MI	• infarct size • mechanical complications (mitral regurgitation, ventricular septal defect, cardiac tamponade) • baseline LV function • to guide further therapy or assess effect of intervention such as drug therapy, ICD implantation, cardiac resynchronisation therapy (CRT) • before coronary artery bypass surgery
Arrhythmia	• clinical suspicion of structural heart disease in proven arrhythmia • assessment of ventricular function for primary prevention of SCD following MI • syncope in a patient with clinically suspected heart disease
Heart failure	• clinical or radiographic signs of heart failure • unexplained shortness of breath in the absence of clinical signs of heart failure if ECG/CXR is abnormal

who present with chest pain, in patients who have chest pain on exertion and in patients with known ischaemic heart disease (Hill & Timmis 2002). The prognostic and diagnostic indicators for ETT are listed in Table 13.4.

The most common method of ETT is for the patient to exercise on a treadmill with progressive increases in the speed and elevation of the treadmill. A 12-lead ECG is recorded during the test, along with continuous monitoring of heart rate, heart rhythm and blood pressure.

The most widely adopted protocol for exercise testing using a treadmill is the Bruce Protocol first described by American cardiologist Robert A. Bruce in 1963. The Bruce protocol has been extensively validated in the assessment of cardiovascular health. The protocol has seven stages, each lasting 3 min, but in clinical practice, patients rarely exercise for the full duration (21 min). Exercise duration is dependent on the age and gender of the patient, and completion of 9–12 min of exercise or reaching 85% of the maximum predicted heart rate (MPHR) is usually satisfactory (Hill & Timmis 2002).

MPHR is defined as:

- 220 minus age for males
- 210 minus age for females

The speed and incline of the treadmill increase with each stage of the protocol. A modified Bruce protocol starts at a lower workload than the standard test and is typically used for exercise testing within 7–10 days of MI and for elderly or sedentary patients.

During exercise, coronary blood flow must increase to meet the higher metabolic demands of the myocardium. For patients with normal coronary arteries, as heart rate and blood pressure increase, the coronary arteries dilate. Coronary flow reserve is maintained in arteries with <70% stenosis. For regions of myocardium that are supplied by an artery with a >70% stenosis, the artery is unable to dilate sufficiently in response to increasing myocardial work, resulting in relative reduction in blood flow to that region (Soine & Hanrahan 2005).

Table 13.4 Diagnostic and prognostic indicators for exercise stress testing.

Diagnostic	Prognostic
• Assessment of chest pain in patients with intermediate probability for coronary artery disease • Arrhythmia provocation • Assessment of symptoms (for example, pre-syncope) occurring during or after exercise	• Risk stratification after MI • Risk stratification in patients with hypertrophic cardiomyopathy • Evaluation of revascularisation or drug treatment • Evaluation of exercise tolerance and cardiac function • Assessment of cardiopulmonary function in patients with dilated cardiomyopathy or heart failure • Assessment of treatment for arrhythmia

Source: Reproduced from Hill and Timmis (2002). With permission from BMJ Publishing Group Ltd.

Key point

Coronary flow reserve is a combined measure of the capacity of the major resistance components (the epicardial coronary artery and the small arteries, arterioles and intramyocardial capillary system that comprise the supplied vascular bed) to achieve maximal blood flow in response to hyperaemic stimulation (Kern et al. 2006).

Limitations to the coronary blood flow due to narrowing or stenosis of coronary arteries may result in changes in the ECG, heart rate, blood pressure and/or the patient can develop angina. Systolic blood pressure should increase to a level of around 225 mmHg as exercis   whilst diastolic blood pressure decreases slightly (Hill & Timmis 2002).

Key point

Beta-blocking and calcium channel blocking agents will lower heart rate and blood pressure and increase exercise tolerance. They should be ceased 24 h prior to a diagnostic ETT if it is clinically safe to do so (Strauss et al. 2002).

Interpretation

Horizontal or down-sloping ST segment depression (see Figure 10.5) or ST segment elevation in adjacent ECG leads is generally a reliable indicator of exercise-induced ischaemia, but it should be noted that ST segment depression has been estimated to occur in up to 20% of normal individuals on ambulatory electrocardiographic monitoring, and this may potentially confound the result of an ETT (Hill & Timmis 2002). A sustained dro p in blood pressure usually indicates coronary artery disease.

Re-polarisation and conduction abnormalities including ST segment abnormalities, bundle branch block, LV hypertrophy, intraventricular conduction defects, paced rhythm, pre-excitation or digoxin effect preclude accurate interpretation of the ETT, and if these abnormalities are present, other forms of ETT should be used.

Key point

Accuracy of the ETT in clinical practice is dependant on a good understanding of the limitations and indications for ETT. The ETT cannot be used to rule in or rule out coronary heart disease (CHD) unless the probability of coronary artery disease in the population tested is taken into account. In a low-risk population, a positive result is more likely to be a false positive and thus is of limited value; whereas in a high-risk population, a negative result cannot rule out ischaemic heart disease, although the results may be of some prognostic value (Hill & Timmis 2002). The predictive accuracy of a positive test in asymptomatic men is in the order of 5–12%, whilst in a man with angina it is approximately 97% (Fleg et al.1990). The greatest diagnostic value is in patients with an intermediate risk of CHD. ETT are less accurate in women than men in predicting coronary artery disease (Weiner 1979).

Safety

The ETT is not without risk, although risk can be minimised by careful selection of patients (see Table 13.5 for contraindications). The rate of serious complications (death or acute MI) is estimated to be around one in 10,000 tests (0.01%), and the incidence of ventricular tachycardia or fibrillation

Table 13.5 Contraindications for exercise testing.

- Acute MI (within 4–6 days)
- Unstable angina (rest pain in previous 48 h)
- Known or suspected severe left main stenosis
- Uncontrolled heart failure
- Acute myocarditis or pericarditis
- Acute systemic infection
- Deep vein thrombosis
- Uncontrolled hypertension (systolic blood pressure >220 mmHg, diastolic >120 mmHg)
- Severe aortic stenosis
- Severe hypertrophic obstructive cardiomyopathy
- Untreated life-threatening arrhythmia, complete heart block or rapid atrial arrhythmia
- Dissecting aneurysm
- Recent aortic surgery
- Hyperthyroidism/thyrotoxicosis

is about 1 in 5,000, if patients are carefully selected. For this reason, it is suggested that patients are informed about the procedure and sign a consent form. Full cardiopulmonary resuscitation (CPR) facilities with personnel trained in provision of CPR must be available (Hill & Timmis 2002).

Key point

ETT is increasingly being performed by experienced cardiac or emergency department nursing staff. In some cases, the ETT is also interpreted by the nurse and there is evidence to suggest that there is similar concordance in interpretation of the ETT between cardiologists and experienced nurse practitioners (Maier et al. 2008).

Myocardial perfusion imaging

A radionuclide stress test is a myocardial perfusion imaging technique that involves intravenous injection of a radiopharmaceutical agent (typically thallium 201 or ^{99m}Technetium sestamibi or ^{99m}Technetium tetrofosmin) to detect the

distribution of nutritional blood flow in the myocardium. These radiopharmaceutical agents (isotopes) are often called 'tracers' because they can be traced as they move through the body. Perfusion imaging provides information about LV chamber size, global and regional LV function, location, size and extent of areas of reduced myocardial blood flow that are associated with ischaemia or infarction and scar. Perfusion can be assessed at rest, during periods of cardiovascular stress (induced by an acute coronary syndrome or exercise) or both.

In diagnostic perfusion imaging with treadmill ETT, nuclear images are obtained in the resting condition, and again immediately following an ETT. The two sets of images are then compared. If there is a blockage in a coronary artery that results in diminished blood flow to a region of the cardiac muscle during exercise, there will be a diminished concentration of the radiopharmaceutical agent in the region of decreased perfusion known as a 'perfusion defect'. Following a period of rest, if coronary perfusion is adequate, the perfusion defect is not obvious. This is known as a 'reversible defect'. Data from the test are presented as views from a number of axes (Figure 13.1). The tracer

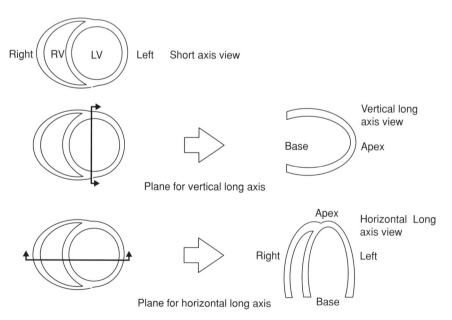

Figure 13.1 Orientation for display of tomographic myocardial perfusion data.
Source: From Strauss et al. (2002).

is injected at peak exercise and the single-photon emission computed tomography (SPECT) images are acquired soon after exercise and at least 4 h after rest. The procedure for the patient is similar to that of a standard ETT but involves two scans and more time. The location and size of a reversible defect guides further treatment strategy in patients with coronary artery disease.

Key point

A 'fixed defect' (unchanged defect, present on both exercise and rest) is likely to represent scar tissue resulting from a previous MI, but it should be noted that in some cases, it may represent viable, under-perfused myocardium (Strauss et al. 2002). Thallium 201 is the most common radionuclide used to distinguish viable or hibernating myocardium from scar (Soine & Hanrahan 2005).

Although radionuclide stress testing is more time-consuming and expensive compared to an ordinary ETT, it greatly enhances the accuracy in diagnosing coronary artery disease and is useful in making decisions regarding coronary revascularisation.

Key point

Imaging can also be performed during acute events, such as during chest pain of unknown aetiology. This is useful to rule out major ischaemia for patients with ongoing chest pain and no evidence ischaemia on the ECG change or rise in cardiac enzymes.

Patient preparation

Ensure that females undergoing this procedure are not pregnant. Patients should fast for 3–6 h prior to the procedure to minimise gastric blood flow and gastric uptake of radionuclides.

Safety

The radiopharmaceuticals used for this procedure have short half lives and used in small amounts;

thus, they pose minimal risk to the patient and the nurse, but nurses should avoid prolonged close-range exposure to the patient following this type of test (Soine & Hanrahan 2005).

Some patients, including those with severe pulmonary disease, arthritis, amputation, neurological disease, may be unable to undertake physical exercise. In this case, the heart can be subjected to chemical 'stressors'. There are two types of pharmacologic agents that are useful to stress the heart to evaluate myocardial perfusion:

- Vasodilator agents (dipyridamole and adenosine) which produce coronary hyperaemia
- Ino/chronotropic adrenergic agents (dobutamine) that increase myocardial oxygen demand (Strauss et al. 2002)

Key point

For patients undergoing pharmacologic stress testing with dipyridamole or adenosine, caffeine-containing beverages should not be taken for at least 12 h before pharmacologic stress imaging. A caffeinated beverage may be used after testing to reverse the effect of dipyridamole. Adenosine is shorter acting and so this is not usually necessary (Strauss et al. 2002).

Stress echocardiography

Stress echocardiography is a particularly useful procedure when a patient has had a prior non-diagnostic ETT or there is a high likelihood of a false-positive result from an ECG stress test. The sensitivity of stress echo is around 80% and the specificity around 90%. This compares favourably to ETT which has a sensitivity of around 70% and a specificity of around 80% (Kaddoura 2002). Stress echocardiography may be conducted with cardiovascular stress induced by exercise, pharmacological agents or temporary cardiac pacing. It is performed using TTE, creating images of the areas of altered myocardial contractility during the stress test to assess myocardial wall motion, myocardial viability, presence of coronary artery disease and prognosis. The normal response of the LV to an increased heart rate (workload) is an increase in regional wall motion, wall thickening and a reduction in end systolic LV cavity size. LV enlargement after stress is a marker of severe ischaemia or other heart muscle disease (Koike et al. 1990). Images are taken at rest, then at peak exercise, or within 1–2 min following exercise as abnormal wall motion will normalise after this time. If abnormalities persist for longer than 30 min, this can be reflective of the severity and duration of ischaemia. Ischaemia occurring at a low workload is associated with a poor prognosis (Ryan et al. 1993). The functional response to stress is also helpful in the management of valvular heart disease and other obstructive lesions. Although stress echocardiography can indicate the presence of severe coronary artery stenosis, it cannot detect instability of coronary plaques.

Key point

Patients with permanent pacemakers are better assessed with stress echocardiography because paced rhythms produce apical and septal wall motion abnormalities. Pharmacologic stress echocardiography is also useful for individuals who have an inability to achieve target heart rate during exercise because of therapy with beta-blocker or calcium channel blocker.

Generally, stress echocardiography is a safe procedure, although it is often performed in elderly patients with multiple co-morbidities that must be considered. The limitations of this procedure are that it is operator-dependant with regard to the quality of the images obtained and subject to inter-interpreter variability.

Magnetic resonance imaging

Magnetic resonance imaging (MRI) is a non-invasive but expensive radiology technique that uses powerful magnets and low-energy radio frequency (RF) signals that allow visualisation of internal body structures without risks of ionising radiation, invasive procedures or potentially nephrotoxic iodinated contrast agents (Levine et al. 2007). Cardiac MRI provides a clear detailed image of the heart as it is beats, creating moving images of the

heart, including chambers and valves, throughout the cardiac cycle. The main indications of cardiac MRI are to assess cardiac structures if echocardiographic images are non-diagnostic, to help in characterisation of congenital heart disease (particularly anomalous coronary arteries) and to determine the extent of myocardial scarring following an infarct, indicating 'non-viability'. It can also be used to assess stress myocardial perfusion and function using pharmacologic stress agents, particularly when other stress imaging methods (stress echo or myocardial perfusion imaging) are non-diagnostic (Alfakih et al. 2004).

The MRI scanner unit is a closed cylindrical magnet (long tube) within which the patient lies as still as possible on a moveable bed within the magnet. The procedure takes generally between 30 and 75 min, depending on the extent of the imaging needed. Most scans involve intravenous injection of MRI contrast (gadolinium) in order to visualise myocardial perfusion, extent of myocardial scarring or fibrosis and proximal coronary arteries. Stress perfusion cardiac MRI involves an injection of gadolinium during pharmacologic stress, typically an adenosine infusion. Types of MRI are listed in Box 13.1.

Risks of MRI

Risks associated with MRI arise from four mechanisms: (1) the static magnetic field; (2) RF energy; (3) gradient magnetic fields and (4) gadolinium contrast. The static magnetic field used by MRI scanners is 30,000–60,000 times the strength of the earth's magnetic field and has the potential to move, rotate, dislodge or accelerate a ferromagnetic object creating a 'projectile effect' towards the magnet that could lead to significant patient injury and damage to the magnetic resonance (MR) system, and alter device function (such as pacemakers and implantable defibrillators; Levine et al. 2007). During MR imaging, RF energy is 'pulsed' into the body to generate the MR image. The body will absorb some of this and will heat up (usually <1°C). Some metallic devices such as pacemaker leads or Swan–Ganz (pulmonary artery) thermodilution catheter can act as an 'antenna' and concentrate this RF energy, leading to local excessive heating particularly at the tip of these devices, and can melt at the skin entry

Box 13.1   Types of MRI

Spin-echo imaging is the most commonly used method to define the structure of the heart and great vessels and provides information about the size of vascular structures and cardiac chambers, ventricular and pericardial wall thickness, cardiac, paracardiac and LV mass, congenital abnormalities and fatty infiltration in arrhythmogenic right ventricular dysplasia (Soine & Hanrahan 2005).

Gradient-echo imaging provides dynamic information on cardiac function and blood flow created with cardiac gating (Soine & Hanrahan 2005).

Coronary magnetic resonance angiography (CMRA) is a method of evaluating coronary arterial blood flow velocity patterns. High-resolution MR has some potential to provide information about plaque composition, fibrous cap thickness and vessel wall morphology, and the quality of information available for evaluation of plaque may improve with newer contrast agents such as Gadoflourine and molecular imaging with contrast tagged fibrin-specific molecules, but this requires further study (Sirineni & Stillman 2007). CMRA does have some drawbacks in that it can take a long period of time to obtain quality images free of distortion caused by the movement during respiratory and cardiac cycles.

site (Levine et al. 2007). Gradient magnetic fields are much weaker than static magnetic fields but are repeatedly turned on and off which can induce electrical currents in electrically conductive devices and cause arrhythmias, and may also excite peripheral nerves (Levine et al. 2007). Although initially thought to be safe, it is now recognised that gadolinium contrast administration can lead to severe nephrotoxicity and even a systemic disorder known as nephrogenic systemic fibrosis, particularly if used in high doses or in patients with at least moderate underlying renal dysfunction.

Having an understanding of how MRI can pose a hazard to patients accentuates the need for careful nursing assessment of the patient prior to them undergoing an MRI. It is important to know if the patient has had any procedures or injuries in the past that have resulted in metal or magnetic implants or devices such as vascular clips used for cerebral aneurysm surgery, embedded metal objects such as shrapnel or bullets, insulin or

narcotic pumps, prosthetic hip joints, implanted nerve stimulators or cochlear implants. Critically ill patients are not good candidates for MRI because of the large amount of equipment such as continuous monitoring systems and life-support ventilators that cannot be bought near the scanner.

Unless the patient has been sedated, there is no recovery time from an MRI. Around 5% of patients will feel claustrophobic and may require some mild sedation.

MRI following device implant

Some implanted devices made from non-ferromagnetic compounds (titanium, titanium alloy or nitinol) that are not subject to MR-related heating concerns are not problematic for patients undergoing MRI. The use of MRI in patients with weakly ferromagnetic devices remains controversial as not all of these devices have been definitively tested under all MRI conditions.

- Most coronary and peripheral vascular stents exhibit non-ferromagnetic or weakly ferromagnetic characteristics. It is advised that for bare-metal stents that are weakly ferromagnetic, the MRI should not take place until 6–8 weeks after stent implantation to allow for tissue ingrowth and anchoring of the stent. It is thought that haemodynamically generated forces from the beating of the heart and blood flow generate forces greater than those associated with MRI. Testing of commonly used drug-eluting stents has shown that there is a lack of ferromagnetic interaction during MRI and MRI can take place immediately after implantation.
- Most endovascular aortic stent grafts have been shown to be safe during MRI, but there are some exceptions and so the manufacturer and type of graft must be checked prior to MRI.
- Prosthetic heart valves, annuloplasty rings and sternal suture wires may exhibit some weak ferromagnetic properties depending on what they are made of, but there is no evidence to suggest they pose a threat to the patient during MRI (Levine et al. 2007).
- There is limited data on the safety of MRI with loop recorders (event monitors). A small study of 10 patients demonstrated no adverse clinical

events or damage to the devices, but excessive artefact on the loop recorder during MRI (Gimbel et al. 2005).

- Implanted pacemakers and internal cardioverter defibrillators (ICDs) potentially could cause harm to a patient undergoing MRI, but as it has been estimated that between 50% and 75% of these patients are likely to have clinical indications for MRI during their lifetime, several studies have been conducted and protocols developed to safely conduct MRI in these patients (Levine et al. 2007).

Key point

Currently used MR scanners are typically superconducting and are always left 'on', so health professionals entering the area must ensure they are free of metal objects.

Computerised tomography

Coronary angiography is the gold standard diagnostic method for assessment of coronary artery disease, but although coronary angiography provides accurate information about the lumen of the coronary artery, it does not reliably detect noncritical disease because of san inability to image the wall of the artery. Thus, significant disease may be present in the coronary arterial wall even though the lumen does not have any significant stenosis owing to positive remodelling of the artery wall (Sirineni & Stillman 2007).

Multidetector row computed tomography (MDCT) and electron-beam computed tomography (EBCT) have a role in non-invasive evaluation of coronary artery disease. MDCT and EBCT are all advances on traditional CT and are often referred to as 'multislice' CT scanning. With multislice scanning, it is possible to acquire high-resolution 3D images of the beating heart and great vessels on a computer screen. MDCT can provide information about the lumen and wall of coronary arteries, and theoretically may be useful in classification of plaques. The sensitivity of calcified plaque detection is high, but sensitivity and specificity for detection of non-calcified plaque are not as high. EBCT

and MDCT are used by some health care providers to calculate a coronary calcium score to stratify asymptomatic individuals for risk of future adverse events such as MI or sudden cardiac death (SCD; Raggi et al. 2000), although this use is controversial. MDCT, with the use of intravenous iodinated contrast agents, is a method currently under investigation for non-invasive visualisation of the coronary arteries (CT angiography) and myocardial perfusion. Concerns regarding radiation exposure to the patient (2–3 times that of invasive coronary angiography) have limited its widespread application thus far. However, MDCT technology is rapidly advancing, and the clinical use of this technique is likely to increase significantly in the near future, particularly in patients with chest pain and a low to intermediate pre-test likelihood of coronary disease.

Computerised tomography is useful in assessing the great vessels, pericardium and myocardial structures, and can accurately detect aortic dissections, aneurysms and pulmonary embolism. CT can also detect pericardial disease such as pericardial effusions, pericardial thickening and calcification. Myocardial abnormalities such as hypertrophy and intraventricular thrombus can be distinctly seen on CT images.

Electrophysiology studies

An electrophysiology study (EPS) is performed to determine a diagnosis of arrhythmia and/or the mechanism of arrhythmia in an individual. Spontaneous and pacing-induced surface and intracardiac electrical signals are recorded of normal timing and sequence of electrical activation, and abnormal timing and electrical activation during arrhythmia. Programmed electrical stimulation may be used to induce arrhythmias. Most EP studies use only the venous system, and commonly used venous access sites are the right and left femoral, subclavian, internal jugular and median cephalic veins (Blancher 2005). The procedure involves the percutaneous introduction of a 12F sheath into a vein through which at least 2 and as many as 10 electrodes are introduced. Catheters are introduced via the sheath, allowing measurement and pacing and recording of the right atrium (RV), right atrial appendage, right ventricular apex, right ventricular outflow tract, coronary sinus and the His bundle region. The left ventricle may be used if VT cannot be induced from the right ventricle (Blancher 2005).

Comprehensive guidelines and indications for an EPS have been published by the American College of Cardiology (ACC), the AHA and the Heart Rhythm Society (HRS). Indications for EPS include symptomatic patients with sinus node dysfunction, patients with conduction defects, patients with long Q-T intervals, asymptomatic patients with a family history of sudden death, unexplained palpitations, symptomatic patients with AV block, diagnosis of tachyarrhythmia, assessment of antiarrythmic drug efficacy, identification of cause of syncope following a cardiac arrest before implantable device insertion, arrhythmia mapping before and during open heart surgery and as part of the procedure of RF ablation treatment.

Patient and procedural considerations

Patients can be very apprehensive about undergoing a diagnostic EPS and so an explanation of the purpose of the procedure potential risks and benefits is essential. Education must be given by the whole team to alleviate patient concerns and to obtain an informed consent.

As in all invasive diagnostic interventions, EPS is not without risk; however, the benefit of choosing a correct treatment once a diagnosis has been obtained is of huge benefit. The patient needs to be aware that the EPS may take several hours and be quite complex and difficult for the operator to obtain the required data and that the test may be negative or equivocal. Sedation may be required if the study takes longer than normal or if the patient proceeds on to having a RF ablation.

Because many EP studies include the intention stimulation of arrhythmias which can cause haemodynamic collapse, it is imperative that emergency equipment is available and that the patient has intravenous access. Defibrillation/pacing electrodes may be placed on the patient prior to study so as not to disrupt sterile field in the event electrical defibrillation is required.

Conclusion

This chapter presents an overview of some of the more commonly used diagnostic techniques that are currently available to assess cardiac structure and function. The determination of which diagnostic procedure to use depends on the clinical condition of the patient, the preference of the patient where there is more than choice and the availability of the test. Information required, expense, availability of expertise and organisational preferences are also factors that influence the choice of procedure.

Major advancements in diagnostic testing in cardiology continue to be made and evaluation of these technologies needs to be closely monitored to ensure patients receive the best options for diagnostic testing and management.

Acknowledgements

We would like to thank Ms Sandra Pennino for reviewing the section on Echocardiography.

References

Alfakih K., Reid S., Jones T., et al. (2004). Assessment of ventricular function and mass by cardiac magnetic resonance imaging. *European Radiology*, **14**:1813–22.

American Heart Association (AHA) (2008). Chest x-ray. Retrieved online 25th August 2008 from http://www.americanheart.org/presenter.jhtml?identifier=3005143

ACC/AHA (2007). Guidelines for the management of patients with unstable angina/non-ST-elevation myocardial infarction: a report of the American College of Cardiology/American Heart Association Task Force on Practice Guidelines (Writing Committee to Revise the 2002 Guidelines for the Management of Patients With Unstable Angina/Non-ST-Elevation Myocardial Infarction): developed in collaboration with the American College of Emergency Physicians, the Society for Cardiovascular Angiography and Interventions, and the Society of Thoracic Surgeons: endorsed by the American Association of Cardiovascular and Pulmonary Rehabilitation and the Society for Academic Emergency Medicine. *Circulation*, **116**:148–304.

Baim, D.S., Knopf, W.D., Hinohara, T., et al. (2000). Suture-mediated closure of the femoral access site after cardiac catheterization: results of the suture to ambulate and discharge (STAND I and STAND II) trials. *American Journal of Cardiology*, **85**:864–9.

Blancher, S. (2005). Cardiac electrophysiology proce-
dures. In: S.L. Woods, E.S.S. Froelicher, S.U. Motzer &
E.J. Bridges (eds), *Cardiac Nursing*, 5th edn. Lippincott
Williams and Wilkins, Philadelphia, pp. 425–38.

Davies, M.K., Gibbs, C.R. & Lip, G.Y.H. (2000). ABC of
heart failure: investigation. *British Medical Journal*,
320:297–300.

Deelstra, M.H. & Jacobson, C. (2005). Cardiac catheteri-
zation. In: S.L. Woods, E.S.S. Froelicher, S.U. Motzer &
E.J. Bridges (eds), *Cardiac Nursing*, 5th edn. Lippincott
Williams and Wilkins, Philadelphia, pp. 459–77.

Dauerman, H.L., Applegate, R.J. & Cohen, D.J. (2007).
Vascular closure devices: the second decade. *Journal
of the American College of Cardiology*, **50**:1617–26.

Duong, M.H., MacKenzie, T.A. & Malenka, D.J. (2004).
N-acetylcysteine prophylaxis significantly reduces
the risk of radiocontrast-induced nephropathy:
comprehensive meta-analysis. *Catheterization and
Cardiovascular Interventions*, **64**:461–79. Retrieved
online 29th August 2008 from http://www3.
interscience.wiley.com.ezlibproxy.unisa.edu.au/
cgi-bin/fulltext/110432702/PDFSTART

Fleg, J., Gerstenblith, G., Zonderman, A., et al. (1990).
Prevalence and prognostic significance of exercise-
induced silent myocardial ischemia detected by
thallium scintigraphy and electrocardiography in
asymptomatic volunteers. *Circulation*, **81**:428–36.

Fox, K., Poole-Wilson, P. & Clayton, T. (2005). 5-year outcome of an interventional strategy in non-ST-elevation
acute coronary syndrome: the British Heart
Foundation RITA 3 randomised trial. *The Lancet*,
366:914–20.

Gimbel, J.R., Zarghami J., Machado, C. & Wilkoff, B.L.
(2005). Safe scanning, but frequent artifacts mim-
icking bradycardia and tachycardia during magnetic resonance imaging (MRI) in patients with an
implantable loop recorder (ILR). *Annals of Noninvasive
Electrocardiology*, **10**:404–8.

GUSTO Angiographic Investigators (1993). The effect
of tissue plasminogen activator, streptokinase, or
both on coronary artery patency, ventricular function
and survival after acute myocardial infarction. *New
England Journal of Medicine*, **329**:1615–22.

Hermiller, J.B., Simonton, C., Hinohara, T., et al. (2006).
The StarClose® vascular closure system: interven-
tional results from the CLIP study. *Catheterization and
Cardiovascular Interventions*, **68**:677–83.

Herring, W. (2007). *Learning Radiology: Recognizing the
Basics*. Elsevier, Philadelphia.

Hill, J. & Timmis, A. (2002). ABC of clinical electrocardiography: exercise tolerance testing. *British Medical
Journal*, **324**:1084–7.

Huseby, J.S. & Ledoux, D. (2005). Radiologic examination of the chest. In: S.L. Woods, E.S.S. Froelicher,
S.U. Motzer & E.J. Bridges (eds), *Cardiac Nursing*, 5th
edn. Lippincott Williams and Wilkins, Philadelphia,
pp. 296–306.

Kaddoura, S. (2002). *Echo Made Easy*, Vol. 1. Churchill
Livingstone, Edinburgh.

Keeley, E.C., Boura, J.A. & Grines, C.L. (2003). Primary
angioplasty versus intravenous thrombolytic therapy
for acute myocardial infarction: a quantitative review
of 23 randomised trials, *The Lancet*; **361**:13–20.

Kern, M.J., Lerman, A., Bech, J., et al. (2006). Physiological
assessment of coronary artery disease in the cardiac
catheterization laboratory: a scientific statement from the
American Heart Association Committee on Diagnostic
and Interventional Cardiac Catheterization, Council on
Clinical Cardiology. *Circulation*, **114**:1321–41. Retrieved
online 30th August 2008 from http://circ.ahajournals.
org/cgi/reprint/CIRCULATIONAHA.106.177276

Koike, A., Itoh, H. & Doi, M. (1990). Beat to beat evaluation of cardiac function during recovery from upright
bicycle exercise in patients with coronary artery disease. *American Heart Journal*, **120**:316–23.

Levine, G.N., Gomes, A.S., Arai, A.E., et al. (2007). Safety
of magnetic resonance imaging in patients with car-
diovascular devices: an American Heart Association
Scientific Statement from the Committee on Diagnostic
and Interventional Cardiac Catheterization, Council on
Clinical Cardiology, and the Council on Cardiovascular
Radiology and Intervention: endorsed by the
American College of Cardiology Foundation, the
North American Society for Cardiac Imaging, and
the Society for Cardiovascular Magnetic Resonance.
Circulation, **116**:2878–91.

Maier, E., Jensen, L., Sonnenberg, B. & Archer, S. (2008).
Interpretation of exercise stress test recordings: con-
cordance between nurse practitioner and cardiologist.
Heart Lung, **37**:144–52.

Nasu, K., Tsuchikane, E. & Sumitsuji, S. (2003). The clinical effectiveness of the Prostar® XL suture-mediated
percutaneous vascular closure device for achievement of hemostasis in patients following coronary
interventions: results of the Perclose AcceleRated
Ambulation and discharge (PARADISE) trials. *The
Journal of Invasive Cardiology*, **15**:251–6.

Olade, R. & Safi, A. (2006). Cardiac catheterization (left
heart). eMedicine. Retrieved online on 30th August 2006
from http://www.emedicine.com/MED/topic2958.htm

Pollard, S.D., Monks, K., Wales, C., et al. (2003). Position
and mobilisation post-angiography study (PAMPAS):
a comparison of 4.5 hours and 2.5 hours bed rest.
Heart, **89**:447–8.

Reading, M. (2002). Chest X-ray quiz. *Intensive and Critical Care Nursing*, **18**(2):131–2.

Raggi, P., Callister, T.Q., Cooil B., et al. (2000). Identification of patients at increased risk of first unheralded acute myocardial infarction by electron-beam computed tomography. *Circulation*, **101**:850–5.

Ryan, T., Segar, D. & Sawanda, S.G. (1993). Detection of coronary artery disease with upright bicycle echocardiography. *Journal of the American Society of Echocardiography*, **6**:186–97.

Sanborn, T.A., Gibbs, H.H., Brinker, J.A., et al. (1993). A multicenter randomized trial comparing a percutaneous collagen hemostasis device with conventional manual compression after diagnostic angiography and angioplasty. *Journal of the American College of Cardiology*, **22**:1273–9.

Scanlon, P.J., Faxon, D.P. & Audet, A. (1999). ACC/AHA guidelines for coronary angiography: executive summary and recommendations : a report of the American College of Cardiology/American Heart Association Task Force on Practice Guidelines (Committee on Coronary Angiography) developed in collaboration with the Society for Cardiac Angiography and Interventions. *Circulation*, **99**:2345–57.

Sirineni, G.K.R. & Stillman, A.E. (2007). Understanding the heart: CT and MRI for coronary heart disease. *Journal of Thoracic Imaging*, **22**:107–13.

Soine, L. & Hanrahan, M. (2005). Nuclear and other imaging studies. In: S.L. Woods, E.S.S. Froelicher, S.U. Motzer & E.J. Bridges (eds), *Cardiac Nursing*, 5th edn. Lippincott Williams and Wilkins, Philadelphia, pp. 319–25.

Strauss, H.W., Miller, D.D., Wittry, M.D., et al. (2002). *Society of Nuclear Medicine Procedure Guideline for Myocardial Perfusion Imaging*. Version 3.0, approved June 15 2002. Retrieved online on 29th August 2008 from http://interactive.snm.org/docs/pg_ch02_0403.pdf

Topol, E.J. (2007). Textbook of cardiovascular medicine. In: J. Thomas (ed.), *Cardiovascular Imaging*. Lippincott Williams & Wilkins, Philadelphia, pp. 778–91.

Wong, E.M.L., Wu, E.B., Chan, W.W.M. & Yu, C.M. (2006). A review of the management of patients after percutaneous coronary intervention. *International Journal of Clinical Practice*, **60**:582–9.

Useful Websites and Further Reading

Aroney, C., Aylward, P., Kelly, A.-M., et al. for the Acute Coronary Syndrome Guidelines Working Group (2006). Guidelines for the management of acute coronary syndromes 2006. *Medical Journal of Australia*, **184**(Suppl.):S1–30. Retrieved 15th October 2007 from http://www.mja.com.au/public/issues/184_08_170406/suppl_170406_fm.pdf (pp. S12–3)

Botti, M.A., Williamson, B. & Steen, K. (2001). Coronary angiography observations: evidence based or ritualistic practice? *Heart & Lung*, **30**:138–45.

Dauerman, H.L., Applegate, R.J. & Cohen, D.J. (2007). Vascular closure devices: the second decade. *Journal of the American College of Cardiology*, **50**. Retrieved online 30th August 2007 from http://www.medscape.com/viewarticle/563855_1

Deelstra, M.H. & Jacobson, C. (2005). Cardiac catheterization. In: S.L. Woods, E.S.S. Froelicher, S.U. Motzer & E.J. Bridges (eds), *Cardiac Nursing*, 5th edn. Lippincott Williams and Wilkins, Philadelphia, pp. 459–77.

Fulton, T.R., Peet, G.I., McGrath, M.A., et al. (2000). Effects of 3 analgesic regimens on the perception of pain after removal of femoral artery sheaths. *American Journal of Critical Care*, **9**:125–9.

Garcia, M.J. (2005). Non invasive coronary angiography: hype or new paradigm? *Journal of the American Medical Association*, **293**:2531–3.

Hogan-Miller, E., Rustad, D., Sendelbach, S. & Goldenberg, I. (1995). Effects of three methods of femoral site immobilization on bleeding and comfort after coronary angiogram. *American Journal of Critical Care*, **4**:143–8.

Levine, G.N., Berger, P.B., Cohen, D.J., et al. (2006). Newer pharmacotherapy in patients undergoing percutaneous coronary interventions: a guide for pharmacists and other health care professionals expert opinion from the American Heart Association's Diagnostic and Interventional Catheterization Committee and Council on Clinical Cardiology, and the American College of Clinical Pharmacy's Cardiology Practice Research Network. *Pharmacotherapy*, **26**:1537–56.

McCabe, P.J., McPherson, L.A., Lohse, C.M. & Weaver A.L. (2001). Evaluation of nursing care after diagnostic coronary angiogram. *American Journal of Critical Care*, **10**:330–40.

O'Rourke, R.A., Brundage, B.H., Froelicher, V.F., et al. (2000). American College of Cardiology/American Heart Association Expert Consensus document on electron-beam computed tomography for the diagnosis and prognosis of coronary artery disease. *Circulation*, **102**:126–40.

Pollard, S.D., Monks, K., Wales, C., et al. (2003). Position and mobilisation post-angiography study (PAMPAS): a comparison of 4.5 hours and 2.5 hours bed rest. *Heart*, **89**:447–8.

Reading, M. (2002). Chest X-ray quiz. *Intensive and Critical Care Nursing*, **18**:131–2.

Sanborn, T.A., Gibbs, H.H., Brinker, J.A., et al. (1993). A multicenter randomized trial comparing a percutaneous collagen haemostasis device with conventional manual compression after diagnostic angio-graphy. *Journal of the American College of Cardiology*, **22**:1273–9.

Sicari, R., Nihoyannopolous, P., Evangelista, A., et al. on behalf of the European Association of Echocardiography (2008). Stress echocardiography consensus statement. *European Journal of Echocardiography*, **9**:415–37.

Weiner, D.A., Ryan, T.J., McCabe, C.H., et al. (1979). Exercise stress testing. Correlations among history of angina, ST-segment response and prevalence of coronary-artery disease in the Coronary Artery Surgery Study (CASS). *New England Journal of Medicine*, **301**:230–235.

14 Sudden Cardiac Death

T. Quinn & P. Gregory

Overview

Sudden cardiac death (SCD), defined as death resulting from abrupt cessation of cardiac function due to cardiac arrest, is a major public health problem, accounting for more than half of deaths worldwide from cardiac disease and responsible for more deaths than stroke, lung and breast cancer, and AIDS combined each year in the United States alone (Seidl & Senges 2003). In the United Kingdom, the Department of Health (2005) has published national standards and quality markers to improve prevention, identification and management of those at risk of SCD. Crucially, these standards encompass counselling, advice, information and psychological support for both individuals and family members.

The principal risk factor for SCD is coronary heart disease (CHD), particularly in the presence of left ventricular (LV) dysfunction with reduced ejection fraction. However, there are several non-CHD conditions placing people at risk of CHD, including genetic factors and structural heart defects, and SCD can occur even if the heart is grossly normal.

Risk-reduction strategies include revascularisation for ongoing ischaemia, beta-blockade and use of implantable cardioverter defibrillators (ICDs), although this list is not exhaustive. A major aspect of care, irrespective of the identified risk factor, is the support for those identified as 'at risk' and their families; for bereaved relatives who have lost a close family member to SCD, further assessment of risk is required together with appropriate therapies and ongoing psychological support.

As this is a very large and complex subject area, it is not possible to cover all aspects in a single chapter. Only the major recommendations of international guidelines – which have considerably informed the writing of this chapter – are included, and the reader is encouraged to access full guidelines for more detailed information. ECG interpretation, arrhythmia recognition and management, and the role and modification of risk factors for cardiovascular disease are discussed elsewhere in this book. Resuscitation from cardiac arrest is discussed in detail in Chapter 15.

Learning objectives

After reading this chapter, you should be able to:

- Discuss the definition of SCD and its limitations.
- Discuss the burden of SCD on patients, their families and the wider society.
- Identify the principal risk factors for SCD.
- List the key aspects of patient assessment and risk stratification and strategies to reduce the risk of SCD.
- Discuss the support needs of 'at risk' patients and their families.

Key concepts

Sudden death; cardiac arrest; arrhythmia; congenital heart disease; structural heart disease

Definitions

The World Health Organization (WHO) defines SCD as unexpected death occurring within 1h of symptom onset (if witnessed), or within 24h of the person last being seen alive and symptom free if unwitnessed (Chugh et al. 2004). However, there is no clear consensus on this definition which is considered by some authorities to lead to misclassification, and the definition used in different epidemiological studies, and a lack of specialist cardiac pathologists, can be seen to influence findings (Zipes et al. 2006). Moreover, there is a clear need to exclude non-cardiac causes, such as acute pulmonary embolism or poisoning, where cardiac arrhythmia may well be the documented mode of death, to avoid over- (or under-) estimating the scale of the problem.

Burden of disease and risk factors for SCD

The global burden of SCD is substantial and accounts for over half of all cardiac deaths. Sudden death may be the first manifestation of underlying CHD and this is particularly the case where there is underlying LV dysfunction with reduced ejection fraction (Solomon et al. 2005). CHD may be present in over two-thirds of cases. The majority of fatal events occur in the community, and most of these in patients' homes. As the population ages and more patients survive acute myocardial infarction, the burden of chronic heart failure increases and with it the risk of SCD associated with reduced ejection fraction. There are differences between men and women, and among ethnic groups, in incidence of SCD. Patients with genetic abnormalities, such as those resulting in long QT syndrome (LQTS), account for a small fraction of the overall population at risk of SCD, but the presence of such abnormalities places the affected individual at very high risk.

Estimated incidence of SCD varies because of the heterogeneity of definitions used as discussed above (Zipes et al. 2006). Overall incidence of SCD in the United States and Europe is 1–2 per 1000 population (0.1–0.2%) annually. Incidence increases with advancing age: the risk is 100-fold less in the under 30 years age group when compared with those over 35 years (Kuisma et al. 1995; Wren 2002). There is a large preponderance of SCD in men when compared with women in young adult and early middle age because of the protection from atherosclerotic disease enjoyed by pre-menopausal women, but even so, SCD is a prominent feature in women, especially as they grow older (Kannel et al. 1998). Racial differences in SCD risk have been suggested in the United States but study findings are conflicting and inconclusive (Gillum 1997).

Comparison of risk factors for SCD with conventional risk factors for CHD and other atherosclerotic diseases has not provided useful patterns to determine individual risk (Zipes et al. 2006). However, family clustering of SCD as a specific manifestation of the disease may lead to identification of specific genetic markers in future. Hypertension is well established as a risk factor for CHD, and ECG and echocardiographic evidence of LV hypertrophy are associated with SCD, as, disproportionately, both are conduction abnormalities such as left bundle branch block (Kannel & Thomas 1982; Eriksson et al. 2005; Wachtell et al. 2007). Meaningful associations with SCD have been seen with other CHD risk factors such as tobacco smoking, obesity and diabetes (Kannel & Thomas 1982). A disproportionate number of SCD events occur in those least physically active individuals performing unaccustomed physical activity. Strategies to reduce SCD risk, including screening before undertaking unaccustomed activity, training gym and other sports personnel in recognition of symptoms and resuscitation, and advising avoidance of high-risk activities, require further study (Thompson et al. 2007).

Social and economic stress has been shown to increase the risk of a coronary event and this is said to be particularly striking in relation to SCD. Behavioural and emotional factors are probable triggers of events in vulnerable individuals, although precise mechanisms and strategies to reduce risk are not yet fully understood (Strike & Steptoe 2005).

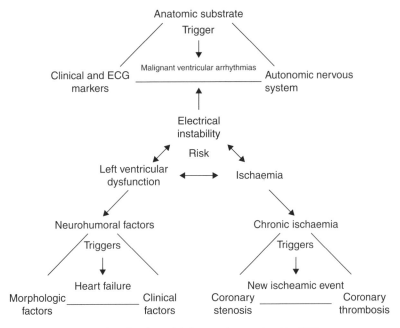

Interplay of various risk factors that can lead to SCD

Figure 14.1   Interplay of risk factors for SCD.
Source: Reprinted with permission from eMedicine.com (2008). Available at http://emedicine.medscape.com/article/151907-overview

The interplay of risk factors for SCD is shown in Figure 14.1. Risk factors and prevention of cardiovascular disease are discussed in more detail in Chapter 5.

Sudden death in the young (including athletes)

Sudden cardiac death is rare in infants, children, adolescents and young adults, but still amounts to many thousands of deaths each year in those under 20 years of age. Athletes are widely regarded as being the epitome of health because of their physical achievements (Basavarajaiah et al. 2007). Despite this, there is a recognised incidence of sudden death in athletes, often highly publicised. The precise incidence is unknown but estimated at 1–2 in 200,000. In athletes aged over 35 years, SCD is most commonly due to CHD. In younger athletes, however, most SCD is attributed to inherent or congenital disorders of the heart that predispose to ventricular arrhythmias. In these younger patients, it is suggested on the

basis of a relatively small study of 158 American athletes by Maron et al. (1996) that death occurs in adolescence (mean age 17.1 years), more often in young black athletes and during or soon after physical exertion. Most deaths in this series were due to inherited cardiomyopathies, with hypertrophic cardiomyopathy (HCM) accounting for up to a third of sudden deaths (Maron et al. 1996); conversely, data from an Italian registry suggest arrhythmogenic right ventricular cardiomyopathy (ARVC) is the most common cause (Thiene et al. 1988). SCD may also result from coronary artery anomalies and acquired causes such as commotio cordis, myocarditis, substance misuse and trauma.

Key point

Identifying the athlete with a cardiac disorder can help to prevent SCD. Major sporting bodies, such as football teams at national and international level, have screening programmes engaging centres of excellence in the diagnosis and treatment of inherited cardiac disorders. In Italy, a screening programme provides mandatory 12-lead ECG annually together with a limited exercise tolerance test. In the United States, pre-participation screening involving a health questionnaire and physical examination is insensitive but said to be cost-effective. In one UK series, the vast majority (more than 80%) of athletes with potentially serious disorders were completely asymptomatic (Basavarajaiah et al. 2007).

While there have been major advances in genetics in the past two decades, a genetic diagnosis is possible currently in less than two-thirds of cases of HCM and even less in congenital LQTS. Diagnosis continues to rely largely on clinical investigations. Aortic stenosis and some patients with HCM can be identified by auscultation, although this alone is somewhat limited. The 12-lead ECG is non-specific if abnormal in 90% of those with heart muscle disorders but can help to identify pre-excitation, Brugada syndrome and LQTS. The exercise ECG lacks sensitivity for myocardial ischaemia in patients with suspected coronary anomalies, but is considered useful in risk stratification in HCM and in suspected LQTS. Echocardiography is regarded as the 'gold standard' investigation in practical terms, but coronary angiography and/or magnetic resonance imaging may also be required subsequently (Zipes et al. 2006).

Structural abnormalities

Studies of survivors of 'aborted' SCD show apparently normal hearts in 5–10%, but the overwhelming majority have cardiac pathology including CHD. At autopsy, most patients with SCD have hypertrophy or scarring, serving as substrate for lethal arrhythmias. Farb and colleagues (1995) reported active coronary lesions at autopsy in around half of SCD cases where myocardial scarring was found in the absence of acute infarction.

Where ventricular arrhythmias are associated with LV dysfunction following myocardial infarction, aggressive management of heart failure and ischaemia, including coronary revascularization, are warranted. Electrophysiological (EP) testing may be warranted if arrhythmias persist following correction of ischaemia. Where revascularisation is not possible (because of anatomy, for instance), then ICDs are considered primary therapy to reduce the risk of SCD in those patients on optimal medical treatment and expected to survive for a year or more with good functional status (Zipes et al. 2006). Decisions about the precise treatment are based on individual characteristics, including whether arrhythmias are sustained, and clinical manifestations of the tachycardia. Those with sustained ventricular tachycardia (VT) that does not precipitate cardiac arrest or severe haemodynamic instability may be at relatively low risk (2% per annum) of SCD (Sarter et al. 1996).

Arrhythmias

The most common electrical event associated with SCD is ventricular fibrillation (VF), often preceded by VT. Since most SCD occurs in the non-monitored patient, the mechanism can only be inferred from limited retrospective series. In a classic report from Bayés de Luna and colleagues (1989), 157 patients had SCD while undergoing ambulatory ECG monitoring. Of these, 8% had primary VF, 62% VT/VF, 13% polymorphic VT or torsades de pointes and 16% bradycardia. Increased premature ventricular beats, preceding the terminal arrhythmia, were observed in 70% of patients, and ST-segment changes associated with myocardial ischaemia were seen in 13%.

In older patients, and those with heart failure, the primary electrical event may be pulseless electrical activity (PEA), (formerly called electromechanical dissociation) or severe bradyarrhythmia. Luu et al. (1989) reported, in contrast to Bayés de Luna et al.'s (1989) observation of VT/VF as the predominant arrhythmia, that hospitalised patients in heart failure were more likely to have non-VT/VF, with 62% suffering severe bradycardia or PEA, and 38% VT/VF. More recently, important insights have been gained from the interrogation of ICDs, with lethal arrhythmias accounting for 20–35% of SCD, and post-shock PEA being a frequent occurrence (Mitchell et al. 2002). These data may be a reflection of the mode of death in the ICD population, who often have underlying poor LV function.

Key point

In out-of-hospital cardiac arrest, asystole may often be the first rhythm observed, but this is probably a marker of the duration of the arrest and delay in getting an ambulance to the patient, rather than an indication of the primary arrhythmia.

Recognition and management of important cardiac arrhythmias are covered in Chapter 23.

Cardiomyopathies and SCD

Dilated cardiomyopathy

Around a third of deaths from dilated cardiomyopathy (DCM) are due to SCD. Incidence of SCD is highest in older patients, and those with more advanced disease and VT/VF are considered common mechanisms for SCD, although as with other patients with heart failure, bradyarrhythmias and PEA account for a significant proportion of deaths. EP testing plays a minor role in risk stratification because of its low predictive value (Grimm et al. 1998). Management is guided by individual features and physician experience (Zipes et al. 2006). Beta-blockers and angiotensin-converting enzyme (ACE) inhibitors may help to reduce SCD risk. ICD therapy is recommended for non-ischaemic DCM patients who have sustained VT or VF (secondary prevention) and those with poor LV function (primary prevention), on optimal medical therapy and expected to survive for a year or more with good functional status (Zipes et al. 2006).

Hypertrophic cardiomyopathy

In a large unselected population community study, HCM was found to be a benign disease with a low incidence (0.6% annually) of SCD (Kofflard et al. 2003). SCD is, however, often the first manifestation of HCM and is usually related to ventricular arrhythmias triggered by ischaemia, obstruction or atrial fibrillation. Risk factors for SCD in this group include family history of SCD, unexplained syncope, abnormal (hypotensive) blood pressure at exercise and echocardiographic evidence

of LV thickness greater than 30 mm together with documented spontaneous VT (whether or not sustained). Risk of SCD is directly related to LV wall thickness (Kofflard et al. 2003). While medical treatment alone does not prevent disease progression (and is not indicated therefore in asymptomatic patients), and no randomised trials of ICD use have demonstrated efficacy in reducing SCD, patients with multiple risk factors are considered at sufficient risk to 'merit consideration' of ICD (Zipes et al. 2006). Genetic testing may contribute to risk stratification and counselling of relatives.

Arrhythmogenic right ventricular cardiomyopathy

Arrhythmogenic right ventricular cardiomyopathy (AVRC), sometimes known as arrhythmogenic right ventricular dysplasia, is typically seen in young men and associated with syncope, pre-syncope and sometimes biventricular failure. As with other conditions, SCD is often the first manifestation, frequently occurring during stress or exertion. Incidence varies from 0.08% to 9% per annum. The ECG may show T-wave inversion in the precordial leads with wide QRS complexes. The role of EP testing in prognostication is unclear, and studies to date of both investigation and management (including medication and ICD use) have been small, therefore the evidence base is limited. Transplantation and ventricular assist devices may be required for patients with severe biventricular failure (Zipes et al. 2006).

Genetic syndromes and SCD

Brugada syndrome

The Brugada syndrome was first described in 1953, but discovery of its genetic basis followed identification by Brugada and Brugada (1992) of a cohort of patients with the characteristically abnormal ECG and high risk for SCD with a structurally normal heart. The syndrome is rare, having a prevalence of less than 5 in 10,000. The ECG in Brugada typically shows incomplete right bundle branch block (RBBB) with ST-segment elevation in leads V1–V3, although there have been reports of

ST-segment elevation in inferior leads. The ECG pattern can be present intermittently, possibly reflecting sporadic periods of vulnerability to SCD. ST-segment elevation can occur spontaneously or be revealed by the administration of drugs such as flecainide, procainamide or ajmaline; those with spontaneously occurring ST-segment elevation are regarded as having a worse prognosis. Patients who have experienced syncope and have spontaneous ECG changes have a sixfold higher risk of cardiac arrest.

Key point

Brugada Syndrome is inherited with autosomal dominance pattern, meaning that men and women are equally likely to inherit the genetic mutation. Clinical expression of the phenotype, however, is modified by gender: 90% of those affected with a diagnostic ECG are men. Syncope or cardiac arrest occurs predominantly in men in their 30s or 40s, often with fever as a predisposing factor. There are reports of cardiac arrest in neonates and children.

Identification of those at risk is highly dependent on symptoms, including syncope, spontaneous ST-segment elevation or sustained ventricular arrhythmia and family history of SCD. However, it is important to note that those without a family history are not at reduced risk, nor are family members of a victim of SCD necessarily at increased risk. The value of EP testing is a matter of debate. The role of genetic testing in determining prognosis is unclear, although analysis might identify silent carriers who can then be closely monitored and counselled (Zipes et al. 2006).

Long QT syndrome

Long QT syndrome is an inherited disease characterised by prolonged ventricular repolarisation and ventricular tachyarrhythmias that can manifest as syncope or SCD (Zipes et al. 2006). The condition can manifest at any age (first to sixth decades) with the average age of 'onset' being 12 years. Arrhythmias may be provoked by stress,

exertion (including swimming) and emotion, but can also occur during sleep (Schwartz et al. 2001).

Of the two identified patterns of inheritance for LQTS, the autosomal dominant syndromes (Romano–Ward and Timothy syndromes) are more common than the often more severe autosomal recessive syndrome (Jervell Lange-Nielsen syndrome). There are eight genetic variants of the disease and these are used alongside factors such as gender and QT interval to inform risk stratification.

Key point

Presentations of LQTS range from near-syncope to syncope and SCD, with the average age of first manifestation being 12 years. Survivors of SCD have a poor outlook with relative risk of further cardiac arrest. Syncope is mostly (but not exclusively) due to malignant ventricular tachyarrhythmias. Torsades de pointes has been identified when ECG monitoring has been available at the time of an attack.

Individuals with LQTS are advised to avoid competitive sports and, for those with the LQT1 form, swimming should only be undertaken with close supervision, if not avoided altogether. Those with LQT2 should be advised to avoid sudden noises such as telephones and alarm clocks. Medications known to prolong QT interval or potassium/magnesium depletion should also be avoided. Beta-blockers may be useful on empiric grounds as prophylaxis against life-threatening arrhythmias (Zipes et al. 2006).

An acquired form of LQTS is well recognised. Drug-induced torsades de pointes is a rare, but potentially lethal, side effect of some commonly prescribed drugs, including many non-cardiac agents such as antihistamines, antipsychotics and some antibiotics (Fitzgerald & Ackerman 2005). There is also evidence that genetic differences in drug metabolism may be a risk factor for acquired LQTS, especially if multiple drugs are involved (Aerssens & Paulussen 2005). Causes for acquired LQTS are shown in Table 14.1.

Table14.1   Causes of acquired LQTS (Sovari 2006).

Drugs	Some drugs can cause LQTS, notably class 1a and III antiarrhythmics
Electrolyte abnormalities	Hypokalaemia, hypomagnesaemia and hypocalcaemia
Cerebrovascular diseases	Intracranial and subarachnoid haemorrhages, stroke and intracranial trauma
Altered nutritional states	Nutritional deficiencies associated with modified starvation diets
	In patients who are obese and on severe weight-loss programmes
Other	Hypothyroidism Altered autonomic status Lesions in the hypothalamus

Conclusion

Sudden Cardiac Death (SCD) is a major public health problem and associated with tragedy affecting hundreds of thousands of individuals and families. While most SCDs are associated with CHD, there are many rarer, but important, associated conditions placing individuals at risk. The evidence base for risk stratification (often based on genetics) and treatment (increasingly involving implantable devices) has grown in recent years. More work is needed to improve access to early diagnosis and treatment, and to appropriate support for individuals and their families.

Learning activity

Does your region have a service aimed at screening athletes for risk factors for SCD? If yes, locate its website and review its referral criteria.

What kind of support is available locally for relatives of patients who have suffered SCD? Identify such support systems, review their websites and discuss with colleagues how best to make use of such services in your practice.

References

Aerssens, J. & Paulussen, A.D. (2005). Pharmacogenomics and acquired long QT syndrome. *Pharmacogenomics*, **6**:259–70.

Basavarajaiah, S., Shah, A. & Sharma, S. (2007). Sudden cardiac death in young athletes. *Heart*, **93**:287–9.

Bayés de Luna, A., Coumel, P. & Leclercq, J.F. (1989). Ambulatory sudden cardiac death: mechanisms of production of fatal arrhythmia on the basis of data from 157 cases. *American Heart Journal*, **117**:151–9.

Brugada, P. & Brugada, J. (1992). Right bundle branch block, persistent ST segment elevation and sudden cardiac death: a distinct clinical and electrocardiographic syndrome. A multicenter report. *Journal of the American College of Cardiology*, **20**:1391–6.

Chugh, S.S., Jui, J., Gunson, K., et al. (2004). Current burden of sudden cardiac death: multiple source surveillance versus retrospective death certificate-based review in a large U.S. community. *Journal of the American College of Cardiology*, **44**:1268–75.

Department of Health (2005). National service framework for coronary heart disease. Chapter 8: Arrhythmias and sudden cardiac death. London. Retrieved online 7th September 2008 from http://www.dh.gov.uk/en/Healthcare/NationalService Frameworks/Coronaryheartdisease/DH_4117048

Eriksson, P., Wilhelmsen, L. & Rosengren, A. (2005). Bundle branch block in middle-aged men: risk of complications and death over 28 years. The primary prevention study in Goteberg, Sweden. *European Heart Journal*, **26**:2300–6.

Farb, A., Tang, A.L., Burke, A.P., Sessums, L., Liang, Y. & Virmani, R. (1995). Sudden coronary death. Frequency of active coronary lesions, inactive coronary lesions, and myocardial infarction. *Circulation*, **92**:1701–9.

Fitzgerald, P.T. & Ackerman, M.J. (2005). Drug-induced torsades de pointes: the evolving role of pharmacogenetics. *Heart Rhythm*, **2**(Suppl.):S30–7.

Gillum, R.F. (1997). Sudden cardiac death in Hispanic Americans and African Americans. *American Journal of Public Health*, **87**:1461–6.

Grimm, W., Hoffmann, J., Menz, V., Luck, K. & Maisch, B. (1998). Programmed ventricular stimulation for arrhythmia risk prediction in patients with idiopathic dilated cardiomyopathy and nonsustained ventricular tachycardia. *Journal of the American College of Cardiology*, **32**:739–45.

Kannel, W.B. & Thomas, H.E. (1982). Sudden coronary death: the Framingham Study. *Annals of the New York Academy of Science*, **382**:3–21.

Kannel, W.B., Wilson, P.W., D'Agostino, R.B. & Cobb, J. (1998). Sudden coronary death in women. *American Heart Journal*, **136**:205–12.

Kofflard, M.J., Ten Cate, F.J., van der Lee, C & van Domburg, R.T. (2003). Hypertrophic cardiomyopathy in a large community-based population: clinical outcome and identification of risk factors for sudden cardiac death and clinical deterioration. *Journal of the American College of Cardiology*, **41**:987–93.

Kuisma, M., Suominen, P. & Korpela, R. (1995). Paediatric out-of-hospital cardiac arrests – epidemiology and outcome. *Resuscitation*, **30**:141–50.

Luu, M., Stevenson, W.G., Stevenson, L.W., Baron, K. & Walden, J. (1989). Diverse mechanisms of unexpected cardiac arrest in advanced heart failure. *Circulation*, **80**:1675–80.

Maron, B.J., Shirani, J., Poliac, L.C., Mathenge, R., Roberts, W.C. & Mueller, F.O. (1996). Sudden death in young competitive athletes. Clinical, demographic, and pathological profiles. *Journal of the American Medical Association*, **276**:199–204.

Mitchell, L.B., Pineda, E.A., Titus, J.L., Bartosch, P.M. & Benditt, D.G. (2002). Sudden death in patients with implantable cardioverter defibrillators: the importance of post-shock electromechanical dissociation. *Journal of the American College of Cardiology*, **39**:1323–8.

Sarter, B.H., Finkle, J.K., Gerszeten, R.E. & Buxton, A.E. (1996). What is the risk of sudden cardiac death in patients presenting with hemodynamically stable sustained ventricular tachycardia after myocardial infarction? *Journal of the American College of Cardiology*, **28**:122–9.

Schwartz, P.J., Priori, S.G., Spazzolini, C., et al. (2001). Genotype–phenotype correlation in the long-QT syndrome: gene-specific triggers for life-threatening arrhythmias. *Circulation*, **103**:89–95.

Seidl, K. & Senges, J. (2003). Worldwide utilization of implantable cardioverter/defibrillators now and in the future. *Cardiac Electrophysiology Review*, 7:5–13.

Solomon, S.D., Anavekar, N., Skali, H., et al. for the Candesartan in Heart Failure Reduction in Mortality (CHARM) Investigators (2005). Influence of ejection fraction on cardiovascular outcomes in a broad spectrum of heart failure patients. *Circulation*, **112**:3738–44.

Sovari, A.A. (2006). Sudden cardiac death. *eMedicine*. Retrieved online 7th September 2008 from http://www.emedicine.com/med/TOPIC276.HTM

Strike, P.C. & Steptoe, A. (2005). Behavioral and emotional triggers of acute coronary syndromes: a systematic review and critique. *Psychosomatic Medicine*, **67**:179–86.

Thiene, G., Nava, A., Corrado, D., Rossi, L. & Pennelli, N. (1988). Right ventricular cardiomyopathy and sudden death in young people. *New England Journal of Medicine*, **318**:129–33.

Thompson, P.D., Franklin, B.A., Balady, G.J., et al. (2007). Exercise and acute cardiovascular events placing the risks into perspective: a scientific statement from the American Heart Association Council on Nutrition, Physical Activity, and Metabolism and the Council on Clinical Cardiology. *Circulation*, **115**:2358–68.

Wachtell, K., Okin, P.M., Olsen, M.H., et al. (2007). Regression of electrocardiographic left ventricular hypertrophy during antihypertensive therapy and reduction in sudden cardiac death: the LIFE Study. *Circulation*, **116**:700–5.

Wren, C. (2002). Sudden death in children and adolescents. *Heart*, **88**:426–31.

Zipes, D.P., Camm, A.J., Borggrefe, M., et al. (2006). ACC/AHA/ESC 2006 guidelines for management of patients with ventricular arrhythmias and the prevention of sudden cardiac death: a report of the American College of Cardiology/American Heart Association Task Force and the European Society of Cardiology Committee for Practice Guidelines (Writing committee to develop guidelines for management of patients with ventricular arrhythmias and the prevention of sudden cardiac death). *Europace*, **8**:746–837.

Useful Websites and Further Reading

Arrhythmia Alliance: http://www.arrhythmiaalliance.org.uk/

Australian Sudden Arrhythmia Deaths Syndrome (SADS) Foundation: http://www.sads.org.au/

Cardiac Risk in the Young: http://www.c-r-y.org.uk/aims.htm

Department of Health, England:http://www.dh.gov.uk/en/Policyandguidance/Healthandsocialcaretopics/Coronaryheartdisease/DH_4117048

National Institute for Health and Clinical Evidence: http://www.nice.org.uk/nicemedia/pdf/word/TA095guidance.doc

National Library for Health: www.library.nhs.uk/cardiovascular

Sovari, A.A. (2006). Sudden cardiac death. *eMedicine*. Retrieved online 7th September 2008 from http://www.emedicine.com/med/TOPIC276.HTM

15 Out-of-Hospital Cardiac Arrest and Automated External Defibrillation

P. Gregory & T. Quinn

Overview

Out-of-hospital cardiac arrest (OHCA) is a major public health problem that incurs significant mortality. Successful resuscitation of victims of OHCA depends upon factors such as associated medical conditions, cardiac rhythm associated with the arrest, whether or not the collapse was witnessed and systems in the community to deal with OHCA (Meyer et al. 2000). Strategies to improve survival from OHCA include education to raise community awareness and response to OHCA. The 'chain of survival' approach has been adopted by many communities; this seeks to promote early recognition and notification of emergency services, early initiation of cardiopulmonary resuscitation (CPR), early defibrillation and early advanced care. The proliferation of automated external defibrillators (AED) in public areas is improving survival from OHCA.

This chapter will cover the major recommendations of international guidelines as they relate to basic life support (BLS, including AED use) in OHCA. The reader is encouraged to access full guidelines for more detailed information, since national guidelines may differ.

Learning objectives

After reading this chapter, you should be able to:

- Establish the aetiology and burden of OHCA.
- Identify hazards to the victim and the rescuer and discuss circumstances that make management of OHCA different to in-hospital resuscitation.
- Recognise cardiac arrest and examine the procedures for performing BLS.
- Establish the value of early defibrillation in the management of ventricular fibrillation (VF) and pulseless ventricular tachycardia (VT).
- Discuss the principles and factors affecting defibrillation.

Key concepts

Prehospital care; basic life support; cardiopulmonary resuscitation; airway management; automated external defibrillation

Out-of-hospital cardiac arrest

OHCA is a major public health problem that accounts for 250,000–350,000 deaths annually in the United States (Sanna et al. 2008) and around 74,000 deaths per annum in the United Kingdom (Norris 1999). About 74% of cardiac arrests occur outside the hospital environment (Norris 1999) and the chances of survival vary according to the availability and quality of interventions carried out immediately following the cardiac arrest. For example, bystander CPR can double or triple survival rates from VF (Larsen et al. 1993; Holmberg et al. 2001) whilst CPR with early prehospital defibrillation can produce survival rates of between 49% and 75% (Handley et al. 2005).

OHCA may be present as asystole, VF, pulseless VT or pulseless electrical activity (PEA) (Nolan et al. 2006). The prognosis for both asystole and PEA is poor despite advanced life support (ALS), but both VF and pulseless VT (which account for between 41% and 70% of cases), can be terminated by defibrillation (Kuisma et al. 2001; Cobb et al. 2002). It has been shown that the time to the first defibrillation shock is a key predictor of outcome with chances of survival to discharge falling by 10–15% for every minute of delay to defibrillation (Weaver et al. 1988; Valenzuela et al. 1997). Unsurprisingly, delays in the initiation of both BLS and ALS have been shown to affect the outcome from prehospital cardiac arrest negatively (Vukmir 2006).

Hazards to the victim and rescuer

Out-of-hospital cardiac arrest differs significantly from in-hospital cardiac arrest in terms of risks to the rescuer and the resources available. These differences need to be considered when managing a cardiac arrest, as failure to do so can lead to suboptimal patient management and unnecessary risk-taking by the practitioner. The practitioner should ensure their own safety, the safety of the patient and the safety of bystanders.

Risks to the rescuer

Perhaps the hazard of greatest concern to the potential rescuer is the perceived risk of infection from performing CPR. There are very few documented cases of rescuers suffering adverse reactions from performing CPR, and only isolated reports of transmission of tuberculosis and severe acute respiratory syndrome (SARS) and no reported incidence of HIV transmission (Handley et al. 2005). Wherever possible, appropriate precautions should be taken to isolate body fluids and related substances; this may necessitate the wearing of impermeable gloves and the use of a pocket mask for artificial ventilation. Where it is known that the patient has a serious infection and full protective precautions are not available, or where the patient has been exposed to poisons such as hydrogen cyanide, mouth-to-mouth should be avoided. It is also imperative that contact with hazardous substances, such as corrosives or poisons that are readily absorbed through the skin, has to be avoided.

Scene safety

Ensuring that the scene is as free from hazards and dangers as possible is always the first step in the management of OHCA and should be a conscious element of the approach to any casualty. A rescuer who becomes injured is less able to help the patient and is likely to increase the work of the Emergency Medical Services (EMS). It may not be possible to eliminate all dangers, so the risks should be assessed and reduced to a level that is acceptable to the individual rescuer. Risk assessment is a very personal assessment and the degree of acceptable risk will vary according to factors such as health care experience (particularly out-of-hospital experience), gender, and age. If the risks cannot be eliminated or brought within the rescuer's own personal scope of safety, then the patient should not be approached and further assistance should be sought. Risk is a fluid situation and circumstances may change; it is essential that the rescuer ensures that there is safe egress from the scene if the risk level increases.

Risks may be inherent in the environment, related to the patient or bystanders on scene, or to the treatments that need to be administered; a few examples are given below.

Environmental hazards

Potential hazards include traffic, gas leaks, electricity, poisons, trip hazards, confined spaces, pets and weather.

Patient/bystander hazards

Occasionally there may be the risk of violence from persons at the scene. This may be related to the stress of the situation, drug or alcohol intoxication, mental illness or another less obvious cause.

Hazards associated with treatment

Defibrillation is a potentially hazardous intervention that may result in injury to any person on scene; it is essential that all appropriate safety procedures are applied when carrying out defibrillation. In addition, it may be necessary to move the patient in order to place them on a firm, flat surface, which produces a risk of injury to both rescuer and patient.

Key point

Advice on manual handling in cardiac arrest can be found at http://www.resus.org.uk/pages/safehand.pdf

---

Circumstances that make OHCA different from hospital resuscitation

Delay

In a hospital, recognition of cardiac arrest and arrival of personnel skilled in resuscitation presents challenges, but these are less complex than for OHCA, where emergency personnel may have to travel several miles to the patient, inevitably delaying definitive treatment. For this reason, guidelines on OHCA management differ in some respects from in-hospital resuscitation. An important difference is in the recommendation that OHCA patients who have not received bystander CPR prior to arrival of the emergency services (or rescuer equipped with a defibrillator) should receive BLS from the trained responder prior to rhythm analysis. This recommendation is based on evidence that survival rates are higher with this strategy compared to immediate defibrillation in a patient who has several minutes 'down time' without CPR before defibrillation is attempted (Cobb et al. 1999).

Resource issues

In OHCA, a nurse may be the only person available with a health care or first aid background and, in such circumstances, will be expected to take the lead in patient management. The problems associated with management of OHCA are often compounded by a lack of the equipment normally available in hospital. It may be that little more than a pocket mask is available or, in many cases, no equipment at all prior to the arrival of emergency services. In order to manage the situation effectively, an action plan is required to overcome these problems.

Learning activity

Create an action plan of how you will manage an OHCA using only the equipment you would normally have with you. Consider the following points:

What considerations would you need to give to ensuring scene safety?

Who you would call and when you would call them – how would you manage if you were in an area with poor mobile phone reception?

How would you manage the airway; what if the patient had vomited?

What are the risks of infection associated with mouth-to-mouth ventilation?

Do you have a pocket mask?

How would you minimise the interruptions to chest compressions?

Recognition of cardiac arrest and BLS

The sequence used for recognition of cardiac arrest will be dependent upon the rescuer's level of training and their experience of assessing respiration and circulation in sick patients. Checking the carotid pulse has been shown to be inaccurate as a method of assessing circulation (Bahr et al. 1997) and it has been demonstrated that health care professionals, as well as lay people, have difficulty in determining the presence or absence of adequate breathing. It should be noted that agonal breathing (described as occasional gasps, slow, laboured or noisy breathing) (Clark et al. 1992) occurs in up to 40% of cardiac arrest cases (Handley et al. 2005) and should not be mistaken for normal respirations.

> **Key point**
>
> Current guidelines suggest that resuscitation should be commenced in an unconscious patient who is not breathing normally (Handley et al. 2005).

Basic life support is a key skill in which every health care professional should be adept. Chest compressions and ventilation of the patient's lungs slow down the rate of deterioration and significantly extend the period for successful resuscitation (Nolan et al. 2006). In addition, CPR increases the likelihood that a shock delivered by a defibrillator will terminate VF and that the heart will resume an effective rhythm after defibrillation, especially where time to shock delivery exceeds 4 min (Cobb et al. 1999). This section is not intended to teach BLS procedures; rather it is designed to provide a rationale for the actions to be taken. The reader is advised to access the published guidelines.

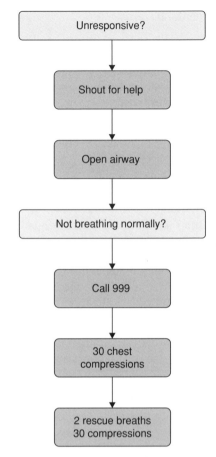

Figure 15.1   Basic life-support algorithm.
Source: From Resuscitation Council UK *2005 Resuscitation Guidelines*.

> **Learning activity**
>
> Basic life-support algorithms from the Resuscitation Council (UK) and the Australian Resuscitation Council are shown in Figures 15.1 and 15.2 respectively. Observe the differences between the two.

> **Key point**
>
> Interruptions in chest compressions have been shown to adversely affect the outcome for patients in cardiac arrest (Eftestol et al. 2002); hence the focus of CPR should be on minimising gaps between compressions.

Continuous compressions can be applied when advanced airway management techniques are available but these are often not accessible in OHCA. Where advanced airway management is not available, effort should be made to resume compressions as quickly as possible; this can be facilitated by:

- Giving rescue breaths over 1 s to reduce delay between compressions
- Placing hands in the centre of the chest rather than measuring for correct position
- Using a ratio of 30:2 compressions:ventilations
- Commencing chest compressions immediately after cardiac arrest is established (in the adult patient) (Resuscitation Council [UK] 2005a)

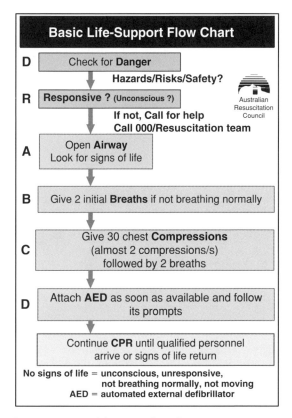

Basic Life-Support Flow Chart

D   Check for **Danger**
    Hazards/Risks/Safety?

Australian
Resuscitation
Council

R   **Responsive ?** (Unconscious ?)
    If not, Call for help
    Call 000/Resuscitation team

A   Open **Airway**
    Look for signs of life

B   Give 2 initial **Breaths** if not breathing normally

C   Give 30 chest **Compressions**
    (almost 2 compressions/s)
    followed by 2 breaths

D   Attach **AED** as soon as available and follow
    its prompts

    Continue **CPR** until qualified personnel
    arrive or signs of life return

No signs of life = **unconscious, unresponsive,**
                   not breathing normally, not moving
          AED = **automated external defibrillator**

Figure 15.2   Basic life-support flow chart.
Source: Copyright Australian Resuscitation Council.

Key point

It has been suggested that compression-only CPR may be effective in eliminating pauses and may be useful for those not wishing to use a mouth-to-mouth technique; however, it is believed that this may only be viable for a period of up to 5 min (Hallstrom et al. 2000) and should not be used routinely by health care professionals.

Automated external defibrillation

Ventricular fibrillation is the most common initial rhythm in OHCA (Kuisma et al. 2001) and has a significantly better outcome than any other cardiac arrest arrhythmia. One large study evaluated over 18,000 victims of OHCA and established survival rates of 10.7% for all rhythm and 21.2% for VF

cardiac arrest (Atwood et al. 2005). The only effective therapy for cardiac arrest caused by VF is the early application of defibrillation which, if applied within 3–5 min of collapse can produce survival rates as high as 49–75% (Handley et al. 2005). The survival benefit to be gained by those treated with CPR plus AED compared with those treated with CPR alone is significant and it is suggested that benefit could be gained by developing public health strategies based on AED use by trained lay-rescuers (Marenco et al. 2001; Capucci et al. 2002; Sanna et al. 2008). Health care professionals should consider the use of an AED as being integral to BLS (Resuscitation Council [UK], 2005b).

Defibrillation is commonly available in EMS systems across the developed world. As CPR and defibrillation need to be administered as early as possible to maximise chances of survival, it is incumbent upon bystanders and health professionals to initiate the opening links of the 'chain of survival'. AEDs use voice and visual prompts to guide the practitioner in the delivery of defibrillatory shocks to patients in cardiac arrest as a result of VF or pulseless VT. They have become more sophisticated and safer over recent years and are suitable for use by lay people as well as health care professionals.

Factors affecting defibrillation

Transthoracic impedance

Transthoracic impedance is the resistance to the passage of electricity created by the chest; it is a key factor in determining the amount of energy that passes through the myocardium during defibrillation. The greater the impedance, the less energy is delivered to the myocardium, which reduces the chances of successful defibrillation. Transthoracic impedance is influenced by factors such as the contact between skin and pad, the size of the pad and the phase of ventilation.

Contact between pad and skin

Chest hair will interfere with electrical contact but hair should be shaved only if excessive, to reduce delay in shock delivery. Often a razor is kept with the AED, but if no razor is immediately available, defibrillation should not be delayed to find one.

Pad position

Successful defibrillation is achieved by the passage of an electrical current between two external electrodes, resulting in a current of sufficient magnitude to defibrillate a critical mass of myocardium. The sternal pad is normally placed to the right of the sternum just below the border of the clavicle; the apical pad should be placed in the mid-axillary line approximately level with the V6 ECG electrode position (Figure 15.3) (Resuscitation Council [UK] 2005b). It is important that the position used is clear of breast tissue; in large-breasted patients it is acceptable to place the apical pad lateral to or underneath the left breast (ILCOR 2005). A further recommendation is that the apical pad be placed in a longitudinal rather than transverse position (Figure 15.4) (Deakin et al. 2003). Most AED defibrillation pads carry a diagram indicating recommended placement. It is not important if the pads are placed in reverse positions.

All new defibrillators deliver shocks using a biphasic waveform, which means that the current

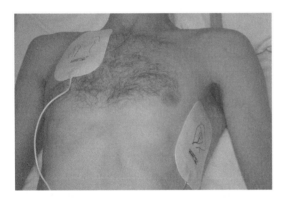

Figure 15.3   Position of the sternal and apical pad.

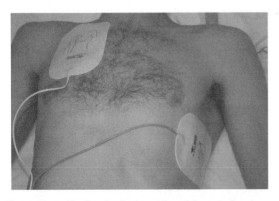

Figure 15.4   The longitudinal position of the apical pad.

flows initially in a positive direction and then, after a predetermined time reverses to a negative direction. Defibrillation energy is predetermined when using an AED, so should not cause any concerns for the rescuer.

Even when all of the above factors are optimal, the survival chances of the victim will be heavily influenced by the delay between defibrillation and recommencement of chest compressions. Two studies have shown a mean postshock delay of 38s between defibrillation and restarting compressions (van Alem et al. 2003; Berg et al. 2005). The use of AEDs will inevitably involve a period of delay whilst rhythms are being analysed but human factors are also associated with postshock delay and should be eliminated from the process. As soon as defibrillation has been delivered, chest compressions should be restarted immediately, irrespective of changes observed in the cardiac rhythm.

Conclusion

Out-of-hospital cardiac arrest is a major public health problem that affects hundreds of thousands of people each year. Programmes that incorporate early BLS and the use of an AED are starting to show significant benefit in terms of survival to discharge from hospital. Health professionals should be competent in performing BLS, should have a strategy for managing OHCA and should be proficient in the use of an AED.

References

van Alem, A.P., Sanou, B.T. & Koster, R.W. (2003). Interruption of cardiopulmonary resuscitation with the use of the automated external defibrillator in out-of-hospital cardiac arrest. *Annals of Emergency Medicine*, **42**:449–57.

Atwood, C., Eisenberg, M.S., Herlitz, J. & Rea, T.D. (2005). Incidence of EMS-treated out-of-hospital cardiac arrest in Europe. *Resuscitation*, **67**:75–80.

Bahr, J., Klingler, H., Panzer, W., et al. (1997). Skills of lay people in checking the carotid pulse. *Resuscitation*, **35**:23–6.

Berg, M.D., Clark, L.L., Valenzuela, T.D., et al. (2005). Post-shock chest compression delays with automated external defibrillator use. *Resuscitation*, **64**:287–91.

Capucci, A., Aschieri, D., Piepoli, M.F., et al. (2002). Tripling survival from sudden cardiac arrest via early defibrillation without traditional education in cardiopulmonary resuscitation. *Circulation*, 106:1065–70.

Clark, J.J., Larsen, M.P., Culley, L.L., et al. (1992). Incidence of agonal respirations in sudden cardiac arrest. *Annals of Emergency Medicine*, 21:1464–7.

Cobb, L.A., Fahrenbruch, C.E., Walsh, T.R., et al. (1999). Influence of cardiopulmonary resuscitation prior to defibrillation in patients with out-of-hospital ventricular fibrillation. *Journal of the American Medical Association*, 281:1182–88.

Cobb, L.A., Fahrenbruch, C.E., Olsufka, M., Copass, M.K. (2002). Changing incidence of out-of-hospital ventricular fibrillation, 1980–2000. *The Journal of the American Medical Association*, 288:3008–13.

Deakin, C.D., Sado, D.M., Petley, G.W. & Clewlow, F. (2003). Is the orientation of the apical defibrillation paddle of importance during manual external defibrillation? *Resuscitation*, 56:15–8.

Eftestol, T., Sunde, K., Steen, P.A. (2002). Effects of interrupting precordial compressions on the calculated probability of defibrillation success during out-of-hospital cardiac arrest. *Circulation*, 105:2270–3.

Hallstrom, A., Cobb, L., Johnson, E. & Copass, M. (2000). Cardiopulmonary resuscitation by chest compression alone or with mouth-to-mouth ventilation. *New England Journal of Medicine*, 342:1546–53.

Handley, A.J., Koster, R., Monsieurs, K., et al. (2005). European Resuscitation Council Guidelines for Resuscitation 2005 Section 2. Adult basic life support and use of automated external defibrillators. *Resuscitation*, 67:S1, S7–23.

Holmberg, M., Holmberg, S. & Herlitz, J. (2001). Factors modifying the effect of bystander cardiopulmonary resuscitation on survival in out-of-hospital cardiac arrest patients in Sweden. *European Heart Journal*, 22:511–9.

International Liaison Committee on Resuscitation (ILCOR) (2005). 2005 International consensus on cardiopulmonary resuscitation and emergency cardiovascular care science with treatment recommendations. Part 3: Defibrillation. *Resuscitation*, 67:203–11.

Kuisma, M., Repo, J. & Alaspää, A. (2001) The incidence of out-of-hospital ventricular fibrillation in Helsinki, Finland, from 1994 to 1999. *The Lancet*, 358(9280):473–4.

Larsen, M.P., Eisenberg, M.S., Cummins, R.O. & Hallstrom, A.P. (1993). Predicting survival from out-of-hospital cardiac arrest: a graphic model. *Annals of Emergency Medicine*, 22:1652–8.

Marenco, J.P., Wang, P.J., Link, M.S., et al. (2001). Improving survival from sudden cardiac arrest: the role of the automated external defibrillator. *Journal of the American Medical Association*, 286:47.

Meyer, A.D.M., Cameron, P.A., Smith, K.L., McNeil, J.J. (2000). Out-of-hospital cardiac arrest. *Tha Medical Journal of Australia*, 172: 73–76.

Nolan, J., Soar, J., Lockey, A. et al. (eds) (2006). *European Resuscitation Council. Advanced Life support Manual: 2006*.

Norris, R.M. on behalf of the UK heart attack study investigators (1999) *Sudden Cardiac Death and Acute Myocardial Infarction in Three British Health Districts the UK Heart Attack Study*. British Heart Foundation, London.

Resuscitation Council UK (2005a). *Adult Basic Life Support*. Resuscitation Council (UK), London.

Resuscitation Council UK (2005b). *The Use of Automated External Defibrillators*. Resuscitation Council (UK), London.

Sanna, T., La Torre, G., de Waure, C., et al. (2008). Cardiopulmonary resuscitation alone vs. cardiopulmonary resuscitation plus automated external defibrillator use by non-healthcare professionals: a meta-analysis on 1583 cases of out-of-hospital cardiac arrest. *Resuscitation*, 76:226–32.

Valenzuela, T.D., Roe, D.J., Cretin, S., et al. (1997). Estimating effectiveness of cardiac arrest interventions: a logistic regression survival model. *Circulation*, 96:3308–13.

van Alem, A.P., Sanou, B.T., Koster, R.W. (2003). Interruption of cardiopulmonary resuscitation with the use of the automated external defibrillator in out-of-hospital cardiac arrest. *Annals of Emergency Medicine*, 42:449–57.

Vukmir, R.B. (2006). Survival from prehospital cardiac arrest is critically dependent upon response time. *Resuscitation*, 69:229–34.

Weaver, W.D., Hill, D., Fahrenbruch, C.E., et al. (1988). Use of the automatic external defibrillator in the management of out-of hospital cardiac arrest. *New England Journal of Medicine*, 319:661–6.

Useful Websites and Further Reading

American Heart Association: http://www.americanheart.org

Australian Resuscitation Council: http://www.resus.org.au

British Heart Foundation: www.bhf.org.uk

European Resuscitation Council: www.erc.edu

Heart Foundation of Australia: http://www.heartfoundation.org.au/index.htm

International Liaison Committee on Resuscitation (ILCOR) C2005 International Consensus on CPR and ECC Science with Treatment Recommendations available from http://circ.ahajournals.org/content/vol112/22_suppl/ #SECTION__

Resuscitation Council (UK): www.resus.org.uk

16 Ethical Issues in Resuscitation

A.M. Kucia & B.F. Williams

Overview

The last few decades have produced a diverse range of pharmacological and technological advancements in health care. The general public are better educated about health care and with this increased understanding comes the higher expectations of health care workers and the health care system. Unfortunately, in the setting of finite resources, there are limitations as to what can be provided in health care, and perhaps, questions about what should reasonably be expected and provided. Ethical tensions exist across the health care spectrum, with resuscitation issues producing some of the most difficult problems faced by health professionals. This chapter discusses some current ethical issues that arise when dealing with end-of-life issues and resuscitation.

Learning objectives

After reading this chapter, you should be able to:

- Discuss the factors in ethical decision-making related to commencing or withholding resuscitation.
- List the clinical signs and symptoms associated with 'futility' in resuscitation.

- Contrast patients' understanding of resuscitation issues with that of the health professional.
- Detail the nature of advanced directives and when they should be used.
- Explore the emotional responses of health professionals in resuscitation situations.

Key concepts

Resuscitation; ethical issues; end-of-life care; autonomy; futility

Guiding ethical principles in resuscitation

Decisions of whether to initiate or withhold resuscitation should incorporate the ethical principles of beneficence (do only good), non-maleficence (do no harm), justice (fairness and equity) and autonomy (self-determination). This statement may seem straightforward, but sometimes the most appropriate application of these principles is not easily discernable. The decision of whether or not to resuscitate must be considered in the context of individual, international and local cultural, legal, traditional, religious, social and economic factors

(Baskett et al. 2005). Death and dying is something that is faced by all of us at some stage, yet the topic provokes much emotive discussion and ethical debate, and there are a number of reasons why this may be so. The general public have high expectations of health providers and their ability to preserve life despite the number of disease processes and multiple co-morbidities that become more prevalent as the population ages. Advances in technology and the ongoing development of new therapies enable the prolongation of life beyond that which could naturally be expected in many circumstances, and may allow some control over when and where one dies. Patients are not always confident that their physicians understand their end-of-life wishes (Heffner & Barbieri 2000) and prefer to be actively involved in resuscitation decisions (Emanuel et al. 1994; Bruce-Jones et al. 1996; Heffner & Barbieri 2000); and preservation of an individual's autonomy in making decisions about health care, including end-of-life choices, should always be upheld wherever possible. However, in the event that a patient is unconscious and requires resuscitation, it is often the health care team that must decide whether or not to initiate life-preserving measures.

Futility

Generally, health professionals are focused on the preservation of life. Fear of litigation and the absence of clear guidelines for circumstances where resuscitation should not be initiated usually result in every effort and available intervention being employed to prevent death, even though these actions may only defer death for a short time and result in added suffering for the patient (Marco et al. 1997).

Resuscitation attempts are unsuccessful in 70–95% of cases (Baskett et al. 2005). In most societies, health care professionals are under no obligation to commence resuscitation that is likely to be futile, but methods of predicting circumstances in which life-saving measures will be futile are not clearly defined (Ebell et al. 1997; Bowker & Stewart 1999; Abrahamson et al. 2001). It is generally accepted that medical futility involves both quantitative and qualitative considerations, such as length and quality of life (Abrahamson et al. 2001).

If the goals of cardiopulmonary resuscitation (CPR) are to preserve life, restore health, relieve suffering and limit disability (Guidelines 2000 for Cardiopulmonary Resuscitation and Emergency Cardiovascular Care 2000), futility may be expressed as the odds of achieving/not achieving these desired results. For example, an intervention may be considered futile if the odds of achieving the desired result are less than 1% (Marco et al. 2000). Specific indicators for likelihood of success or failure of an intervention should be based on current scientific evidence.

Key point

There is some evidence to suggest that CPR is unlikely to be successful in the absence of (1) spontaneous circulation at any time during 25–30min of advanced life support, (2) recurrent or refractory ventricular fibrillation or tachycardia during resuscitation, (3) exposure to a toxic agent likely to mask recovery of the central nervous system and (4) hypothermia prior to the arrest (Bonnin et al. 1993). Following in-hospital cardiac resuscitation, patients are unlikely to survive hospital discharge if (1) the arrest was unwitnessed, (2) there was no pulse after 10min of resuscitation and (3) the initial cardiac rhythm was not ventricular tachycardia or fibrillation (Van Walraven et al. 1999). Although there does seem to be some predictors for non-survival after attempted resuscitation, we do not yet have sufficient evidence to develop guidelines for all resuscitation decisions.

Rights of the individual versus the needs of society

Where patients are considered competent to make decisions, their wishes are the major consideration in end-of-life decision-making in Western societies. There is, however, escalating debate over whether the patient should have total autonomy in decision-making regarding resuscitation if a positive outcome is unlikely. In an environment of spiralling health care costs and shrinking resources, there is a need to consider fair distribution of economic resources that will yield the greatest benefit for society at large (Abrahamson et al. 2001; Khalafi et al. 2001). It has been argued that physicians should not be required to provide treatment that they consider to be futile or harmful because of a patient's (or relative's) unrealistic expectations (Paris & Reardon 1992) and that CPR should not be provided as standard care where poor outcomes are expected (Jecker & Pearlman 1992; Murphy & Finucane 1993; Baskett et al. 2005).

Patient perceptions of resuscitation

Patients have a very poor understanding of what resuscitation involves (Heyland et al. 2006). They lack 'real life' exposure to resuscitation scenarios and rely on unrealistic media portrayal of CPR practices and success rates to guide their decision-making (Diem et al. 1996; Gordon et al. 1998; Leonard et al. 1999). A review of televised hospital dramas suggests that most dramatised cardiac arrests occurred in children or young adults, were caused by trauma, had unrealistic survival to hospital discharge rates and generally resulted in death or complete recovery (Diem et al. 1996). Consequently, the general public are not exposed to the reality of prolonged suffering, severe neurological impairment or undignified death that may result from resuscitation attempts (Leonard et al. 1999; Agård et al. 2000).

There is little community awareness of what do-not-resuscitate (DNR) orders entail. Patients may choose to be actively resuscitated because of uncertainty and fear that a decision not to be resuscitated may result in withdrawal of all treatment and care. This fear is not entirely unfounded, given that there is often disagreement within the health care team about the inclusiveness of DNR orders. Baskett et al. (2005) state that DNR orders simply mean that CPR will not be performed in the event of cardiac or respiratory arrest and that other treatment, particularly pain relief and sedation, should be continued. Other measures such as therapy to support ventilation and oxygenation, nutrition, hydration, circulation and treatment of infection should be continued if they contribute to comfort and quality of life. Many DNR orders now list each of these measures with the option to withhold them according to the individual's (or loved ones) wishes.

Introducing the DNR conversation

Patients and their families often rely upon the expertise of health professionals to recommend appropriate therapy (Jecker & Pearlman 1992), particularly in emergencies requiring rapid assessment and initiation of treatment (Marco et al. 2000). Yet, many health care professionals are uncomfortable about proactively initiating discussion about resuscitation with patients, particularly when it comes to describing what resuscitation actually involves, potential consequences and likelihood of success. The personal values of health care workers have the potential to influence their decision-making regarding resuscitation, and it must be remembered that patients and their families, particularly those from a different cultural background, may not share the same opinions as to what odds of a successful outcome make a treatment worth trying (Marco et al. 2000). Health care workers must ensure that their personal opinions do not bias information presented to the patient and/or their family in order to manipulate them into choosing a particular course of action (Tulsky et al. 1996). Decisions regarding the potential benefit of an intervention should take into account scientific evidence, societal consensus and professional standards rather than individual bias involving subjective measures such as quality of life (Marco et al. 2000).

Witnessed resuscitation

Traditionally, patients' relatives have been excluded from witnessing resuscitation. This is partly to protect relatives from the immediate and long-term impact of witnessing distressing events (Rosenczweig 1998), but the practice of removing relatives from their loved ones at the time of resuscitation has been challenged (Rosenczweig 1998; Tsai 2002). Booth et al. (2004) claim that it is common practice in emergency departments in the United Kingdom for relatives to witness resuscitation, particularly that of children. Family members seldom ask to be present unless they are specifically encouraged to do so (Tsai 2002). It has been suggested that family members of patients with cardiac arrest would prefer to be offered the opportunity to stay during resuscitation efforts

(Barratt & Wallis 1998; Meyers et al. 2004). In studies where relatives have been able to stay during resuscitation, the majority report that it has helped them to adjust to the death and aided in the grieving process (Tsai 2002). Resuscitation in the setting of an acute coronary syndrome is usually an unexpected event; thus it is difficult to predict how family members will respond to witnessed resuscitation efforts. If the event is unexpected, it is unlikely that there will be time to ascertain whether it will be psychologically harmful or beneficial to individual family members. Resuscitation procedures can be traumatic to watch, and although most people have been exposed to medical dramas on the television, it does not prepare relatives for the reality of these procedures being performed on a loved one.

Although relatives witnessing resuscitation is supported by some health professionals (Grice et al. 2003), others may not wish relatives to be present during resuscitation procedures because they fear that relatives may physically interfere with the procedures (Crisci 1994; Scilling 1994). Resuscitation often involves frantic activity with many people in a confined space, and relatives may unintentionally hamper resuscitation efforts by obstructing access to the patient or equipment. The presence of relatives may also influence a decision to prolong futile resuscitation efforts or cease them prematurely at the request of relatives (Rosenczweig 1998). The presence of relatives during resuscitation may result in a heightened awareness amongst health care professionals of litigation potential and may change the focus of care away from what is in the best interests of the patient to what is the best way of avoiding litigation.

Advanced directive

'Advanced directive' is a term used to describe a person's expressed end-of-life preferences. The most common form of advanced directive is verbally expressed wishes or thoughts to family, friends or physicians, but may be more formalised in written directives, such as living wills, or durable power of attorney. A living will provides an indication of what a person desires in terms of medical treatment should they become terminally ill and unable to make decisions. Durable power of attorney allows a designated person, usually a family member or friend, to make decisions about treatment on a person's behalf if they are unable to do so themselves (Guidelines 2000 for Cardiopulmonary Resuscitation and Emergency Cardiovascular Care 2000). Advanced care planning allows a patient to express their wishes (or choose a surrogate to carry out their wishes) regarding medical care if they are unable to do so.

There is evidence to suggest that patients who have had a prior cardiac event or are at high risk of cardiac arrest would prefer to learn about end-of-life care and would welcome an opportunity to discuss advance planning with physicians (Agård et al. 2000; Heffner & Barbieri 2000). Advance directives allow health care providers to respect a patient's autonomy should they lose their decision-making capacity; however, following advance directives is not a legal requirement in many countries.

Very few people have developed advanced directives in case of serious illness. Few people anticipate the occurrence of an acute coronary event and potential life-threatening sequelae. Discussions about end-of-life care between patients and families, or patients and their medical practitioners, do not happen often enough (Mirza et al. 2005), leaving physicians and families unaware of patients' wishes regarding CPR and other life-prolonging therapies. Even where discussion has taken place with friends, family or a physician about hypothetical situations that can occur in serious illness, it is unlikely that all eventualities will have been covered to enable a surrogate to confidently make resuscitation decisions. A patient's perception of quality of life and desired duration of life often changes as they decline or recover from an illness. Patients who have chosen not to be resuscitated often show a strong desire to survive when faced with imminent death, and patients who are acutely ill and have expressed a wish to die are grateful that death has been postponed when their symptoms have been alleviated. Several studies have demonstrated that patients change their mind about what treatment they want over time (Silverstein et al. 1991; Teno et al. 1991; Danis et al. 1994; Emanuel et al. 1994; Puchalski et al. 2000) or when they are given incremental information (Schonwetter et al. 1991; O'Brien et al.

1995). Other studies suggest that most patients would prefer that their families and physicians make resuscitation decisions for them if they lose their decision-making capacity, rather than following their own stated resuscitation preferences (Puchalski et al. 2000), and that desire for autonomy in health care decisions seems to decline with severity of illness and advancing age (Ende et al. 1989; Puchalski et al. 2000). However, there is often poor agreement between what a physician or family member thinks a patient would want and the patient's expressed preference (Heyland et al. 2006). Moreover, expressed preferences cannot be accepted as informed decisions in the absence of a good understanding of the potential benefits and burdens of CPR, and there is often confusion in an emergency situation about whether or not to honour advance directives (Marco et al. 1997).

Health professionals must be aware that a patient's wishes about resuscitation may change over time, and patients should be made aware that they can make changes to their advance directives whenever they wish. Advanced directives should be reviewed periodically and with each hospital admission or change in the patient's condition in an effort to ensure that the patients' wishes about resuscitation are implemented with consideration given to their current health status.

Withdrawal of treatment

There is often reluctance in the hospital setting to withdraw life-sustaining treatment once it has been instituted, and this may result from the fear of litigation rather than the exercising of ethical judgment (Darr 1991). Patients may be denied potentially beneficial therapies if there is fear that a therapy once started cannot be withdrawn (American College of Physicians 1998). Realistically, a therapy may be tried for a predefined period of time, at the end of which an assessment is made of whether or not the therapy has been therapeutically beneficial. In this way, health care workers, the patients and their families know that every effort has been made to preserve life.

The decision to withdraw life-sustaining treatment often is left entirely with the patent's family, who may not have a realistic understanding of the limitations of current therapies, and thus feel they are not qualified to make this decision. Compounding this are feelings of grief and guilt if the family members feel they have made a wrong decision. One approach to this problem is that the decision to withdraw life-sustaining treatment is made by the health care team, based on the evidence available and the patient's wishes if known. This decision is then presented to the family along with the rationale for treatment withdrawal. This gives the family the chance to object and participate in revising the treatment plan if they wish so, but it also relieves them of the burden of responsibility and feelings of guilt that may be involved in making a decision to withdraw treatment from a loved one.

Employment of medical devices to preserve life and quality of life issues

Employment of medical devices in the acute situation to preserve life may appear to be the appropriate action if a patient's wishes regarding treatment options are not known. The withdrawal of external devices offering ventilatory or circulatory support in a patient who is showing no sign of improvement or potential for survival without support from these devices in the long term is justified, and generally is no more problematic than withdrawal of pharmacotherapy. Implantation of a device on a more permanent basis following an acute event may be more ethically problematic to withdraw.

Implantable cardioverter defibrillators (ICDs) have been shown to be superior to antiarrhythmic therapy in prolonging survival for patients with a history of sustained ventricular tachycardia or ventricular fibrillation (Connolly et al. 2000), and evidence now supports the conceptual use of ICDs in most patients with severe left ventricular dysfunction (Kadish 2005). A number of studies have addressed the quality of life issues for patients with ICDs (Irvine et al. 2002; Schron et al. 2002; Sears & Conti 2002). It is unclear whether the mood disturbances that seem to be prevalent in patients with ICDs (Pycha et al. 1990; Chevalier et al. 1996; Hegel et al. 1997; Heller et al. 1998) are purely due to quality of life with an ICD, or whether other factors, such as associated health problems, have an impact. Frequency of shocks may also be a factor: patients receiving numerous shocks seem to report an impaired quality of life compared to those with fewer or no shocks following ICD implant (Irvine et al. 2002). In practice, patients who frequently receive shocks from ICDs may find that the treatment is unbearable and that they would rather risk death from a lethal arrhythmia than continue to sustain frequent shocks. Every avenue should be explored to limit the number of shocks a patient has, but if there is nothing further to offer the patient, their wishes should be considered, providing that they understand the consequences of ICD withdrawal. Similarly, terminally ill patients, such as those with severe heart failure, may wish to have ICD or pacemaker support withdrawn. Death following withdrawal of unwanted medical support in the setting of terminal illness may be seen as due to the patient's underlying pathology rather than euthanasia or physician-assisted suicide (Mueller et al. 2003). Withdrawal of ICD or pacemaker support requires careful consultation with the patient (and relatives) and the medical team, with due consideration given to the patient's current circumstances and expected prognosis.

Organ donation

Organ donation is not as prevalent in the setting of acute coronary syndromes as it may be in other situations, such as that of acute trauma, as patients with acute coronary syndromes are not generally suitable donors. However, given the increasing need for organs and tissues, the issue may arise. The number of people waiting for donated organs and tissues by far outnumbers those available, despite public awareness of the organ shortage (Waldby 2007). Efforts to increase donations using strategies such as presumed consent laws and mandated choice have had minimal effect to date (Youngner & Arnold 1993; Ozark & DeVita 2001), probably because they are not enforced.

Training and research with the newly dead

In some countries, the newly dead are used for teaching techniques such as endotracheal intubation, CPR and evaluation of pharmacologic treatments and mechanical devices (Abrahamson et al. 2001). It has been argued that the practice of using the newly dead for training in endotracheal intubation is justifiable because it is non-mutilating, brief and an effective teaching technique that ultimately is beneficial to others. In many cases, endotracheal intubation training takes place without consent from the patient prior to death, or the family following death. It has been claimed by some that obtaining consent for this practice from the family is unnecessary because corpses are 'non-persons' and thus have no autonomy (Abrahamson et al. 2001). Others argue a case for 'presumed consent' which implies that a reasonable person would give consent to being involved in this practice under the same circumstances. Consent for this practice is desirable, but the feelings of the deceased person's family should be considered. The process of obtaining consent for this practice may distress the family and place considerable stress on the staff seeking the consent (Abrahamson et al. 2001).

As with issues of organ transplantation, the use of newly dead persons for training and research should be the topic of community debate to raise awareness about the issue and perhaps encourage individuals to make their wishes known.

Learning activity

A resuscitation emergency is called and we automatically start to perform our various roles and tasks. After calling for help, someone commences cardiac massage and someone else starts ventilating the patient and assisting the anaesthetist to intubate. Someone takes over the task of defibrillation whilst others draw up and administer medications, infusions and assist with central lines. We look for signs that the efforts we are employing are meeting with success, or, more likely, we realise that all efforts are meeting with failure. Treadway (2007) records her observations of what happens when resuscitation is unsuccessful.

> We all stopped what we were doing, and then, as though the whole episode had been some minor distraction in our otherwise packed day, we filed out of the room. We were no longer involved. We left to others the jobs of cleaning up the mess we'd created and of notifying the patient's doctor and family. We returned to our rounds, picking up as though nothing had happened.

Treadway (2007) believes that if we thought about the true significance of what we were doing, the profound event taking place, seeing the person as a mother/father/son/daughter minute by minute, in every action we took, we would not be able to do our jobs. The trick is not to lose these feelings altogether – rather, put them away and come back to them later, when you have time to think about them. Reflect upon how nurses cope emotionally following an unsuccessful resuscitation attempt. Nurses are very good about debriefing with each other – perhaps it is because they feel that other nurses will understand. Obtain and read the article below which explores the realities of CPR and accounts of the emotions experienced by nurses in response.

References

Abrahamson, N., de Vos, R., Fallat, M.E., et al. (2001). Ethics in emergency cardiac care. *Annals of Emergency Medicine*, **37**:S196–200.

Agård, A., Hermerén, G. & Herlitz, J. (2000). Should cardiopulmonary resuscitation be performed on patients with heart failure? The role of the patient in the decision-making process. *Journal of Internal Medicine*, **248**:279–86.

American College of Physicians (1998). Ethics manual, 4th edn. *Annals of Internal Medicine*, **128**:576–94.

Barratt, F. & Wallis, D.N. (1998). Relatives in the resuscitation room: their point of view. *Journal of Accident and Emergency Medicine*, **15**:109–11.

Baskett, P.J.F., Steen, P.A. & Bossaert, L. (2005). European Resuscitation Council Guidelines for Resuscitation 2005: Section 8. The ethics of resuscitation and end-of-life decisions. *Resuscitation*, **67**(Suppl. 1):S171–80.

Bonnin, M.J., Pepe, P.E., Kimball, K.T., et al. (1993). Distinct criteria for termination of resuscitation in the out of hospital setting. *Journal of the American Medical Association*, **270**:1457–62.

Booth, M.G., Woolrich, L. & Kinsella, J. (2004). Family witnessed resuscitation in UK emergency departments: a survey of practice. *European Journal of Anaesthesiology*, **21**:725–8.

Bowker, L. & Stewart, K. (1999). Predicting unsuccessful cardiopulmonary resuscitation (CPR): a comparison of three morbidity scores. *Resuscitation*, **40**:89–95.

Bruce-Jones, P., Roberts, H., Bowker, L., et al. (1996). Resuscitating the elderly: what do the patients want? *Journal of Medical Ethics*, **22**:154–9.

Chevalier, P., Verrier, P., Kirkorian, G., et al. (1996). Improved appraisal of the quality of life in patients with automatic implantable cardioverter defibrillator: a psychometric study. *Psychotherapy & Psychosomatics*, **65**:49–56.

Connolly, S.J., Hallstrom, A.P. & Cappato, R., on behalf of the investigators of the AVID, CASH and CIDS studies (2000). Meta-analysis of the implantable cardioverter defibrillator secondary prevention trials. *European Heart Journal*, **21**:2071–8.

Crisci, C. (1994). Local factors may influence decision [letter]. *British Medical Journal*, **309**:406.

Danis, M., Garrett, J., Harris, R. & Patrick, D.L. (1994). Stability of choices about life-sustaining treatments. *Annals of Internal Medicine*, **120**:567–73.

Darr, K. (1991). *Ethics in Health Services*, 2nd edn. Health Professions Press, Baltimore.

Diem, S.J., Lantos, J.D.& Tulsky, J.A. (1996). Cardiopulmonary resuscitation on television: miracles and misinformation. *New England Journal of Medicine*, **334**:1578–82.

Ebell, M.H., Kruse, J.A., Smith, M., et al. (1997). Failure of three decision rules to predict the outcome of in-hospital cardiopulmonary resuscitation. *Medical Decision Making*, **17**:171–7.

Emanuel, L.L., Emanuel, E.J., Stoeckle, J.D., et al. (1994). Advance directives: stability of patients' treatment choices. *Archives of Internal Medicine*, **154**:209–17.

Ende, J., Kazis, L., Ash, A. & Moskowitz, M.A. (1989). Measuring patients' desire for autonomy: decision making and information-seeking preferences among medical patients. *Journal of General Internal Medicine*, **4**:23–30.

Gordon, P.N., Williamson, S. & Lawler, P.G. (1998). As seen on TV: observational study of cardiopulmonary resuscitation in British television medical dramas. *British Medical Journal*, **317**:780–3.

Grice, A.S., Picton, P. & Deakin, C.D.S. (2003). Study examining attitudes of staff, patients and relatives to witnessed resuscitation in adult intensive care units. *British Journal of Anaesthetics*, **91**:820–4.

Guidelines 2000 for cardiopulmonary resuscitation and emergency cardiovascular care: International Consensus on Science (2000). *Circulation*, **102**(Suppl. I):12–21.

Heffner, J.E. & Barbieri, C. (2000). End-of-life preferences of patients enrolled in cardiovascular rehabilitation programs. *Chest*, **117**:1474–81.

Hegel, M.T., Griegel, L.E., Black, C., et al. (1997). Anxiety and depression in patients receiving implanted cardioverter-defibrillator: a longitudinal investigation. *International Journal of Psychiatric Medicine*, **27**:57–69.

Heller, S.S., Ormont, M.A., Lidagoster, L., et al. (1998). Psychosocial outcome after ICD implantation: a current perspective. *Pacing and Clinical Electrophysiology*, **21**:1207–15.

Heyland, D.K., Frank, C., Groll, D., et al. (2006). Understanding cardiopulmonary resuscitation decision making: perspectives of seriously ill hospitalized patients and family members. *Chest*, **130**:419–28.

Irvine, J., Dorian, P., Baker, B., et al. (2002). Quality of life in the Canadian Implantable Defibrillator Study (CIDS). *American Heart Journal*, **144**:282–9.

Jecker, N.S. & Pearlman, R.A. (1992). Medical futility: who decides? *Archives of Internal Medicine*, **152**:1140–4.

Kadish, A. (2005). Prophylactic defibrillator implantation – toward an evidence-based approach. *New England Journal of Medicine*, **352**:285–7.

Khalafi, K., Ravakhah, K. & West, B.C. (2001). Avoiding the futility of resuscitation. *Resuscitation*, **50**:161–6.

Leonard, C.T., Doyle, R.L. & Raffin, T.A. (1999). Do-not-resuscitate orders in the face of patient and family opposition. *Critical Care Medicine*, **27**:1045–7.

Marco, C.A., Bessman, E.S., Schoenfeld, C.N., et al. (1997). Ethical issues of cardiopulmonary resuscitation: current practice among emergency physicians. *Academic Emergency Medicine*, **4**:898–904.

Marco, C.A., Larkin, G.L., Moskop, J.C. & Derse, A.R. (2000). Determination of "futility" in emergency medicine. *Annals of Emergency Medicine*, **35**:604–12.

Meyers, T.A., Eichhorn, D.J., Guzzetta, C.E., et al. (2004). Family presence during invasive procedures and resuscitation. *American Journal of Nursing*, **100**:32–43.

Mirza, A., Kad, R. & Ellison, N.M. (2005). Cardiopulmonary resuscitation is not addressed in the admitting medical records for the majority of patients who undergo CPR in the hospital. *American Journal of Hospice and Palliative Care*, **22**:20–5.

Mueller, P.S., Hook, C.C. & Hayes, D.L. (2003). Ethical analysis of withdrawal of pacemaker or implantable cardioverter-defibrillator (ICD) support at the end of life. *Mayo Clinic Proceedings*, **78**:959–63.

Murphy, D.J. & Finucane, T.E. (1993). New do-not-resuscitate policies: a step in cost control. *Archives of Internal Medicine*, **152**:1641–8.

O'Brien, L.A., Grisso, J.A., Mailin, G., et al. (1995). Nursing home residents' preferences for life-sustaining treatments. *Journal of the American Medical Association*, **274**:1775–9.

Ozark, S. & DeVita, M. (2001). Non-heartbeating organ donation: ethical controversies and medical considerations. *International Anesthesiology Clinics*, **39**:103–16.

Paris, J.J. & Reardon, F.E. (1992). Physician refusal of requests for futile or ineffective interventions. *Cambridge Q Healthcare Ethics*, **2**:127–34.

Puchalski, C.M., Zhong, Z., Jacobs, M.M., et al. (2000). Patients who want their family and physician to make resuscitation decisions for them: observations from SUPPORT and HELP. *Journal of the American Geriatric Society*, **48**:S84–90.

Pycha, C., Calabrese, J.R., Gulledge, D., et al. (1990). Patient and spouse acceptance and adaptation to implantable cardioverter defibrillators. *Cleveland Clinic Journal of Medicine*, **57**:441–4.

Rosenczweig, C. (1998). Should relatives witness resuscitation? Ethical issues and practical considerations. *Canadian Medical Association Journal*, **158**:617–20.

Schonwetter, T.S., Teasdale, T.A., Taffet, G., et al. (1991). Educating the elderly: cardiopulmonary resuscitation decisions before and after an intervention. *Journal of the American Geriatric Society*, **39**:372–7.

Schron, E.B., Exner, D.V., Yao, Q., et al. (2002). Quality of life in the antiarrhythmics versus implantable defibrillators trial: impact of therapy and influence of adverse symptoms and defibrillator shocks. *Circulation*, **105**:589–94.

Scilling, R.J. (1994). No room for spectators [letter]. *British Medical Journal*, **309**:406.

Sears, S.F., Jr. & Conti, J.B. (2002). Quality of life and psychological functioning of ICD patients. *Heart*, **87**:488–93.

Silverstein, M.D., Stocking, C.B., Antel, J.P., et al. (1991). Amyotrophic lateral sclerosis and life-sustaining therapy: patient's desires for information, participation in decision making, and life-sustaining therapy. *Mayo Clinical Proceedings*, **66**:906–13.

Teno, J., Mor, V. & Fleishman, J. (1991). Stability of preferences among patients with HIV-related disease. *Clinical Research*, **40**:632A.

Treadway, K. (2007). The code. *New England Journal of Medicine*, **357**:1273–5.

Tsai, E. (2002). Should family members be present during cardiopulmonary resuscitation? *New England Journal of Medicine*, **346**:1019–21.

Tulsky, J.A., Chesney, M.A. & Lo, B. (1996). How do medical residents discuss resuscitation with patients: timing and truth-telling. *Chest*, **9**:11–2.

Van Walraven, C., Forster, A.J. & Stiell, I.G. (1999). Derivation of a clinical decision rule for discontinuation of in-hospital cardiac arrest resuscitations. *Archives of Internal Medicine*, **159**:129–34.

Waldby, C. (2007). The big donor shortage. Retrieved online 17th September 2007 from http://www.news-medical.net/?id=26389

Youngner, S. & Arnold, R. (1993). Ethical, psychosocial, and public policy implications of procuring organs from non-heart-beating cadaver donors. *Journal of the American Medical Association*, **269**:2769–74.

Useful Websites and Further Reading

Ardagh, M. (2000). Futility has no utility in resuscitation medicine. *Journal of Medical Ethics*, **26**:396–9.

McCrary, S.V., Swanson, J.W., Youngner, S.J., et al. (1994). Physicians' quantitative assessments of medical futility. *Journal of Clinical Ethics*, **5**:100–5.

Page, S. & Meerabeau, L. (1996). Nurses' accounts of cardiopulmonary resuscitation. *Journal of Advanced Nursing*, **24**:317–25.

Solomon, M.Z. (1993). How physicians talk about futility: making words mean too many things. *Journal of Law and Medical Ethics*, **21**:231–7.

Van Norman, G.A. (2003). Another matter of life and death: what every anesthesiologist should know about the ethical, legal and policy implications of the non-heart-beating cadaver organ donor. *Anesthesiology*, **98**:763–73.

17 Pathogenesis of Acute Coronary Syndromes

A.M. Kucia & J.D. Horowitz

Overview

Traditionally, it was believed that the severity (degree of obstruction) of atherosclerotic stenosis in the coronary artery was the deciding factor in transition from stable to unstable coronary artery disease (CAD). More recently, serial angiographic studies have demonstrated that coronary arteries with more severe stenoses do not cause the majority of acute myocardial infarctions (MIs) and many acute MIs occurred in arteries that had not previously demonstrated any stenosis (Libby et al. 2006). Moreover, a study reported by Hackett et al. (1988) of 60 patients who underwent coronary angiography following thrombolytic therapy for acute MI found that once the clot was lysed, the residual stenosis was non-critical in around half of the patients studied.

Our understanding of the processes involved in the pathogenesis of CAD and development of acute coronary syndromes (ACSs) has increased dramatically in the past decade. Where atherosclerosis was once considered to be primarily a cholesterol storage disease, the primary cause is now thought to be inflammation. The understanding of the nature of atherosclerotic plaque lesions has now evolved to encompass the concept of stable lesion versus vulnerable lesion and the likelihood of plaque rupture and development of ACS. This chapter describes the current understanding of the processes involved in the development of ACS.

Learning objectives

After reading this chapter, you should be able to:

- Describe the factors related to the process of atherogenesis.
- Discuss the differences between stable and vulnerable plaques.
- Describe the process of thrombogenesis and the factors related to thrombus formation at the site of a plaque rupture.
- Discuss the contribution of vasoconstriction to the development of ACSs.
- Demonstrate an understanding of the role of endothelium and the role of endothelial dysfunction in the development of ACSs.

Key concepts

Atherosclerosis; vulnerable plaque; endothelial dysfunction; thrombogenesis; vasoconstriction

Acute coronary syndrome

The term 'acute coronary syndromes' refers to a range of conditions associated with symptomatic CAD that result in myocardial ischaemia or infarction. The pathogenesis of ACS usually involves atherosclerotic plaque rupture, platelet activation and thrombus formation. Although the range of conditions from unstable angina pectoris (UAP) to ST-segment elevation myocardial infarction (STEMI) share a common pathophysiological base, these conditions differ in severity and outcome, according to the severity of the contributing factors discussed below.

Atherosclerosis

Acute coronary syndrome generally results from atherosclerosis, which causes plaque formation in the inside lumen of medium- and large-sized coronary arteries. Plaque may cause partial obstruction of the coronary artery, or, in the setting of plaque rupture and associated thrombosis, progress to total occlusion. Atherosclerosis is a progressive disease that probably begins in adolescence, with progression depending upon a number of factors including age, gender, genetic make-up and other risk factors (Libby 2000). In some people, atherosclerosis may progress rapidly from their third decade, whilst in others it may not become apparent until later years. Some individuals with atherosclerosis will never experience symptoms or complications from this disease, whilst others may have chronic symptoms. Others may experience sudden acute symptoms with no prior warning which may have serious consequences, including death (Libby 2000).

Currently, atherogenesis is understood to result from a complex interaction of cardiovascular risk factors, inflammation and endothelial dysfunction (Libby & Theroux 2005). Factors such as hypercholesterolaemia, hypertension, smoking and diabetes cause damage to the arterial endothelium and initiate the atherosclerotic process (Cannon & Braunwald 2003). Certain bacterial products have also been implicated in this process (Libby & Theroux 2005). When the endothelium is damaged, macrophages bind to the dysfunctional endothelial wall and can infiltrate the endothelial cell. Low-density lipoproteins (LDL) also infiltrate the endothelial cell where they are digested by macrophages, becoming foam cells, and thus creating a lipid-filled atherosclerotic plaque. Foam cells produce large amounts of tissue factor derived from macrophages (Libby 1995). Tissue factor is a small-molecular-weight glycoprotein that initiates the extrinsic clotting cascade and is believed to be a regulator of coagulation, haemostasis and thrombosis (Moreno et al. 1996). Over time, fats, cholesterol, platelets, cellular debris and calcium are deposited in the damaged artery wall. Smooth muscle proliferation occurs in response to cytokines secreted by the damaged endothelial cells, resulting in the formation of a dense, fibrous extracellular matrix (connective tissue) cap covering the plaque. The integrity of the fibrous cap determines the stability of the atherosclerotic plaque: once the fibrous cap is breached, the thrombogenic lipid core comes into contact with the blood (Fernandez-Ortiz et al. 1994; Toschi et al. 1997; Badimon et al. 1999; Mallat et al. 1999).

Endothelial dysfunction

Endothelial dysfunction is associated with most forms of cardiovascular disease, including hypertension, CAD, chronic heart failure, peripheral artery disease, diabetes and chronic renal failure (Endemann & Schiffrin 2004). Endothelium lines the walls of blood vessels and has a role in the regulation of the anti-inflammatory, mitogenic (cell division) and contractile activities of the vessel wall, and the haemostatic process within the vessel lumen (Bonetti et al. 2003) and produces biologically active compounds, including prostacyclin, nitric oxide and endothelin, that influence the diameter of the blood vessel. It also mediates haemostasis, cell proliferation and inflammatory mechanisms in the cell wall (Klabunde 2005). Dysfunction of the endothelium is an important early event in the pathogenesis of atherosclerosis, significantly contributing to plaque initiation and progression. It is characterized by a change in the normal functioning of the endothelium towards reduced vasodilation, a proinflammatory state and prothrombic properties (Endemann & Schiffrin 2004).

Plaque disruption

Four mechanisms of plaque disruption have been described: (1) plaque rupture, (2) plaque erosion,

(3) erosion of a calcified nodule in the fibrous cap and (4) intra-plaque haemorrhage. Of these mechanisms, plaque rupture is the most common and accounts for up to 75% of deaths due to acute MI. Plaque erosion is thought to be responsible for between 20% and 25% of deaths due to acute MI (Libby et al. 2005). Calcium nodule rupture and intra-plaque haemorrhage appear to be uncommon causes of death due to acute MI, but it is not known if they occur more commonly in non-fatal MI.

Plaque rupture

Some plaques are more prone to rupture than others. Plaques that form a relatively thick covering over the fatty core, due to either fibrosis (scarring) or calcification, are considered to be stable plaques. In comparison, unstable plaques have a larger fatty core and more white blood cells encased within a thinner, softer, more unpredictable coating that can rupture at any time without warning. The term 'vulnerable plaque' is used to describe these unstable plaques. The location, size and consistency of the plaque, as well as circumferential wall stress and blood flow characteristics, particularly at the proximal aspect of the plaque, contribute to the likelihood of plaque rupture (Falk et al. 1995).

Macrophages are capable of degrading extracellular matrix by phagocytosis or secretion of proteolytic enzymes, leaving the fibrous cap more vulnerable to rupture (Moreno et al. 1994; Libby 1995). Macrophage-rich areas of plaque are more commonly found in patients with ACS than in those with stable angina, which suggests that macrophages may be a marker of unstable atherosclerotic plaques and that macrophages may play a significant role in the pathophysiology of ACS (Moreno et al. 1996). It is not unusual for patients with ACS to have more than one plaque rupture and it is thought that this may reflect an underlying inflammatory process as a precipitant of plaque rupture (Hong et al. 2004).

Plaque erosion

Plaque erosion is a less frequent pathological cause of ACS and is defined by an acute thrombus in direct contact with the intima, in an area of absent endothelium (Virmani et al. 2006). In the setting of plaque erosion, the intimal plaque tends to be rich in smooth muscle cells and proteoglycan matrix (Farb et al. 2000). Macrophages and lymphocytes are few in number or absent altogether and the lesions tend to be eccentric and occasionally they are calcified. The underlying plaque in erosions consists of pathologic intimal thickening or fibrous cap atheroma (Virmani et al. 2006).

Inflammation

Levels of the inflammatory marker C-reactive protein (CRP) have been correlated with the presence and severity of atherosclerosis (Heinrich et al. 1995; Ridker et al. 1997) and a strong correlation has been observed between elevated levels of CRP and coronary events (Liuzzo et al. 1994; Thompson et al. 1995; Haverkate et al. 1997; March et al. 1997; Ridker 1998; Rebuzzi et al. 1998; Ferreiros et al. 1999; Abdelmouttelab et al. 1999) including death (Kuller et al. 1997; Lindahl et al. 2000). Multiple mechanisms, including infection, have been proposed as possible causative factors in the inflammatory component of ACS. It has been suggested that acute or chronic infection may have a role in the process of atherosclerosis by exerting direct local effects on the coronary endothelium, vascular smooth muscle cells and macrophages within the atherosclerotic lesion, and that infection may also produce systemic effects through an increase in circulating cytokines that compromise the anti-thrombotic and vasodilator properties of the endothelium (Maseri 1999). *Chlamydia pneumoniae* (Buja 1996; Muhlestein et al. 1996) and cytomegalovirus (Buja 1996) have been identified within atherosclerotic plaques, and there is some evidence to suggest that seropositivity for *C. pneumoniae* may be linked to CAD (Saikku et al. 1988; Thom et al. 1992; Linnanmaki et al. 1993; Patel et al. 1995), by association if not by causality, although some studies have not demonstrated this (Wald et al. 2000). A diverse range of pathogens have been found in atherosclerotic plaques of people with CAD at post-mortem (Ott et al. 2006).

Thrombosis

The majority of acute coronary events are due to rupture of an atherosclerotic plaque with associated intra-luminal thrombosis (Libby & Theroux 2005). When an atherosclerotic plaque ruptures, the thrombogenic materials within it are exposed to circulating blood, leading to activation of the clotting cascade and platelet adhesion, activation and aggregation. The resulting thrombus may compromise the lumen of the affected artery.

In ACS most thrombi are largely composed of platelets, and are often multiple and multi-layered, causing persistent thrombogenic stimuli and recurring inflammation causing or contributing to plaque instability that may persist over a period of days or weeks (Maseri 1999).

Local risk factors for thrombogenesis include the degree of plaque erosion or ulceration, the degree of stenosis, tissue substrate (lipid-rich plaque has high thrombogenicity), recurrent thrombus and vasoconstriction (Fuster et al. 1999).

Vasoconstriction

In the setting of acute plaque rupture and thrombosis, vasoconstriction can further impair coronary blood flow. Although it is transient, it can cause significant disruption to myocardial oxygen supply (Maseri & Sanna 1998). Vasoconstriction in ACS is due to pre-existing endothelial dysfunction near the culprit lesion, and also occurs in response to locally released serotonin and thromboxane A_2 (from platelets), which affects smooth muscle cells at the site of de-endothelialisation due to arterial damage or plaque disruption (Willerson et al. 1989).

Conclusion

Understanding of pathophysiological processes related to atherosclerosis and the development of ACS has progressed significantly over the past two decades and continues to evolve. With this further understanding, we can target those individuals at greatest risk for preventative therapies and develop new therapies that may target newly understood pathophysiological processes inherent in the onset of ACS.

Learning activity

Consider the processes of thrombosis and vasoconstriction in ACS: what pharmacotherapies do we use in ACS that directly target these processes?

Reflect upon the number of clinical trials in ACS – what aspect of the pathophysiological process is usually targeted by novel pharmacological agents?

References

Abdelmouttaleb, I., Danchin, N., Ilardo, C., et al. (1999). C-reactive protein and coronary artery disease: additional evidence of the implication of an inflammatory process in acute coronary syndromes. *American Heart Journal*, **137**:346–51.

Badimon, J.J., Lettino, M., Toschi, V., et al. (1999). Local inhibition of tissue factor reduces the thrombogenicity of disrupted human atherosclerotic plaques: effects of tissue factor pathway inhibitor on plaque thrombogenicity under flow conditions. *Circulation*, **99**:1780–7.

Bonetti, P.O., Lerman, L.O. & Lerman, A. (2003). Endothelial dysfunction: a marker of atherosclerotic risk. *Arteriosclerosis, Thrombosis and Vascular Biology*, **23**:168–75.

Buja, L.M. (1996). Does atherosclerosis have an infectious etiology? *Circulation*, **94**:872–3.

Cannon, C.P. & Braunwald, E. (2003). The spectrum of myocardial ischaemia. In: C.P. Cannon (ed.), *Management of Acute Coronary Syndromes*, 2nd edn. Humana Press, New Jersey.

Endemann, D.H. & Schiffrin, E.L. (2004). Endothelial dysfunction. *Journal of the American Society of Nephrology*, **15**:1983–92.

Falk, E., Shah, P.K. & Fuster, V. (1995). Coronary plaque disruption. *Circulation*, 92:657–71.

Farb, A., Burke, A.P., Kolodgie, F.D., et al. (2000). Platelet-rich intramyocardial thromboemboli are frequent in acute coronary thrombosis, especially plaque erosions. *Circulation*, **102**:II774.

Fernandez-Ortiz, A., Badimon, J.J., Falk, E., et al. (1994). Characterization of the relative thrombogenicity of atherosclerotic plaque components: implications for consequences of plaque rupture. *Journal of the American College of Cardiology*, **23**:1562–9.

Ferreiros, E.R., Boissonnet, C.P., Pizarro, R., et al. (1999). Independent prognostic value of elevated C-reactive protein in unstable angina. *Circulation*, **100**:1958–63.

Fuster, V., Fayad, Z.A. & Badimon, J.J. (1999). Acute coronary syndromes: biology. *The Lancet*, **353**(Suppl II):5–9.

Fuster, V., Moreno, P.R., Fayad, Z.A., Corti, R. & Badimon, J.J. (2005). Atherothrombosis and high-risk plaque: Part I: evolving concepts. *Journal of the American College of Cardiology*, **46**:937–54.

Hackett, D., Davies, G. & Maseri, A. (1988). Pre-existing coronary stenoses in patients with first myocardial infarction are not necessarily severe. *European Heart Journal*, **9**:1317–23.

Haverkate, F., Thompson, S.G., Pyke, S.D.M., et al. (1997). Production of C-reactive protein and risk of coronary events in stable and unstable angina. *The Lancet*, **349**:462–6.

Heinrich, J., Schulte, H., Schonfield, R., et al. (1995). Association of variables of coagulation, fibrinolysis and acute-phase with atherosclerosis in coronary and peripheral arteries and those supplying the brain. *Thrombosis and Haemostasis*, **73**:374–8.

Hong, M.-K., Mintz, G.S., Lee, C.W., et al. (2004). Comparison of coronary plaque rupture between stable angina and acute myocardial infarction: a three-vessel intravascular ultrasound study in 235 patients. *Circulation*, **110**:928–33.

Klabunde, R.E. (2005). *Cardiovascular Physiology Concepts*. Lippincott, Williams and Wilkins, Philadelphia.

Kuller, L.H., Tracy, R.P., Shaten, J. & Meilahn, E.N. (1996). Relation of C-reactive protein and coronary heart disease in the MRFIT nested case-control study. *American Journal of Epidemiology*, **144**:537–47.

Libby, P. (1995). Molecular bases of the acute coronary syndrome: from bench to bedside. *Circulation*, **91**:2844–50.

Libby, P. (2000). Changing concepts of atherogenesis. *Journal of Internal Medicine*, **247**:349–58.

Libby, P. & Theroux, P. (2005). Pathophysiology of coronary artery disease. *Circulation*, **111**:3481–8.

Libby, P., Cook, J., van der Steen, A.F.W. & Gloffke, W. (2005). Inflammatory aspects and detection of vulnerable plaque: clinical impact of assessment. Retrieved online on 10th September 2008 from http://www.arc-mesa.org/iavp//monograph.pdf

Libby, P. (2006). Atherosclerosis: disease biology affecting the coronary vasculature. *American Journal of Cardiology*, **98**:S3–9.

Lindahl, B., Toss, H., Siegbahn, A., Venge, P. & Wallentin, L. (2000). Markers of myocardial damage and inflammation in relation to long-term mortality in unstable coronary artery disease. *New England Journal of Medicine*, **343**:1139–47.

Linnanmaki, E., Leionen, M., Mattila, K., et al. (1993). Chlamydia pneumonia-specific circulating immune complexes in patients with chronic coronary heart disease. *Circulation*, **87**:1130–4.

Liuzzo, G., Biasucci, L.M., Gallimore, J.R., et al. (1994). Prognostic value of C-reactive protein and serum amyloid A protein in severe unstable angina. *New England Journal of Medicine*, **331**:417–24.

Mallat, Z., Hugel, B., Ohan, J., et al. (1999). Shed membrane microparticles with procoagulant potential in human atherosclerotic plaques: a role for apoptosis in plaque thrombogenicity. *Circulation*, **99**:348–53.

March, F., Lovis, C., Gaspoz, J.M., et al. (1997). C-reactive protein as a marker for acute coronary syndromes. *European Heart Journal*, **18**:1897–902.

Maseri, A. & Sanna, T. (1998). The role of plaque fissures in unstable angina: fact or fiction? *European Heart Journal*, **19**(Suppl K):K2–4.

Maseri, A. (1999). Antibiotics for acute coronary syndromes: are we ready for megatrials? Editorial. *European Heart Journal*, **20**:89–92.

Moreno, P.R., Falk, E., Palacios, I.F., Newell, J.B., Fuster, V. & Fallon, J.T. (1994) Macrophage infiltration in acute coronary syndromes. Implications for plaque rupture. *Circulation*, **90**:775–8.

Moreno, P.R., Bernardi, V.H., Lopez-Cuellar, J., et al. (1996). Macrophages, smooth muscle cells and tissue factor in unstable angina: implications for cell-mediated thrombogenicity in acute coronary syndromes. *Circulation*, **94**:3090–7.

Muhlestein, J.B., Hammond, E.H., Carlquist, J.F., et al. (1996). Increased incidence of chlamydia species within the coronary arteries of patients with symptomatic atherosclerosis versus other forms cardiovascular disease. *Journal of the American College of Cardiology*, **27**:1555–61.

Ott, S.J., El Mokhtari, N.E., Musfeldt, M., et al. (2006). Detection of diverse bacterial signatures in atherosclerotic lesions of patients with coronary heart disease. *Circulation*, **113**:920–2.

Patel, P., Mendall, M.A., Carrington, D., et al. (1995). Association of helicobacter pylori and chlamydia pneumoniae infections with coronary heart disease and risk factors. *British Medical Journal*, **311**:711–4.

Rebuzzi, A.G., Quaranta, G., Liuzzo, G. et al. (1998). Incremental prognostic value of serum levels of Troponin T and C-reactive protein on admission in patients with unstable angina. *American Journal of Cardiology*, **82**:715–9.

Ridker, P.M., Cushman, M., Stamper, M.J., et al. (1997). Inflammation, aspirin, and the risk of cardiovascular disease in apparently healthy men. *New England Journal of Medicine*, **336**:973–9.

Ridker, P.M. (1998). Inflammation, infection, and cardiovascular risk: how good is the clinical evidence? *Circulation*, **97**:2007–11.

Saikku, P., Leinonen, M., Mattila, K., et al. (1988). Seroloical evidence of an association of a novel Chlamydia, TWAR, with chronic coronary heart disease and acute myocardial infarction. *The Lancet*, **ii**: 983–6.

Thom, D.H., Grayston, J.T., Siscovik, D.S., et al. (1992). Association of prior infection with chlamydia pnuemoniae and angiographically demonstrated coronary artery disease. *Journl of the American Medical Association*, **268**:68–72.

Thompson, S.G., Kienast, J., Pyke, S.D.M., et al. (1995). Hemostatic factors and the risk of myocardial infarction or sudden death in patients with unstable angina pectoris. *New England Journal of Medicine*, **332**:635–41.

Toschi, V., Gallo, R., Lettino, M., et al. (1997). Tissue factor modulates the thrombogenicity of human atherosclerotic plaques. *Circulation*, **95**:594–9.

Virmani, P., Burke, A.P., Farb, A. & Kolodgie, F.D. (2006). Pathology of the vulnerable plaque. *Journal of the American College of Cardiology*, **47**:13–8.

Wald, N.J., Law, M.R., Morris, J.K., et al. (2000). Chlamydia pneumoniae infection and mortality from ischaemic heart disease: large prospective study. *British Medical Journal*, **321**:204–7.

Willerson, J.T., Gobrao, P., Fidr, J., et al. (1989). Specific platelet mediators and unstable coronary lesions: experimental evidence and potential clinical implications. *Circulation*, **80**:198–205.

Useful Websites and Further Reading

Boudi, F.B. & Ahsan, C.H. (2006). Atherosclerosis. *eMedicine*. Available from http://www.emedicine.com/med/topic182.htm

CVspectrum.org Pathophysiology of atherosclerosis: http://www.cvspectrum.org/cms/templates/ce_activity.aspx?articleid=2507&zoneid=44

Fenton, D.E. (2008). Acute coronary syndrome. *eMedicine*. Available from http://www.emedicine.com/EMERG/topic31.htm

18 Presentations of Acute Coronary Syndromes

A.M. Kucia & J.F. Beltrame

Overview

Coronary heart disease (CHD) is a major cause of morbidity and mortality in communities across the globe, and arises from disease and/or dysfunction involving the coronary circulation. This coronary dysfunction may involve the large epicardial coronary arteries (coronary artery disease [CAD]) or the network of microvascular resistance vessels (microvascular dysfunction), resulting in myocardial ischaemia. The most common clinical manifestation of myocardial ischaemia is chest pain, which is typically referred to as 'angina pectoris'. This chapter will examine the common presentations of acute coronary syndromes (ACSs), including symptoms and clinical findings.

Learning objectives

After reading this chapter, you should be able to:

- Discuss current global trends in ACS presentations.
- Describe typical features of chest pain associated with ACSs.
- Describe electrocardiogram (ECG) changes associated with myocardial ischaemia and infarction and their diagnostic application.

- Describe serum cardiac enzymes associated with ACSs and their diagnostic application.
- Discuss signs and symptoms of atypical presentations with ACSs and groups of patients in whom these atypical presentations are most likely.

Angina pectoris

Angina is the most common manifestation of CHD and a common presenting complaint to general practitioner's (GP's) surgeries and hospital emergency departments. Angina may be stable or unstable: both result from a perfusion-dependent imbalance between myocardial oxygen supply and demand, but the mechanisms differ.

The classical description of angina pectoris by William Heberden remains as accurate today as the day he penned it in 1772. In his landmark paper entitled 'Some account of a disorder of the breast' he wrote:

> They who are afflicted with it, are seized while they are walking, (more especially if it be up hill, and soon after eating) with a painful and most disagreeable sensation in the breast, which seems as if it would extinguish life, if it were to increase or to continue; but the moment they stand still, all this uneasiness vanishes.

Table 18.1   ACC/AHA/ACP-ASIM clinical classification of chest pain.

Type	Definition
Typical angina	(a) sub-sternal discomfort with characteristic quality and duration that is (b) provoked by exertion or emotional stress and (c) relieved by rest or sub-lingual nitrates
Atypical angina	pain with ≥2 of the above features
Non-anginal chest pain	≤1 of the above features fulfilled

Source: From Gibbons et al. (1999).

This description captures the essential features of chronic stable angina, namely its constrictive sensation and relationship to exertion. The clinical classification of chest pain according to the American College of Cardiology (ACC), American Heart Association (AHA), American College of Physicians (ACP) and the American Society of Internal Medicine (ASIM) (Gibbons et al. 1999) is summarised in Table 18.1.

Stable angina

Stable angina is not classed as an ACS but is worth mentioning here as it may progress to an unstable phase. The chest pain described by Heberden and summarised in Table 18.1 reflects a predictable pattern of chest pain that occurs in response to a provocative physiological stimulus such as exercise, sexual activity and emotional stress that increases heart rate/blood pressure, and thus myocardial oxygen demand, resulting in ischaemia in the region of myocardium that is supplied by a vessel with an obstructive lesion. Symptoms including pain, shortness of breath, sweating, nausea, vomiting, palpitationsand weakness are usually relieved by rest. Symptoms seem to be worse early in the morning, after a heavy meal or in cold weather (Quinn et al. 2003).

As this pain is predictable and usually self-limiting once the provocative stimulus has been removed, it is referred to as *stable angina*. Patients with this form of angina have a reasonable

prognosis with an annual risk of infarction of 1% per year. A change in pattern of stable angina may herald progression to unstable angina (UA). Patients may describe their angina as becoming more frequent, more severe, lasting longer or occurring with less exertion than has previously been the case. It may occur at rest with no obvious precipitating factors and may wake them from sleep. They may describe symptoms limiting their activity that are not responsive to rest or nitroglycerine (Quinn et al. 2003).

> **Key point**
>
> Although unstable phases of ischaemic heart disease carry a more severe short-term prognosis than chronic stable phases, people with stable angina are at greater risk of developing an ACS or sudden death when compared to individuals without anginal symptoms (Crea et al. 1997; Verheught 1999).

The acute coronary syndromes

The term 'acute coronary syndromes' has evolved over time to encompass a group of patients who have prolonged acute myocardial ischaemia which may rapidly progress on to myocardial infarction (MI). Compared with patients who have stable angina, these patients have the same characteristic chest pain but usually without a physiologically provocative stimulus, and symptoms persist on the removal of the stimulus. Hence these patients typically experience angina at rest rather than exertional angina such as occurs in stable angina. Moreover, these patients are at much higher risk of cardiac death.

Acute coronary syndrome encompasses the clinical syndromes of UA and MI. These two syndromes are characterised on the basis of rest angina and the presence/absence of myocardial necrosis as reflected by cardiac markers. Previously this has been creatine kinase (CK), but more recently a more sensitive marker of myocardial necrosis has been adopted, namely troponin (Tn). Thus in contemporary practice, rest angina without an increase in Tn is considered to be UA whereas in the presence of an abnormal Tn, MI is diagnosed.

Unstable angina pectoris

The diagnosis of unstable angina pectoris (UAP) suggests that symptoms are of new onset, or depart from the usual pattern of angina (Theroux & Fuster, 1998), occur in the absence of physical or emotional stress and last more than 20 min. Like stable angina, UA is due to an imbalance between myocardial oxygen supply and demand, but the mechanism is usually a reduction in coronary perfusion due to plaque rupture leading to coronary thrombosis.

Key point

Variant (Prinzmetal) angina is a form of myocardial ischaemia due to coronary artery spasm that should be mentioned here. Variant angina may present with rest pain in the absence of a primary component of underlying atherothrombosis, but it is a relatively rare disorder in Caucasians (Pristipino et al. 2000) and requires specific vasodilation therapy (nitrates and calcium channel blockers).

Acute MI

The pathogenesis of UAP and acute MI (AMI) are the same (Fuster et al. 1999), and it is not clear which individuals will develop one or the other. AMI may occur with no prior warning, or may be preceded by a short period of instability characterised by angina at rest for 24–48 h (Hochman et al. 1999). A precipitating factor such as vigorous physical exercise, emotional stress or medical/surgical illness can be present in those who develop AMI, but symptoms often appear at rest. Frequency of AMI seems to be highest in the morning, within a few hours of waking (Antman & Braunwald 2001). AMI is characterised by ischaemic pain which is usually prolonged and severe, with symptoms as described earlier.

Patients with MI have now been sub-categorised into ST elevation myocardial infarction (STEMI) and non-ST elevation myocardial infarction (NSTEMI), on the basis of their presentation ECG findings (Table 18.2). Studies undertaken more than 25 years ago demonstrated that patients presenting with an AMI who had ST elevation on their presentation ECG, frequently had an occluded epicardial coronary artery, whereas those without ST elevation often did not. Strategies to open the occluded vessel in patients with acute ST elevation have developed with substantial success. However, these same strategies, thrombolysis and immediate angiography, appear to be less effective in those patients without ST elevation.

The definition of STEMI and NSTEMI requires knowledge of the presenting symptoms, ECG and Tn. Urgent management of ACS, particularly STEMI, is of paramount importance for patient prognosis. However, the Tn may not be rapidly available and may not rise for several hours

Table 18.2   Clinical classification of ACSs.

Syndrome	Abbreviation	Clinical definition
Unstable angina	UA	• rest angina >20 min • ECG changes present or absent
Non-ST elevation acute coronary syndrome	NSTE-ACS	• rest angina >20 min • ST/T changes but no ST elevation • Tn result pending (patients may evolve to UA or NSTEMI)
ST elevation acute coronary syndrome	STE-ACS	• rest angina >20 min • ST elevation • Tn result pending (most patients will progress to STEMI)
Non-ST elevation myocardial infarction	NSTEMI	• rest angina >20 min • ST/T changes but no ST elevation • Positive Tn
ST elevation myocardial infarction	STEMI	• rest angina >20 min • ST-segment elevation • positive Tn

after the initial presentation; thus, it is not always possible to make an immediate diagnosis of STEMI/NSTEMI. As a result, two equivalent terms have evolved to define patients on the basis of clinical symptoms and ECG alone. Patients with an ST elevation acute coronary syndrome (STE-ACS) present with rest angina and ST elevation. Most of these patients will evolve into a STEMI and are managed as per STEMI protocols. Patients with a non-ST elevation acute coronary syndrome (NSTE-ACS) will subsequently be classified as NSTEMI if the Tn is positive, or UA if the Tn is negative (Table 18.2). Hence, the diagnoses of NSTE-ACS and STE-ACS are of particular use in the early acute care setting. Furthermore, the term NSTE-ACS is often used to categorise UA and NSTEMI together with the exclusion of STEMI.

Global trends in ACS presentations

More than a million patients with ACS are admitted to coronary care units in the United States alone each year. The proportion of NSTE-ACS to STEMI patients has changed in recent years, although this is difficult to quantitate due to the changing definition of AMI with the development of the Tn assay. Currently, the rate of NSTE-ACS is higher than STEMI with 3 NSTE-ACS admissions occurring per 1,000 inhabitants. The initial aggressive management with STEMI patients has impacted on prognosis, although 1-month mortality remains higher than NSTE-ACS,

being 7% versus 5% respectively. However, by 6 months, the mortality is similar between STEMI and NSTE-ACS, that is, 12% versus 13%. Thus, cardiac events occur early in the course of STEMI whereas they occur late in NSTE-ACS (Bassand et al. 2007).

A universal definition of 'MI' has recently been proposed which is based on differences in pathophysiology, including MI related to percutaneous intervention (PCI) or coronary bypass graft surgery (CABG) (Table 18.3) (Thygesen et al. 2007). This definition may be useful in refining guidelines for management of MI according to causal mechanism, and in describing or categorising MI in epidemiological studies and clinical trials.

Clinical history in ACS

Typical clinical presentations

Chest pain is the most common presenting symptom for ACS. Several clinical presentations have been particularly distinguished (Bassand et al. 2007), including:

- Rest angina: prolonged angina at rest persisting >20 min
- De novo severe angina: new onset angina which markedly limits ordinary physical activity (e.g. inability to walk around the block)
- Destabilised stable angina: patients with chronic stable angina who are increasingly

Table 18.3 Proposed clinical classification of types of MI.

Type	Description
1	Spontaneous MI related to ischaemia due to a primary coronary event such as plaque erosion and/or rupture, fissuring or dissection
2	MI secondary to ischaemia due to either increased oxygen demand or decreased oxygen supply (in conditions such as coronary artery spasm, coronary embolism, anaemia, arrhythmias, hypertension or hypotension)
3	Sudden unexpected cardiac death, including cardiac arrest: • often with symptoms suggestive of myocardial ischaemia accompanied by presumably new ST-segment elevation or new left bundle branch block, or • evidence of fresh thrombus in a coronary artery by angiography and/or at autopsy, but death occurring before blood samples could be obtained or at a time before the appearance of cardiac biomarkers in the blood
4a	MI associated with percutaneous intervention
4b	MI associated with stent thrombosis as documented by angiography or at autopsy
5	MI associated with CABG

Source: Reprinted from Thygesen et al. (2007). Copyright 2007, with permission from Elsevier.

limited by their angina (rapidly deteriorating exercise tolerance)

- Post-infarct angina: angina in a patient with a recent MI

The features of chest pain in ACS are similar to those described by Heberden, although the relationship with exertion is often less evident. The pain is usually described as tightness, pressure, heaviness, ache or may be mistaken for indigestion. The location of pain can vary, but usually involves the chest and may be central or left sided. It may also involve the epigastrium, left or both arms, and/or the throat, and may radiate to the jaw, back or shoulder. According to Pope and Selker (2003a), the exact location of chest pain is not significantly different in patients with ischaemic and non-ischaemic chest pain, but radiation to the arms

or neck does increase the likelihood of myocardial ischaemia. Chest pain related to myocardial ischaemia is not usually altered by changes in posture or position, and is not exacerbated by movement in the region of pain localisation or by deep inspiration. Symptoms that may be associated with the chest pain include dyspnoea, nausea and vomiting, diaphoresis and dizziness. Typical symptoms of myocardial ischaemia are listed in Table 18.4.

Patients who present with AMI are often anxious and distressed due to severe pain. Associated diaphoresis and peripheral coolness may be present. Although haemodynamic observations may be initially within normal limits, around 25% of patients with anterior wall AMI have associated sympathetic nervous system hyperactivity (tachycardia and/or hypertension), whereas up to half of patients presenting with inferior wall AMI have

Table 18.4 Typical symptoms of myocardial ischaemia.

Stable angina	Unstable angina	Acute myocardial infarction

Typical symptoms:
- pain
  most typically:
  –central or left-sided chest
  –left arm
  –jaw
  may involve or radiate to:
  –both arms
  –epigastrium
  –back
  –throat
	Typical symptoms:
	- As for stable angina but may be more severe
		Typical symptoms:
		- As for stable angina but may be more severe and involve a wider range of the symptoms listed

May also have: - shortness of breath - nausea and vomiting - sweating - palpitations - weakness - anxiety		
Typically provoked by: - exercise - sexual activity - emotional stress - angina is often provoked by the same types of activities and may be predictable	*Typically provoked by:* - may occur during exercise, stress or at rest - provoking factors are usually unpredictable	*Typically provoked by:* - may occur during exercise, stress or at rest
Typically occurs: - in the morning - after a heavy meal - in cold weather	*Typically occurs:* - can occur at any time - may occur with increasing frequency	*Typically occurs:* - can occur at any time

Table 18.4   *(cont'd)*

Stable angina	Unstable angina	Acute myocardial infarction
Typical duration: • 2–10 min	*Typical duration:* • usually <30 min • episodes may come and go frequently over a period of time • patients may describe having had pain for 2 or 3 days, but in fact the pain is not constant – it comes and goes	*Typical duration:* • >30 min
Alleviating factors: • rest • sub-lingual nitrate	*Alleviating factors:* May require • intravenous nitrates • anticoagulation • beta-blockers or calcium channel blockers	*Alleviating factors:* • Reperfusion (PCI or thrombolysis)

associated parasympathetic activity (bradycardia and/or hypotension) (Antman & Braunwald 2001).

Atypical presentations

Approximately 8% of ACS patients do not experience chest pain (Brieger et al. 2004). The major presenting symptoms in these patients include dyspnoea (49%), diaphoresis (26%), nausea/vomiting (24%) and pre-syncope/syncope (19%) (Brieger et al. 2004). Other less-common presentations may result from sudden loss of consciousness, confusion or profound weakness, which may occur as a result of impaired ventricular function or arrhythmia (Antman & Braunwald 2001). Patients with an atypical presentation frequently have poorer outcomes with increased in-hospital mortality (Brieger et al. 2004), and thus an increased vigilance is required for these presentations. Atypical ACS presentations are more likely to occur in women and those with a history of diabetes, heart failure or hypertension. It has been suggested that the elderly and those with high alcohol intake may also have an atypical presentation (Canto et al. 2000).

Patients presenting without chest pain are sometimes considered to have 'silent ischaemia'. The mechanism(s) responsible for silent ischaemia is (are) unclear. Somatic pain sensitivity and endorphins do not appear to be causal agents in the phenomenon (Glusman et al. 1996), nor does there seem to be an associated psychological bias against reporting pain in these individuals (Freedland et al. 1996). It has been suggested that abnormal central processing of afferent pain messages from the heart may play a role in silent myocardial ischaemia (Rosen et al. 1996).

Key point

Not all presentations with ACS experience typical symptoms: these atypical presentations may obscure the diagnosis.

Physical examination in ACS patients

The physical examination is an important component in the assessment of patients with an ACS, although it may often be unremarkable. The experienced clinician will rapidly identify the characteristic features of a patient with an AMI from the 'end of the bed'. These patients will appear pale, sweaty and sit/lie motionless often clutching their chest. If associated with dyspnoea, then significant left ventricular dysfunction should be suspected. Examination of the pulse and blood pressure will identify the presence of arrhythmias or shock. This later finding is especially essential, as urgent therapy of shock states is imperative. Examination of the precordium is important to ascertain the presence of ACS haemodynamic consequences (such as acute mitral regurgitation or ventricular septal rupture) or other previous cardiac abnormalities which may impact on management strategies (for instance, severe aortic stenosis). Also, assessment for the presence of cardiac failure is important.

Besides defining the characteristic of the ACS presentation, the clinical examination is useful in considering alternate diagnoses for the presenting chest pain. For example, differential blood pressures between each arm and an aortic regurgitant murmur may indicate aortic dissection. The presence of a pericardial or pleural rub may suggest pericarditis or pleuritis respectively. Refer to Chapter 9 for more detailed information on physical assessment.

The 12-lead electrocardiogram in ACS

The ECG is a fundamental clinical tool in the assessment of the ACS patient in many cases, and can be instrumental in providing an instantaneous indication as to what the immediate management strategy should be. It should be remembered, however, that electrocardiography does have some limitations: an ECG may suggest that a patient's heart is entirely normal when, in fact, severe and widespread CAD is present. Less than half of patients presenting to hospital with an AMI will have the typical and diagnostic electrocardiographic changes present on their initial ECG, and as many as 20% of patients will have a normal, or near normal ECG (Channer & Morris 2002). Nevertheless, the ECG has stood the test of time to remain one of the most useful clinical tools available in diagnosing abnormal cardiac conditions.

In ACS, acute and evolving ECG changes may provide information that assists the clinician to identify the likely culprit coronary artery; estimate the timing of the ischaemic event in MI and estimate the amount of myocardium at risk according to coronary artery dominance, collateralisation, size and distribution of arterial segments, and location, extent, and severity of coronary stenoses (Thygesen et al. 2007). Characteristic changes on the 12-lead ECG indicative of myocardial ischaemia and infarction involve the ST segment, T wave and the QRS complex.

ST segment

The ST segment can become elevated or depressed in myocardial ischaemia/infarction.

ST-segment depression

ST-segment depression usually indicates sub-endocardial ischaemia. If ST-segment depression is new, persistent and marked, there is an increased likelihood that it will be related to AMI (Pope & Selker 2003b). Marked ST-segment depression in the precordial leads, particularly in leads V4 and V5, is often due to extensive ischaemia as a result of stenosis of the left main coronary artery and/or to triple vessel disease, and may produce life-threatening haemodynamic disturbance, both systolic and diastolic (Sclarovsky et al. 1986).

Key point

ST-segment depression has been shown in several studies to be a predictor of poor clinical outcome in terms of recurrent myocardial ischaemia, AMI and death (Patel et al. 1996; Anderson et al. 1996; Cannon et al. 1997; Boersma et al. 2000).

ST-segment elevation

Taken in context with a patient history and examination, ST-segment elevation is likely to indicate AMI and requires the urgent application of a reperfusion strategy to minimise myocardial damage.

T waves

T waves may increase in amplitude, become flattened, biphasic or inverted during episodes of myocardial ischaemia. The first ECG sign of sudden narrowing or obstruction of an epicardial artery is often tall, peaked (hyperacute) T waves (Chesebro et al. 1991) that precede the elevation of the ST segment (Thygesen et al. 2007). Biphasic T waves generally are associated with an acute ischaemic episode, and biphasic pattern (terminal T-wave inversion) will usually progress to deep symmetrical T-wave inversion, best seen in the anterior precordial leads (Channer & Morris 2002). 'Pseudonormalisation' or 'normalisation' of the T wave is a phenomenon where the T wave has become inverted following an ischaemic event, and a recurrent ischaemic event results in the

Table 18.5 ECG localisation of the culprit artery in ACS.

Culprit artery	12-lead ECG ST changes
Right coronary artery (RCA)	• Lead II, III and aVF • ST depression in V1–2 and ST elevation in incremental leads V7–9 (posterior infarct) • Lead aVR or incremental lead V4$_R$ (right ventricular infarction)
Cx	• Lead V5–6 • May be electrographically silent
Left anterior descending (LAD)	• Lead V2–4 and may involve I, aVL, V5–6 • Isolated Lead I & aVL (suggestive of diagonal branch disease)
Left main coronary artery (LMCA)	• ST depression with T inversion in V1–2

inverted T wave first becoming biphasic and then returning to what appears to be a normal configuration. This is usually followed by ST-segment elevation if the ischaemia is not resolved.

The QRS complex

Pathological Q waves (initial downward deflection of ≥40 ms in duration in any lead except III and aVR) is the most characteristic ECG finding of transmural MI of the left ventricle (AHA 2007), but are of limited value in the acute setting as the age of the Q wave is often indeterminate (Pope & Selker 2003b).

A pattern of poor R-wave progression in the precordial leads may indicate an anterior MI, but as with Q waves, the age of the infarction may be indeterminate. Observing the pattern of R-wave progression is useful though in patients with a normal ECG but other clinical indicators of AMI, as progressively reduced R-wave amplitude occasionally is seen on serial ECGs in anterior infarction as the only electrocardiographic indicator of recent MI.

Key point

ST-segment and T-wave changes can occur for a number of reasons unrelated to myocardial ischaemia. Refer to Chapter 11 for more detailed information about the ECG.

The 12-lead ECG assists not only in the identification of the presence of myocardial ischaemia,

but also its coronary territory. This is of major importance in the management of the ACS patient as it assists in identifying the culprit coronary artery responsible for the ACS presentation. Common patterns are described in Table 18.5.

Cardiac markers in ACS

Traditionally CK, or its isoenzyme CK-MB, has been used as the primary biomarker of myocardial injury in ACS. However, in contemporary cardiac practice, Tn is the diagnostic marker of myocardial injury in ACS, given its greater sensitivity and specificity. Furthermore, troponins have been shown to be the best biomarkers for predicting 30-day MI and death. In a patient with MI, a Tn rise is evident within 3–4 h of its onset and may persist up to 2 weeks. Two Tn biomarkers are available, namely Troponin T (TnT) and Troponin I (TnI). Although differences between assay accuracy have been reported in the literature, expert consensus is that there is no fundamental difference between the assays (Bassand et al. 2007).

Clinical assessment and risk stratification in ACS

The fundamental purpose of assessing a patient with an ACS is to determine their risk for further events. This is best undertaken by considering the clinical presentation, ECG findings and Tn levels. Several ACS risk stratification models have been established and these are further discussed in the next chapter.

Another important consideration is the immediate assessment of the ACS patient when they arrive at the emergency department and triaged by the triage nurse. This is an important consideration which must be rapidly undertaken without the immediate availability of the standard diagnostic investigations listed earlier. The role of the nurse in risk assessment and triage is detailed in Chapters 19 and 20. Summarised guidelines for the triage nurse in the rapid assessment of those at risk of ACS are summarised in Table 18.6.

Key point

Telephone triage

Health practitioners frequently receive telephone calls from patients who are seeking information or reassurance about symptoms that they are experiencing, such as chest pain or discomfort. Patients with symptoms that suggest possible ACS should be referred to a facility that allows evaluation by a physician, recording of a 12-lead ECG and blood tests for cardiac markers to be taken. Patients with known CAD who report a worsening should be advised to go directly to an emergency department, preferably by ambulance (Gibbons et al. 2003).

Table 18.6. Triage nurse guidelines for the identification of ACS patients.

Presenting complaint
- Chest pain
    Location: central, sub-sternal, epigastric
        Type: compressing, crushing, tightness, heaviness, pressure, cramping, aching pain
    Radiation: neck, jaw, shoulders
- Associated dyspnoea, nausea/vomiting or diaphoresis

Prior medical history
- Previous heart attack, bypass, angioplasty
- Regular use of sub-lingual nitrates
- Diabetes, hypertension, smoking, high cholesterol

Special considerations
- Women – frequently have atypical pain
- Diabetics – may have no chest pain
- Elderly – may have atypical presentation such as confusion, lethargy

Source: From Braunwald et al. (2000).

Conclusion

Acute coronary syndromes represent a wide spectrum of coronary disorders with variable prognosis and management. The clinical presentation is fundamental in the assessment of these patients, and therefore important in their management.

Learning activity

Arthur Dodd is a 70-year-old male who presents to the emergency department with chest pain. He has a past history of peptic ulcer disease but no other significant medical problems. His only regular medication is omeprazole, but he tells you that he has taken aspirin in the last few days because he hurt his back whilst digging in the garden. He says that over the last few days, he has had a lot of epigastric discomfort and burning. This morning, he was awoken from sleep by a different type of pain in his chest which radiated to his jaw. He said that he had palpitations and gave a typical description of ischaemic chest pain. His ECG shows atrial fibrillation at a rate of 180 beats per minute with 1 mm of ST-segment depression in the anterior leads. His cardiac enzymes are pending, and the only other abnormality is a low haemoglobin (98 g/dL).

What is his working diagnosis at this point in time according to the definitions and descriptions of ACS that you have read?

Arthur's cardiac enzymes are now available and his Tn is elevated. He will be transferred to the coronary care unit.

What is his diagnosis now?

Looking at the 'universal definition' of MI, what sort of MI has Arthur had?

References

American Heart Association (AHA) (2007). Myocardial injury, ischaemia and infarction. Retrieved online 6th November 2007 from http://www.americanheart.org/presenter.jhtml?identifier=251

Anderson, K., Eriksson, S.V., Dellborg, M. (1996). Non-invasive risk stratification within 48 hours of hospital admission in patients with unstable coronary disease. *European Heart Journal*, **18**:780–8.

Antman, E. & Braunwald, E. (2001). Acute myocardial infarction. In: E. Braunwald (ed.), *Braunwald: Heart Disease: A Textbook of Cardiovascular Medicine*, 6th edn, Vol. 2. W.B. Saunders, St. Louis, pp. 1114–231.

Bassand, J.P., Hamm, C.W., Ardissino, D., et al. (2007). Guidelines for the diagnosis and treatment of non-ST-segment elevation acute coronary syndromes: the task force for the diagnosis and treatment of non-ST-segment elevation acute coronary syndromes of the European Society of Cardiology. *European Heart Journal*, **28**:1598–660.

Boersma, E., Pieper, K.S., Steyerberg, E.W., et al. for the PURSUIT Investigators (2000). Predictors of outcome in patients with acute coronary syndromes without persistent ST-segment elevation. *Circulation*, **101**:2557–67.

Braunwald, E., Antman, E.M., Beasley, J.W., et al. (2000). ACC/AHA guidelines for the management of patients with unstable angina and non-ST-segment elevation myocardial infarction. A report of the American College of Cardiology/American Heart Association Task Force on Practice Guidelines (Committee on the Management of Patients With Unstable Angina). *Journal of the American College of Cardiology*, **36**:970–1062.

Brieger, D., Eagle, K.A., Goodman, S.G., et al. (2004). Acute coronary syndromes without chest pain, an underdiagnosed and undertreated high-risk group: insights from the Global Registry of Acute Coronary Events. *Chest*, **126**:461–9.

Cannon, C.P., McCabe, C.H., Stone, P.H., et al. (1997). The electrocardiogram predicts one-year outcome of patients with unstable angina and non-Q-wave myocardial infarction: results of the TIMI III Registry ECG Ancillary Study: thrombolysis in myocardial ischaemia. *Journal of the American College of Cardiology*, **30**:133–40.

Canto, J.G., Shlipak, M.G., Rogers, W.J., et al. (2000). Prevalence, clinical characteristics, and mortality among patients with myocardial infarction presenting without chest pain. *Journal of the American Medical Association*, **283**:3223–9.

Channer, K. & Morris, F. (2002). ABC of clinical electrocardiography: myocardial ischaemia. *British Medical Journal*, **324**:1023–6. Available online at http://www.bmj.com/cgi/reprint/324/7344/1023

Chesebro, J.H., Zolhelyi, P. & Fuster, V. (1991). Pathogenesis of thrombosis in unstable angina. *American Journal of Cardiology*, **68**:B2–10.

Crea, F., Biasucci, L.M., Buffon, L, et al. (1997). Role of inflammation in the pathogenesis of unstable coronary artery disease. *American Journal of Cardiology*, **80**(Suppl.):10E–16.

Freedland, K.E., Carney, R.M., Krone, R.J., et al. (1996). Psychological determinants of anginal pain perception during exercise testing of stable patients after recovery from acute myocardial infarction or unstable angina pectoris. *American Journal of Cardiology*, **77**:1–4.

Fuster, V., Fayad, Z.A. & Badimon, J.J. (1999). Acute coronary syndromes: biology. *The Lancet*, **353** (Suppl. II):5–9.

Gibbons, R.J., Chatterjee, K., Daley, J., et al. (1999). ACC/AHA/ACP-ASIM guidelines for the management of patients with chronic stable angina: a report of the American College of Cardiology/American Heart Association Task Force on Practice Guidelines (Committee on Management of Patients With Chronic Stable Angina). *Journal of the American College of Cardiology*, **33**:2092–197.

Gibbons, R.J., Alpert, J.S. & Antman, E.M. (2003). ACC/AHA 2002 guideline update for the management of patients with chronic stable angina: a report of the American College of Cardiology/American Heart Association Task Force on Practice Guidelines (Committee to update the 1999 Guidelines for the Management of Patients With Chronic Stable Angina). *Circulation*, **107**:149–58, doi:10.1161/01.CIR.0000047041.66447.29

Glusman, M., Coromilas, J., Clark, W.C., et al. (1996). Pain sensitivity in silent myocardial ischemia. *Pain*, **64**:477–83.

Heberden, W. (1772). Some account of a disorder of the breast. *Medical Transactions*, **2**:59.

Hochman, J.S., Sleeper, L.A., Webb, J.G., et al. for the Should We Emergently Revascularize Occluded Coronaries for Cardiogenic Shock (SHOCK) Investigators (1999). Early revascularization in acute myocardial infarction complicated by cardiogenic shock. *New England Journal of Medicine*; **341**:625–34.

Patel, D.J., Holdright, D.R., Knight, C.J., et al. (1996). Early continuous ST segment monitoring in unstable angina: prognostic value additional to the clinical characteristics and the admission electrocardiogram. *Heart*, **75**:222–8.

Pope, J.H. & Selker, H.P. (2003a). Diagnosis of acute cardiac ischemia. *Emergency Medical Clinics of North America*, **21**:27–59.

Pope, J.H. & Selker, H.P. (2003b). Emergency department presentations of acute myocardial ischaemia. In: C.P. Cannon (ed.), *Management of Acute Coronary Syndromes*, 2nd edn. Human Press Inc, New Jersey, pp. 121–55.

Pristipino, C., Beltrame, J.F., Finocchiaro, M.L., et al. (2000). Major racial differences in coronary constrictor response between Japanese and Caucasians with recent myocardial infarction. *Circulation*, **101**:1102–8.

Quinn, T., Webster, R. & Hatchett, R. (2003). Coronary heart disease: angina and acute myocardial infarction. In: R. Hatchett & D. Thompson (eds), *Cardiac Nursing*. Churchill Livingstone, Edinburgh.

Rosen, S.D., Paulesu, E., Nihoyannopoulos, P., et al. (1996). Silent ischemia as a central problem: regional brain activation compared in silent and painful myocardial ischemia. *Annals of Internal Medicine*, **124**:939–49.

Sclarovsky, S., Davidson, E., Strasberg, B., et al. (1986). Unstable angina: the significance of ST segment elevation or depression in patients without evidence of increased myocardial oxygen demand. *American Heart Journal*, **112**:463–7.

Theroux, P. & Fuster, V. (1998). Acute coronary syndromes: unstable angina and non-Q-wave myocardial infarction. *Circulation*, **97**:1195–206.

Thygesen, K., Alpert, J.S. & White, H.D. on behalf of the Joint ESC/ACCF/AHA/WHF Task Force for the redefinition of myocardial infarction (2007). *Journal of the American College of Cardiology*, 50:2173–95.

Verheugt, F.W.A. (1999). Acute coronary syndromes: interventions. *The Lancet*, **353**(suppl II):16–19.

Useful Websites and Further Reading

Antman, E.M., Anbe, D.T., Armstrong, P.W., et al. (2004). ACC/AHA guidelines for the management of patients with ST-elevation myocardial infarction – executive summary. A report of the American College of Cardiology/American Heart Association Task Force on Practice Guidelines (Writing Committee to revise the 1999 guidelines for the management of patients with acute myocardial infarction). *Journal of the American College of Cardiology*, **44**:671–719.

Bassand, J.P., Hamm, C.W., Ardissino, D., et al. (2007). Guidelines for the diagnosis and treatment of non-ST-segment elevation acute coronary syndromes: the task force for the diagnosis and treatment of non-ST-segment elevation acute coronary syndromes of the European Society of Cardiology. *European Heart Journal*, **28**:1598–660.

Braunwald, E., Antman, E.M., Beasley, J.W., et al. (2000). ACC/AHA guidelines for the management of patients with unstable angina and non-ST-segment elevation myocardial infarction. A report of the American College of Cardiology/American Heart Association Task Force on Practice Guidelines (Committee on the Management of Patients with Unstable Angina). *Journal of the American College of Cardiology*, **36**:970–1062.

Channer, K. & Morris, F. (2002). ABC of clinical electrocardiography: myocardial ischaemia. *British Medical Journal*, **324**:1023–6. Available online at http://www.bmj.com/cgi/reprint/324/7344/1023

Edhouse, J., Brady, W.J. & Morris, F. (2002). ABC of clinical electrocardiography: myocardial infarction – Part II. *British Medical Journal*, **324**:963–6. Available online at http://www.bmj.com/cgi/reprint/324/7343/963

Goldman, L. & Kirtane, A.J. (2003). Triage of patients with acute chest pain and possible cardiac ischemia: the elusive search for diagnostic perfection. *Annals of Internal Medicine*, **139**:987–95. Available online at http://www.annals.org/cgi/content/full/139/12/987

Lee, H.T. & Goldman, L (2000). Evaluation of the patient with chest pain. *New England Journal of Medicine*, **342**:1187–95.

Morris, F. & Brady, W.J. (2002). ABC of clinical electrocardiography: myocardial infarction – Part I. *British Medical Journal*, **324**:831–4. Available online at http://www.bmj.com/cgi/reprint/324/7341/831

The Joint European Society of Cardiology/American College of Cardiology Committee (2000). Myocardial infarction redefined. A consensus document of The Joint European Society of Cardiology/American College of Cardiology Committee for the redefinition of Myocardial Infarction. *European Heart Journal*, **21**:1502–13.

Thygesen, K., Alpert, J.J., White, H.D., et al. (2007). Universal definition of myocardial infarction. *Circulation*, published online 19 October 2007, DOI: 10.1161/CIRCULATIONAHA.107.187397. Available at http://circ.ahajournals.org/cgi/reprint/CIRCULATIONAHA.107.187397v1.pdf

19 Risk Stratification in Acute Coronary Syndromes

A. Day, C. Ryan & T. Quinn

Overview

Acute coronary syndromes (ACS) are a major health problem resulting in high rates of hospital attendance. For patients who present with ischaemic symptoms and evidence of ST-segment elevation acute myocardial infarction (STEMI), treatment should progress rapidly following standard reperfusion protocols. In the absence of ST-segment elevation, early risk assessment is required to guide specific treatment to reduce the likelihood of an adverse outcome. There is growing recognition that patients with non-ST segment elevation presentations of ACS are at increased risk of death, and that, moreover, the vast majority of presentations with acute chest pain result in a non-cardiac diagnosis. The challenge for the nurse, as part of the team assessing patients presenting with chest pain or other symptoms suggestive of ACS, is to help identify those patients who need prompt access to specialised (and costly) cardiac care, as well as those who are sufficiently at low risk to be discharged or cared for in a lower dependency area.

Learning objectives

After reading this chapter, you should be able to:

- Discuss the burden of both ACS and undifferentiated chest pain.

- Discuss the importance of risk stratification in ACS.
- Describe the key elements of the assessment of patients with suspected ACS.
- Examine the role of chest pain units and pathways in dealing with patients with ACS and compare this with your current clinical facility.
- Identify and compare risk scoring systems for ACS patients.

Key concepts

Risk stratification; chest pain protocols; algorithms

Introduction

Non-ST elevation presentations of ACS are common, with an estimated 1,200,000 hospital admissions in the United Kingdom alone each year (British Cardiac Society 2001). Discharge diagnoses of unstable angina exceed those for myocardial infarction (MI) with a ratio of 2:1 (Fox et al. 2000). Six-month mortality and incidence of non-fatal MI is around 12%. When refractory angina or re-admission for unstable angina is included, the overall rate of adverse events at 6 months is

30%. A three- to fivefold increase in risk of death or new MI is seen in elderly (>75 years) patients and those with ST depression or bundle branch block, in comparison to younger patients and those presenting with a normal ECG. The elevated risk is sustained at 4-year follow-up (Collinson et al. 2000). Non-ST elevation ACS is not a benign condition.

Identification of the 'true positive' ACS patient from the vast numbers presenting with chest pain is a challenge. In one UK study, only 1 in 18 patients with acute chest pain calling for an ambulance had a final diagnosis of ACS (Deakin et al. 2006). Moreover, of around 700,000 patients attending emergency departments with acute chest pain in England and Wales each year (around 6% of adult attendances), one-third had a clinical diagnosis of ACS without clear ECG changes (Goodacre et al. 2005), further illustrating the need for robust assessment processes to safeguard patients from inappropriate discharge.

Risk stratification

When a patient presents with chest pain or other symptoms suggestive of ACS, assessment must progress rapidly. While chest pain is conventionally regarded as the principal symptom suggesting ACS, and is the focus of this chapter, it is important that the nurse should be aware of the significant minority of patients who present atypically.

Patients with suspected ACS fall into three main categories: (1) those with objective evidence of ischaemia (ST-segment deviation) who need prompt admission and treatment; (2) those with a clear non-cardiac cause and (3) those who require a diagnostic process to rule out ACS (Christenson et al. 2006). The evaluation of a patient with suspected ACS is challenging because chest discomfort has many causes and even 'bona fide' ACS may present in atypical fashion. The differential diagnosis of chest pain is broad and includes pulmonary, musculoskeletal, gastrointestinal, dermatological, psychiatric and cardiovascular conditions. Life-threatening differential diagnoses include pulmonary embolism, tension pneumothorax and aortic dissection, which require rapid diagnosis and interventions that are very different from ACS therapies (Swap & Nagurney 2005).

Patients with suspected ACS should undergo a brief focused history, physical examination and 12-lead ECG. ST-segment elevation myocardial infarction (STEMI) patients are usually identified early because of characteristic electrocardiograph changes. The majority of 'suspected ACS' patients encountered in emergency department practice present with 'undifferentiated chest pain', non-ST elevation MI (NSTEMI) or unstable angina. Diagnosis can be especially difficult if the patient is pain free on presentation, with a normal 12-lead ECG and normal baseline cardiac markers. An unstructured approach to management may lead, on the one hand, to inappropriate discharge and a 'missed' MI in 1–5%, or to unnecessary or prolonged hospitalisation in up to 50% of patients with chest pain (Aroney et al. 2003). Mortality in patients discharged with missed MI is four times greater than in those admitted to hospital (Herren et al. 2001).

The health professional must assess the likelihood that symptoms result from acute ischaemia caused by coronary artery disease (CAD). Traditional risk factors for CAD, such as hypertension, hypercholesterolaemia and smoking, are only weakly predictive of the likelihood of acute ischaemia and are much less significant than the duration of symptoms, ECG findings and biomarker levels (Pollack & Gibler 2001). Patients with likely ACS are subsequently stratified into high, intermediate or low short-term risk of death or non-fatal MI, using validated tools discussed later in this chapter.

The application of risk stratification models to the patient with chest pain is consistent with the emerging focus on safety of the overall management strategy, rather than merely establishing a diagnosis (Boufous et al. 2003). High-risk patients require close monitoring and therapeutic interventions. Intermediate-risk patients are common. Confirmed low-risk patients can often safely be discharged home and managed subsequently in the outpatient setting. An attempt to determine which chest pain patients admitted to cardiac care unit (CCU) could be safely transferred to a lower dependency area reported the poor performance of a consensus-derived algorithm based on ECG and clinical features alone (Quinn et al. 2000).

Rapid, efficient and accurate evaluation of the patient who presents with chest pain optimises care from an individual, as well as public health, economic and (institutional and professional) liability perspective (Ng et al. 2001; Mitchell et al. 2006). With improved availability and access to interventional cardiology, reperfusion and antiplatelet drugs, patients with ACS now have improved outlook compared to earlier years. Treatment benefits are dependent upon early identification and initiation of definitive therapies (Kucia et al. 2001).

Key points

There are three major components to the risk stratification of patients presenting with chest pain.

1 Assessment of the likelihood that symptoms are related to ACS
2 Evaluation of the short-term risk of death, MI or other adverse events
3 Frequent re-evaluation for the development of high-risk features in patients initially assessed as having intermediate- or low-risk presentations

Risk stratification guidelines

The European Society of Cardiology (ESC) (2007) recommends that diagnosis and short-term risk stratification of ACS patients should be based on a combination of clinical history, symptoms, ECG biomarkers and risk score results. These tests help triage the patient and place them on the most appropriate route within the clinical pathway. Physical examination and chest X-ray are often normal but essential to exclude non-cardiac causes of chest pain (such as pulmonary embolism or musculoskeletal pain), and provides the health care professional with a baseline to work from.

The 12-lead ECG is quick and non-invasive. ECG changes compatible with ischaemia usually confirm the diagnosis of an acute coronary syndrome, but the initial ECG in patients with acute MI can be normal or non-diagnostic in many patients. A normal ECG does not exclude ACS (Gamon et al. 2007).

Continuous 12-lead ST-segment monitoring is recommended because ECG changes can be dynamic, reflecting the nature of coronary thrombosis and

myocardial ischaemia. Ischaemic episodes may be clinically silent in up to two-thirds of cases and, therefore, not detectable by standard resting ECG. About 15–30% of patients with non-ST elevation ACS have transient episodes of ST-segment changes, predominantly ST-segment depression. These patients have an increased risk of subsequent cardiac events (European Society of Cardiology [ESC] 2007).

Biomarkers reflect myocardial cell injury, inflammation, platelet activation or neurohormonal activation. Troponins (cTnT or cTnI) are the preferred markers of injury, and have better sensitivity and specificity than traditional cardiac enzymes. Troponins are released into the blood within 3h of injury, peak at 12–24h and remain elevated for 14 days. Around 50% of patients with acute MI will have a positive troponin 6h after the onset of chest pain, but 12h may be required for these markers to become reliably positive in 99% of cases (Jowett & Thompson 2007). Myoglobin is typically released within 1–3h after MI, peaking at 4–8h before returning to normal within 24h. It is important to recognise the many other conditions in which troponin elevation occurs (Ammann et al. 2004), as listed in Box 19.1. Several novel biomarkers have been the subject of research in recent years, although prospective evaluation is required before these become available for use in routine clinical practice. Bedside ('point of care') testing has some advantages, enabling adequately trained staff to obtain information rapidly. However, point of care testing is observer dependent and where there is doubt about the accuracy of interpretation, such tests should be repeated and verified in the laboratory. Biomarker results, as with any other investigation, require interpretation in the context of careful history taking and other assessment.

Exercise tolerance tests (ETT) are often conducted if biomarkers are negative and allow identification of low-risk patients who might avoid hospital admission. The main aims are:

• To provoke symptoms such as chest pain and dyspnoea
• To demonstrate ECG changes with progressive workload
• To determine maximum workload
• To assess prognosis

Box 19.1   Conditions other than ACS that are associated with troponin elevation

Amyloidosis
Aortic dissection
Aortic valve disease
Apical ballooning syndrome
Burns
Cardiac ablation
Cardiac biopsy
Cardiac contusion
Cardiomyopathy
Cardioversion
Cardiac pacing
Drug toxicity
Heart failure
Hypothyroidism
Renal failure
Respiratory failure
Rhabdomyolysis
Snake envenomation
Sepsis
Stroke
Sub-arachnoid haemorrhage
Severe heart failure

Immediate ETT of low-risk patients with chest pain, who would otherwise have been admitted to hospital, is an effective way to risk-stratify this group into patients who can be discharged and those who require admission. ETT is a relatively safe procedure, with a mortality rate of 1 in 50,000 and non-fatal MI rate of <4 in 10,000 (Arnold & Goodacre 2007). Nevertheless, advanced life support–trained staff must be available. A positive ETT predicts a sixfold increase in risk of adverse events over the 6 months following attendance. ETT testing is useful before discharge in patients with non-diagnostic ECG provided there is no pain, no signs of heart failure and serial biomarkers are normal. Early exercise testing has a high negative predictive value (ESC 2007) but does have some limitations.

Other means of evaluating the ACS patient include echocardiography to assess left ventricular function, and to exclude aortic dissection or pulmonary embolism. Echocardiography facilities should be available as part of the facilities for acute chest pain assessment. Stress echocardiography, stress scintigraphy and magnetic resonance imaging may also be useful in assessing viability of the myocardium. Angiography remains the 'gold standard' for assessing coronary anatomy, and while there is growing interest in use of cardiac computed tomography (CT), this imaging modality is not currently recommended because of sub-optimal diagnostic accuracy and the potential to add delay to percutaneous intervention should this be required (ESC 2007).

Risk scores

In recent years, a systematic approach to risk stratification of patients with ACS has been promoted with several risk scores developed through analysis of clinical trial and registry data. The key variables for each score are shown in Box 19.2. Performance of risk scores has been evaluated in two recent series, employing 'real world' data from large national ACS registries. Yan et al. (2007) compared the TIMI, PURSUIT and GRACE scores for non-STEMI ACS patients, using data from the Canadian ACS II Registry. While all three risk scores were found to confer additional, important, prognostic value beyond global risk assessment by physicians, the PURSUIT and GRACE risk scores were found to allow superior discrimination for hospital and 1-year mortality in patients with a wide range of ACS presentations, compared to TIMI. In the United Kingdom, Gale et al. (2009) compared five risk models – PURSUIT, GUSTO-1, GRACE, Simple Risk Index and EMMACE – using data from the Myocardial Infarction National Audit Project (MINAP). While all models maintained their performance in the categories of patients for whom they had originally been designed, they performed less well in higher risk 'super groups' including diabetes, renal failure or prior angina. Simpler models were considered to be more useful for case-mix adjustment, whereas the more complex models such as GRACE were more useful for assisting decision-making about individual patients. These findings confirm that 'simpler is not necessarily better' (Yan et al. 2007) when deciding on the most appropriate risk score for use in the 'real world' setting.

Box 19.2   Risk models

Risk model	Key variables	
PURSUIT (Boersma et al. 2000)	Age, HR, SBP, ST depression, heart failure, biomarkers	Predicts 30-day death and composite of death or MI in non-STEMI ACS
GUSTO-1 (Califf et al. 2000)	Age, weight, Killip class, SBP, HR, QRS duration, smoking, hypertension, cerebrovascular disease and arrhythmia	Predicts 1-year survival in 30-day survivors of STEMI
GRACE (Fox et al. 2006)	Age, HR, SBP, creatinine, Killip class, ST depression, biomarkers, cardiac arrest	Predicts in-hospital and 6-month deaths (all cause) in STEMI and non-STEMI ACS
Simple risk index (Morrow et al. 2001)	Age, SBP, HR	Predicts 30-day mortality in STEMI
EMMACE (Dorsch et al. 2001)	Age, SBP, HR	Predicts 30-day mortality in STEMI
TIMI (Antman et al. 2000)	Age, risk factors for CAD, recent ASA use, known coronary artery stenosis, angina in past 24 h, ST-segment deviation, biomarkers	Predicts risk of cardiac events (death, MI, urgent revascularisation) at 14 days in non-STEMI ACS

HR, heart rate; SBP, systolic blood pressure; CAD, coronary artery disease; ASA, aspirin.

Chest pain units

When CCUs were originally conceived almost half a century ago, there was little awareness of the high morbidity and mortality of non-ST segment ACS. Care for ACS patients has now embraced new technologies, greatly improved diagnostic and risk stratification strategies, and new therapeutic options. Analysis of a large national registry in the United Kingdom has reported that only two-fifths of patients with non-ST elevation ACS were admitted to CCU and recommended a redefinition of the role of the CCU so that such high-risk patients gain access to specialist care (Quinn et al. 2005).

Recognising the limited number of CCU beds available, chest pain assessment units are growing in popularity and feature in many cardiac clinical pathways, particularly in the United States. There is limited experience of such units in the United Kingdom (Goodacre & Dixon 2005) where services have been developed in an ad hoc and disorganised fashion (Cross et al. 2007). Chest pain units

are systems aimed at providing standardised and efficient care, utilising dedicated and appropriately trained clinical staff with access to diagnostic testing, resulting in rapid patient assessment. Redesigned services for this group of patients have the potential to safely discharge low- to medium-risk patient within 24 h of admission, improving efficiency and avoiding unnecessary admission. Careful, patient-specific, risk assessment aids decision-making regarding therapeutic interventions, triage to alternative levels of hospital care and allocation of clinical resources (Lee & Goldman 2000; Morrow et al. 2000).

Ideally, assessment units should be located within or adjacent to the emergency department, medical admission unit and cardiac care unit to enable easy transfer of the patient between areas. Facilities should be designated for this role and offer ECG telemetry monitoring (including continuous ST-segment monitoring) and resuscitation equipment, especially defibrillation. Diagnostic testing including ETT, pathology and radiology must be readily accessible. To improve efficiency and promote seamless care, nursing staff should be highly trained and should be able to practice according to patient group directions and pre-agreed chest pain protocols/pathways, able to perform venipuncture and intravenous cannulation, and should be advanced life-support providers.

A randomised trial of chest pain observation units in the United Kingdom has reported that of the 79–89% of patients discharged home after assessment, adverse events were uncommon, and that patient anxiety and depression were reduced, and patient-reported quality of life and satisfaction were high compared to standard chest pain assessment (Arnold et al. 2007).

Conclusion

Identification of patients presenting with suspected ACS, and particularly those at high risk of adverse events, is a key priority for nurses in acute cardiac care. The development and use of clinical pathways and new models of care supported by evidence-based guidelines is essential to ensure safe and effective care.

Learning activities

Locate your hospital's agreed pathway for patients with suspected ACS. Review the pathway to determine the evidence base for the pathway.

Find out which ACS risk score is used in your hospital. Use the risk score on your next ACS patient and discuss the outcome with a senior colleague.

References

Ammann, P., Pfisterer, M., Fehr, T. & Rickli, H. (2004). Raised cardiac troponins. *British Medical Journal*, **328**:1028–9.

Antman, E.M., Cohen, M. & Bernink, P.J. (2000). The TIMI risk score for unstable angina/non-ST elevation MI: a method for prognostication and therapeutic decision making. *Journal of the American Medical Association*, **284**:835–42.

Arnold, J. & Goodacre, S. (2007). Should exercise treadmill testing be provided in the emergency department? *Emergency Medicine Journal*, **24**:151.

Arnold, J., Goodacre, S. & Morris, F. on behalf of the ESCAPE research trial (2007). Structure, process and outcomes of chest pain units established in the ESCAPE trial. *Emergency Medicine Journal*, **24**:262–6.

Aroney, C., Dunlevie, H. & Bett, J. (2003). Use of an accelerated chest pain assessment protocol in patients at intermediate risk of adverse cardiac events. *Medical Journal of Australia*, **178**:370–4.

Boersma, E., Pieper, K.S., Steyerberg, E.W., et al. (2000). Predictors of outcome in patients with acute coronary syndrome without persistent ST-segment elevation. Results from an international trial of 9461 patients. *Circulation*, **101**:2557–67.

Boufous, S., Kelleher, P. & Pain, C. (2003). Impact of a chest-pain guideline on clinical decision-making. *Medical Journal of Australia*, **128**:375–80.

British Cardiac Society (2001). Guideline for the management of patients with acute coronary syndromes without persistent ECG ST segment elevation British Cardiac Society Guidelines and Medical Practice Committee, and Royal College of Physicians Clinical Effectiveness and Evaluation Unit. *Heart*, **85**:133–42.

Califf, R.M., Pieper, K.S., Lee, K.L., et al. (2000). Prediction of 1-year survival after thrombolysis for acute myocardial infarction in the global utilization of streptokinase and TPA for occluded coronary arteries trial. *Circulation*, **101**:2231–8.

Christenson, J., Innes, G., McKnight, D., et al. (2006). A clinical prediction rule for early discharge of patients with chest pain. *Annals of Emergency Medicine*, **47**:1–9.

Collinson, J., Flather, M.D., Fox, K.A.A., et al. (2000). Clinical outcomes, risk stratification and practice patterns of unstable angina and myocardial infarction without ST elevation: prospective registry of acute ischaemic Syndromes in the UK (PRAIS-UK). *European Heart Journal*, **21**:1450–7.

Cross, E., How, S. & Goodacre, S. (2007). Development of acute chest pain services in the UK. *Emerg Emergency Medicine Journal*, **24**:100–102

Deakin, C.D., Sherwood, D.M., Smith, A. & Cassidy, M. (2006). Does telephone triage of emergency (999) calls using Advanced Medical Priority Dispatch (AMPDS) with Department of Health (DH) call prioritisation effectively identify patients with an acute coronary syndrome? An audit of 42,657 emergency calls to Hampshire Ambulance Service NHS Trust. *Emergency Medicine Journal*, **23**:232–5.

Dorsch, M.F., Lawrance, R.A., Sapsford, R.J., et al. (2001). A simple benchmark for evaluating quality of care of patients following acute myocardial infarction. *Heart*, **86**:150–4.

Fox, K.A., Cokkinos, D.V., Deckers, J., et al. (2000). The ENACT study: a pan-European survey of acute coronary syndromes. *European Heart Journal*, **21**:1440–9.

Fox, K.A., Dabbous, O.H., Goldberg, R.J., et al. (2006). Prediction of risk of death and myocardial infarction in the six months after presentation with acute coronary syndrome: prospective multinational observational study (GRACE). *British Medical Journal*, **333**:1091–4.

Gale, C.P., Manda, S.O., Weston, C., et al. (2009). Evaluation of risk scores for risk stratification of acute coronary syndromes in the Myocardial Infarction National Audit Project (MINAP) database. *Heart*, **95**:221–7. Heart Online First 10.1136/hrt.2008.144022.

Gamon, R. Quinn, T. & Parr, B. (2007). *Emergency Care of the Patient with a Heart Attack*. Elsevier, Philadelphia, p. 37.

Goodacre, S. & Dixon, S. (2005). Is a chest pain observation unit likely to be cost effective at my hospital? Extrapolation of data from a randomised controlled trial. *Emergency Medicine Journal*, **22**:418–22.

Goodacre, S., Cross, E. & Arnold, J. (2005). The health care burden of acute chest pain. *Heart*, **91**:22930.

European Society of Cardiology (ESC) (2007). Guidelines for the diagnosis and treatment on non ST segment elevation acute coronary syndromes. *European Heart Journal*, **28**:1598–660.

Herren, K., Mackway-Jones, K., Richards, C., et al. (2001). Is it possible to exclude a diagnosis of myocardial damage within six hours of admission to an emergency department? Diagnostic cohort study. *British Medical Journal*, **323**:372–4.

Jowett, N. & Thompson, D. (2007). *Comprehensive Coronary Care*, 4th edn. Elsevier, Philadelphia.

Kucia, A.M., Taylor, K.T. & Horowitz, J.D. (2001). Can a nurse trained in coronary care expedite emergency department management of patients with acute coronary syndromes? *Heart Lung*, **30**:186–90.

Lee, T. & Goldman, L. (2000). Evaluation of the patient with acute chest pain. *New England Journal of Medicine*, **342**:1187–95.

Mitchell, A., Garvey, L., Chandra, A., et al. (2006). Prospective multicenter study of quantitative pretest probability assessment to exclude acute coronary syndrome for patients evaluated in emergency department chest pain units. *Annals of Emergency Medicine*, **47**:438–47.

Morrow, D., Antman, E., Charlesworth, A., et al. (2000). TIMI risk score for ST-elevation myocardial infarction: a convenient, bedside, clinical score for risk assessment at presentation. *Circulation*, **102**:2031–7.

Morrow, D.A., Antman, E.M. & Giugliano, R.P. (2001). A simple risk index for rapid initial triage of patients with ST-segment elevation myocardial infarction: an InTime II substudy. *The Lancet*, **358**:1571–5.

Ng, S., Krishnaswamy, P., Morissey, R., et al. (2001). Ninety-minute accelerated critical pathway for chest pain evaluation. *American Journal of Cardiology*, **88**:611–7.

Pollack, C. & Gibler, W. (2001). Advances create opportunities: implementing the major tenets of the new unstable angina guidelines in the emergency department. *Annals of Emergency Medicine*, **38**:241–7.

Quinn, T., Thompson, D.R. & Boyle, R.M. (2000). Determining chest pain patients' suitability for transfer to a general ward following admission to a cardiac care unit. *Journal of Advanced Nursing*, **32**:310–17.

Quinn, T., Weston, C., Birkhead, J., et al. (2005). Redefining the coronary care unit: an observational study of patients admitted to hospitals in England and Wales in 2003. *Quarterly Journal of Medicine*, **98**:797–802.

Swap, C.J. & Nagurney, J.T. (2005). Value and limitations of chest pain history in the evaluation of patients with suspected acute coronary syndromes. *Journal of the American Medical Association*, **294**:2623–9.

Yan, A.T., Yan, R.T., Tan, M., et al. (2007). Risk scores for risk stratification in acute coronary syndromes: useful but simpler is not necessarily better. *European Heart Journal*, **28**:1072–8.

Useful Websites and Further Reading

TIMI Study Group: http://www.timi.org/
This site includes free access to an online risk calculator together with an abundance of further reading material.
CRUSADE: http://www.crusadeqi.com/Main/AboutUs.shtml
CRUSADE is a US national quality improvement initiative, designed to increase the practice of evidence-based medicine for patients diagnosed with non-ST segment elevation acute coronary syndromes (NSTE ACS) (i.e. unstable angina or NSTE myocardial infarction).
GRACE – Global Registry of Acute Coronary Events: http://www.outcomes-umassmed.org/grace/bibliography.cfm
The GRACE is an international database designed to track outcomes of patients presenting with ACS.

20 Reducing Time to Treatment

T. Quinn & A. Day

Overview

The importance of time in relation to coronary occlusion, the main cause of acute ST-segment elevation myocardial infarction (STEMI), has been recognised for almost three decades. Reimer and colleagues described the 'wavefront phenomenon' of myocardial ischaemic cell death in animal models in 1979. In humans, a meta-analysis of hospital-based thrombolytic trials (Fibrinolytic Therapy Trialists' [FTT] Collaborative Group 1994) demonstrated a direct linear effect of time delay on mortality, infarct size and ejection fraction. Boersma et al. (1996) added to the evidence base for a time-dependent relationship for thrombolysis by incorporating results from pre-hospital trials into a further meta-analysis, suggesting a 'golden hour' from symptom onset when reperfusion treatment might be most effective. The advantage of early treatment extends to percutaneous reperfusion.

This chapter examines some of the mechanisms resulting in treatment delays for patients with acute coronary syndromes (ACSs) and the strategies for reducing such delays once patients present to health services.

Learning objectives

After reading this chapter, you should be able to:

- Discuss the time-dependent nature of emergency cardiac care.
- Identify the key areas of delay in community and hospital settings.
- Discuss the limitations of community-wide efforts to expedite help-seeking behaviour.
- Discuss the principles of reducing treatment delays once patients present to health services.

Key concepts

Time to treatment; treatment delay; 'golden hour'; 'door-to-needle time'; 'door-to-balloon inflation'

Benefits of early reperfusion

Following early studies that reported a direct linear effect of time delay on mortality, infarct size and ejection fraction, Boersma (2006) reported findings of a further meta-analysis of 25 trials comparing thrombolysis and primary percutaneous coronary intervention (PPCI). He concluded that PPCI was associated with significantly lower 30-day mortality relative to thrombolytic treatment, regardless of treatment delay. In contrast, Asseburg et al. (2007) concluded from meta-analysis that while PPCI was superior for 1-month outcomes if treatment delays were 30–90 min, the benefits of PPCI over thrombolysis at a 6-month follow-up were dependent on time to treatment, suggesting that for treatment delays of around 90 min, thrombolysis may be the preferred option, with considerable uncertainty remaining for longer delays. These latter findings are consistent with the findings of the very large (192,509 patients in 645 hospitals) study from the US National Registry of Myocardial Infarction (NRMI), in which mortality advantage of PPCI over thrombolytic treatment declined as delays to PPCI increased (Pinto et al. 2006). Thus, irrespective of the mode of reperfusion therapy (drug or balloon), time is of the essence.

Smaller, individual trials have also provided indications of time-dependent outcomes, although for thrombolysis these seem to accrue mostly within the first 2–3 h from symptom onset (Chareonthaitawee et al. 2000). It has been suggested that for STEMI patients presenting within the first 2 h of onset, each minute's delay in administering thrombolysis equates to 11 days of lost life expectancy (Rawles 1997).

A key message arising from these and other studies is that the 'ideal' reperfusion strategy for STEMI depends on logistical considerations such as the efficiency of emergency medical services and hospital cardiology departments in ensuring rapid assessment and treatment, together with (by extension) factors outside the control of health professionals, namely help-seeking behaviour and geography. But, overall, the goal must be to reduce to a minimum the delay from onset to initiating reperfusion therapy, irrespective of which therapeutic strategy is employed.

Time is also critically important for patients with suspected STEMI because of the even more time-critical nature of cardiac arrest. In the United Kingdom Heart Attack Study (UKHAS), the relationship between time-of-symptom onset and the MI patient coming under ambulance and hospital

care was examined in relation to 30-day mortality and lives saved by resuscitation and thrombolytic treatment. Delay was found to be strongly related to outcome, with a fivefold reduction in 30-day fatality in those coming under care within an hour of onset compared to those delayed for more than 12 h. Importantly, 80% of the mortality reduction was attributed to resuscitation compared to other treatments. Importantly, survival to 30 days following out-of-hospital cardiac arrest was highest (40%) in MI patients who 'arrested' in the presence of ambulance staff: powerful arguments for ensuring patients with symptoms suggestive of MI receive a rapid emergency response (Norris et al. 1998). Time as a crucial factor in determining outcome from out-of-hospital cardiac arrest has been confirmed in the Swedish Cardiac Arrest Registry involving 33,453 patients (Herlitz et al. 2005). Out-of-hospital cardiac arrest is covered in more detail in Chapter 14.

Identifying and addressing delays

In the United States, the National Heart Attack Alert Program Co-ordinating Committee (NHAAP 1994) introduced the concept of the '4 D's' denoting measurable time intervals (Door, Data, Decision and Drug). This concept could be used by hospital managers and clinicians to help improve systems for in-hospital care of patients with suspected MI and reduce the 'door-to-needle' time for thrombolysis. This concept was taken a stage further by Quinn & Thompson (1995) to encompass delays occurring before the patient reached hospital with the addition of 'D0', denoting 'domicile'. More recently, similar efforts have begun to address delays in access to PPCI.

D0: Domicile

Entry into the health care system is an essential prerequisite to obtaining appropriate clinical assessment and treatment – not least resuscitation in the event of cardiac arrest; thus, efforts are required to identify and address symptom recognition and help-seeking behaviour amongst patients with symptoms suggestive of ACSs, their families and wider community members. Patients often delay hours, and sometimes days, before seeking medical help, and the reasons for this are complex and multifaceted. McKinley et al. (2004) conducted an observational study comparing help-seeking delays in 595 MI patients in the United States, England, Japan and Korea. Most patients developed symptoms at home and where an ambulance was called, either by the patient themselves or by a relative/bystander, patients reached the hospital 2–3 times sooner than if an alternative route was taken to access care, such as calling the general practitioner or driving to hospital. Multiple logistic regression was used to determine factors which might serve as predictors of pre-hospital delay. Only one factor – symptoms perceived as 'serious' – was positively associated with seeking help; patients who attributed symptoms to something other than a heart problem, and those who simply waited to see if symptoms would resolve, delayed longer in seeking help. Patients from England had the shortest time from onset to treatment. In a recent Australian study, 105 MI patients were interviewed to investigate predictors of ambulance use; less than half (46%) called an ambulance when symptoms developed, and multivariate analysis identified self-administered nitrates, sharp chest pain and onset while at home as independent predictors of ambulance use (Kerr et al. 2006).

Efforts to expedite help-seeking behaviour in patients with symptoms suggestive of a heart attack have yielded suboptimal results. The Rapid Early Action for Coronary Treatment (REACT) community trial tested a multicomponent community-based intervention in 20 American communities over a 2-year period, but the results were disappointing, with only modest increases in public knowledge of what the authors describe as the 'complex constellation of heart attack symptoms' (Goff et al. 2004). A systematic review of the literature concluded not only that media and public education campaigns fail to increase the proportion of patients with MI that call for help early, but that such campaigns can increase the burden on emergency services (Kainth et al. 2004). An unintended consequence of such campaigns may be reflected in the findings of Deakin et al. (2006) who reported that only 5% of patients calling an ambulance for chest pain had a final diagnosis of ACS. Targeting messages about help-seeking behaviour at patients with known coronary disease or with key risk factors for MI might be a more appropriate

strategy (Roberts & Timmis 2007), although the effectiveness of such an approach has yet to be confirmed in a robust study.

Improving ambulance response times appears to be a cost-effective means of reducing death from MI. Improving the ambulance response so that 75% of calls receive a response within 8 min has been shown in a UK study to save 57 life years per million per year, at an incremental cost per life year saved of £8500 over a 20-year period. This compares favourably with the estimated 15 life years saved per million per year at a cost of £10,150–54,230 over 20 years gained by reducing hospital door-to-needle times for thrombolysis to 20 min. The combined benefits of reducing both ambulance and door-to-needle times resulted in 70 life years saved per million (Chase et al. 2006) and supports government policy to improve ambulance performance (Department of Health 2000, 2005). Time to arrival of a defibrillator is an important determinant of outcome as demonstrated by Norris et al. (1998), and over 10,000 'community first responders' (CFRs) have been recruited, covering most ambulance services in England, to help reduce the time taken for a defibrillator to reach the patient. However, CFRs respond to less than 2% of the 5 million 999 calls received by ambulance services annually (Healthcare Commission 2007).

Shortening the pre-hospital delay by improving ambulance performance has other consequences apart from reducing delays to defibrillation and reperfusion. A paradoxical deterioration in hospital mortality has been suggested, particularly if there is underutilisation of reperfusion therapy in the hospital the patient is taken to. This phenomenon is explained by very sick patients – who presumably would otherwise have died in the community – surviving to reach hospital because of better pre-hospital care (Wilkinson et al. 2002).

D1: Door

In order to reflect the rapidly changing face of acute cardiac care, with the traditional role of the cardiac care unit (CCU) in the early management of suspected MI being largely devolved to emergency services (Quinn et al. 2005) and the increased use of PPCI as the reperfusion strategy of choice, 'Door' can mean different things in different health systems. For example, where pre-hospital thrombolysis is used, then 'Door' refers to the time of arrival of the ambulance crew with the patient. Conversely, where PPCI or (becoming less common) hospital-administered thrombolysis is used, then 'Door' applies to the reception of the patient in hospital. Practice guidelines may use the term 'First Medical Contact' to denote the point where process measures (e.g. time to initiation of reperfusion treatment) commence.

Irrespective of which health professionals (ambulance, emergency department or cardiology staff) first assess the patient, time remains the essence for the reasons discussed earlier in this chapter. Rapid assessment of the patient is undertaken, with resuscitation initiated if required. The presence of a defibrillator is mandatory. Supplementary oxygen may be required, although the evidence that this widely used treatment is effective and safe in patients with ACS is uncertain (Nicholson 2004). Pain relief is an important consideration, as is ensuring that the often terrified patient and family receive appropriate information, reassurance and compassion. The patient should be assessed and managed in an appropriate clinical space such as a dedicated 'chest pain bay' or resuscitation room (in hospital) or, in the pre-hospital setting, moved into the ambulance at the earliest opportunity. Every effort should be made to reduce delay irrespective of the setting.

D2: Data

In this context, 'data' refers to the information required to determine the eligibility for reperfusion or other treatments and to begin the process of risk stratification (see Chapter 21). As already discussed, the vast majority of patients who call an ambulance because of chest pain do not have ACS, and it is important that reperfusion and other treatments, which carry their own risks, and the relatively expensive facilities provided by a CCU, are reserved for patients who can benefit from them. While detailed assessment of the cardiac patient is covered in Chapter 9, the hallmark of decision-making in relation to reperfusion treatment and risk stratification is the 12-lead ECG. This very common test is universally available in emergency departments and increasingly on ambulances (in the United Kingdom, all emergency

ambulances are equipped with 12-lead ECG machines). Recent guidelines recommend widespread implementation of pre-hospital ECG programmes (Garvey et al. 2006; Antman et al. 2008).

The benefit of PPCI or thrombolysis is proven in patients with ECG evidence of ST-segment elevation or (presumed new) left bundle branch block (LBBB). Patients without these characteristics but with ST-segment depression have high mortality risk but do not benefit from reperfusion treatments. It has been suggested recently that the distinction between the two ECG manifestations of STEMI – pre-infarction syndrome (PIS) and evolving MI (EMI) – distinguished by T-wave polarity and the presence of pathological Q waves, may help determine whether PPCI or thrombolysis is the preferred treatment strategy, but more research is required (Eskola et al. 2007).

In practical terms, it is important that nurses and other team members understand the importance of recording a 12-lead ECG at the earliest opportunity where a patient presents with possible ACS, and know how to obtain a high quality recording and recognise ST-segment elevation and LBBB (as a minimum) so that appropriate therapeutic decisions can be made. Studies in the United Kingdom (Quinn et al. 1998) and Australia (Kremser & Lyneham 2007) have reported accurate and safe recognition of STEMI patients based largely on nurse interpretation of the 12-lead ECG. Moreover, the involvement of an appropriately trained nurse in the early assessment of suspected ACS patients has been shown to reduce both the time taken to obtain the initial ECG (Purim-Shev-Tov et al. 2007) and reperfusion treatment delays (Wilmshurst et al. 2000; Kucia et al. 2001).

D3: Decision

The ECG is not the only information required to assess a patient's suitability for reperfusion. An assessment is required of the presenting complaint, duration from onset and the presence of any contraindications for treatment. The latter is particularly important if thrombolysis is being considered because of the risk of haemorrhage. For example, there is debate about whether warfarin should be considered a contraindication to thrombolysis (Stanley et al. 2006). In both hospital and ambulance settings, it may be helpful to provide checklists and other *'aides memoir'* to guide decision-making, with the provision of rapid senior advice if there are any concerns or if the patient is particularly complex. It is important that a health professional competent and empowered to make decisions regarding reperfusion is available promptly. This professional does not necessarily need to be a cardiologist – thrombolysis decisions are frequently made by emergency department staff and paramedics; and in the case of PPCI, there is growing evidence that paramedics are able to safely identify patients who need to go straight to a cardiac catheter laboratory, and if needs be, bypassing a local hospital (Le May et al. 2006; Van 't Hof et al. 2006; Afolabi et al. 2007). The successful implementation of such initiatives is not, however, universal: Vaught et al. (2006) reported that initial gains from transmission of the ECG from the ambulance to the emergency department to reduce the door-to-balloon time for PPCI were not sustained, although this appears to have been a result of suboptimal processes within the hospital rather than the ambulance.

D4: Drug or destination

Once a decision has been made about the appropriate treatment for an individual patient, taking into account the findings of the clinical assessment and ECG data, together with the available facilities and logistical considerations, it is vital that treatment commences as soon as possible. This means that, where thrombolysis is the available treatment, it should be administered immediately after the decision is made, without having to move the patient to a different clinical setting. Thus, pre-hospital thrombolysis is given by paramedics in the ambulance rather than waiting for the patient to reach the hospital – unless there are contraindications or the ambulance crew are not appropriately trained. The newer bolus-administered thrombolytic agents (reteplase and tenecteplase) are easy to administer and have ensured that prompt administration to eligible patients is not only feasible but also a reality, reducing delay and improving outcomes in modern clinical practice (Chittari et al. 2005; Bjorklund et al. 2006).

Where pre-hospital thrombolysis is administered, there are other important considerations: thrombolysis is not the end of the emergency treatment of the STEMI patient. Every effort must be made to start a heparin infusion (where enoxaparin is not in use) to reduce the risk of re-infarction. The delay in reaching hospital following pre-hospital thrombolysis has been implicated in higher re-infarction rates and subsequent mortality (Horne et al. 2008). Thus, the nurse receiving a patient into an emergency department or CCU following pre-hospital thrombolysis needs to be aware of the urgent need to commence a heparin infusion. The administration of aspirin may also be time dependent (Zijlstra et al. 2002).

Where PPCI is available within a timely fashion – within 90 min of first medical contact – then this is the preferred treatment (Van de Werf et al. 2003; Antman et al. 2008). As discussed above, time remains the essence, and reports have suggested that many centres find achievement of this standard challenging: in the US NRMI, only 35% of patients had a door-to-balloon time of less than 90 min (McNamara et al. 2006). Patients who are transferred from another hospital for PPCI, and those presenting 'out of hours', are at most risk of delay (Nallomothu et al. 2007).

There is a growing literature on the subject of reducing delays to PPCI. This mirrors in part efforts to reduce 'call to needle' time for thrombolysis reported in earlier series (Quinn et al. 2003). Bradley et al. (2006) surveyed 365 US hospitals to identify strategies being employed to reduce PPCI delay. Six strategies were significantly associated with faster door-to-balloon times, although these were in use in only a minority of hospitals:

- Activation of the catheter laboratory by emergency department staff
- Use of a central pager system ('crash bleep') to activate catheter laboratory
- Activation of the catheter laboratory while the patient was en route to the hospital rather than waiting until assessment in the emergency department (based on pre-hospital ECG)
- Setting targets for catheter laboratory staff to be in place within 20 min of the pager alert
- Having 24/7 on-site availability of a senior cardiologist
- Using real-time data to feedback on performance to emergency department and catheter laboratory staff

Bradley et al. (2006) have added further to our knowledge of how best to reduce delays to PPCI by summarising the published evidence from 13 studies. From this review of largely observational studies, they concluded that three were supported by strongest evidence: activation of the catheter laboratory by emergency department staff rather than cardiologists, effective use of the pre-hospital 12-lead ECG and provision of data monitoring and feedback on performance.

Conclusion

Time matters in the care of patients with suspected STEMI, irrespective of the particular reperfusion strategy employed in a particular health system, and for improving the chances of resuscitation should cardiac arrest occur. Delays in help-seeking behaviour remain a major challenge but there is little evidence that media or public information campaigns reduce delay, instead adding to the burden on already stretched emergency services. Introduction of 12-lead ECGs on ambulances has helped to expedite both thrombolytic treatment and PPCI provided appropriate systems are in place to ensure that appropriate feedback is given to all appropriate staff to foster continuing improvements where 'minutes mean myocardium'.

Learning activity

Help-seeking or treatment-seeking behaviour is a substantial component of treatment delay in many cases. A number of variables contribute to delay in seeking treatment, and demographic characteristics are amongst these. Dracup & colleagues (1995) list some of these as being older age (>55 years), female gender, low socioeconomic status and history of angina or diabetes. Think about the particular population that you work with. Do you think these characteristics are associated with delay in your population and can you think of any additional factors specific to your target population?

References

Afolabi, B.A., Novaro, G.M., Pinski, S.L., et al. (2007). Use of the prehospital ECG improves door to balloon times in ST segment elevation myocardial infarction irrespective of the day of the week. *Emergency Medical Journal*, **24**:588–91.

Antman, E.M., Anbe, D.T., Armstrong, P.W., et al. (2008). 2007 focused update of the ACC/AHA 2004 guidelines for the management of patients with ST elevation myocardial infarction: a report of the American College of Cardiology/American Heart Association Task Force on practice guidelines. *Circulation*, **117**:296–329

Asseburg, C., Vergel, Y.B., Palmer, S., et al. (2007). Assessing the effectiveness of primary angioplasty compared with thrombolysis and its relationship to time delay: a Bayesian evidence synthesis. *Heart*, **93**:1244–50.

Bjorklund, E., Stenestrand, U., Lindback, J., et al. (2006). Pre-hospital thrombolysis delivered by paramedics is associated with reduced time delay and mortality in ambulance-transported real-life patients with ST elevation myocardial infarction. *European Heart Journal*, **27**:1146–52.

Boersma, E., Mass, A.C.P., Deckers, J.W. & Simoons, M.L. (1996). Early thrombolytic treatment in acute myocardial infarction: reappraisal of the golden hour. *The Lancet*, **348**:771–5.

Boersma, E. and The Primary Coronary Angioplasty vs. Thrombolysis (PCAT)-2 Trialists' Collaborative Group. (2006). Does time matter? A pooled analysis of randomized clinical trials comparing primary percutaneous coronary intervention and in-hospital fibrinolysis in acute myocardial infarction patients. *European Heart Journal*, **27**:779–88.

Bradley, E.H., Herrin, J., Wang, Y., et al. (2006). Strategies for reducing the door-to-balloon time in acute myocardial infarction. *New England Journal of Medicine*, **355**:2308–20.

Chareonthaitawee, P., Gibbons, R.J., Roberts, R.S., et al. (2000). The impact of time to thrombolytic treatment on outcome in patients with acute myocardial infarction. For the CORE investigators (Collaborative Organisation for RheothRx Evaluation). *Heart*, **84**:142–8.

Chase, D., Roderick, P., Cooper, K., et al. (2006). Using simulation to estimate the cost-effectiveness of improving ambulance and thrombolysis response times after myocardial infarction. *Emergency Medicine Journal*, **23**:67–72.

Chittari, M.S., Ahmad, I., Chambers, B., et al. (2005). Retrospective observational case-control study comparing pre-hospital thrombolytic therapy for ST-elevation myocardial infarction with in-hospital thrombolytic therapy for patients from same area. *Emergency Medical Journal*, **22**:582–5.

Deakin, C.D., Sherwood, D.M., Smith, A. & Cassidy, M. (2006). Does telephone triage of emergency (999) calls using Advanced Medical Priority Dispatch (AMPDS) with Department of Health (DH) call prioritisation effectively identify patients with an acute coronary syndrome? An audit of 42,657 emergency calls to Hampshire Ambulance Service NHS Trust. *Emergency Medical Journal*, **23**:232–5.

Department of Health (2000). *National Service Framework for Coronary Heart Disease*. Department of Health, London.

Department of Health (2005). *Taking Healthcare to the Patient*. Department of Health, London.

Dracup, K., Moser, D.K., Eisenberg, M., et al. (1995). Causes of delay in seeking treatment for heart attack symptoms. *Social Science Medicine*, **40**:379–92.

Eskola, M.J., Holmvang, L., Nikus, K.C., et al. (2007). The electrocardiographic window of opportunity to treat vs. the different evolving stages of ST-elevation myocardial infarction: correlation with therapeutic approach, coronary anatomy, and outcome in the DANAMI-2 trial. *European Heart Journal*, **28**:2985–91.

Fibrinolytic Therapy Trialists' (FTT) Collaborative Group. (1994). Indications for fibrinolytic therapy in suspected acute myocardial infarction: collaborative overview of early mortality and major morbidity results from all randomised trials of more than 1000 patients. *The Lancet*, **343**:311–22.

Garvey, J.L., MacLeod, B.A., Sopko, G., et al. (2006). Pre-hospital 12 lead electrocardiography programs. A call for implementation by emergency medical systems providing advanced life support – National Heart Attack Alert Program (NHAAP) Co-ordinating Committee. *Journal of the American College of Cardiology*, **47**:485–91.

Goff, D.C. Jr., Mitchell, P., Finnegan, J., et al. REACT Study Group (2004). Knowledge of heart attack symptoms in 20 US communities. Results from the rapid early action for coronary treatment community trial. *Preventive Medicine*, **38**:85–93.

Healthcare Commission (2007). *The Role and Management of Community First Responders*. Commission for Healthcare Audit and Inspection, London.

Herlitz, J., Engdahl, J., Svensson, L., Angquist, K.A., Young, M. & Holmberg, S. (2005). Factors associated with an increased chance of survival among patients suffering from an out-of-hospital cardiac arrest in a national perspective in Sweden. *American Heart Journal*, **149**:61–6.

Horne, S., Weston, C., Quinn, T., et al. (2008). The impact of prehospital thrombolytic treatment on reinfarction rates: analysis of the myocardial infarction national audit project (MINAP). *Heart*, **95**:559–63.

Kainth, A., Hewitt, A., Snowden, A., et al. (2004). Systematic review of interventions to reduce delay in patients with suspected heart attack. *Emergency Medical Journal*, **21**:506–8.

Kerr, D., Holden, D., Smith, J., et al. (2006). Predictors of ambulance use in patients with acute myocardial infarction in Australia. *Emergency Medical Journal*, **23**:948–52.

Kremser, A.K. & Lyneham, J. (2007). Can Australian nurses safely assess for thrombolysis on EKG criteria? *Journal of Emergency Nursing*, **33**:102–9.

Kucia, A.M., Taylor, K.T. & Horowitz, J.D. (2001). Can a nurse trained in coronary care expedite emergency department management of patients with acute coronary syndromes? *Heart Lung*, **30**:186–90.

Le May, M.R., Davies, R.F., Dionne, R., et al. (2006). Comparison of early mortality of paramedic-diagnosed ST elevation myocardial infarction with immediate transport to a designated primary percutaneous coronary intervention center to that of similar patients transported to the nearest hospital. *American Journal of Cardiology*, **98**:1329–33.

McKinley, S., Dracup, K., Moser, D.K., et al. (2004). International comparison of factors associated with delay in presentation for AMI treatment. *European Journal of Cardiovascular Nursing*, **3**:225–230.

McNamara, R.L., Wang, Y., Herrin, J., et al. (2006). Effect of door-to-balloon time on mortality in patients with ST-segment elevation myocardial infarction. *Journal of the American College of Cardiology*, **47**:2180–6.

Nallomothu, B.K., Bradley, E.H. & Krumholz, H.M. (2007). Time to treatment in primary percutaneous intervention. *New England Journal of Medicine*, **357**:1631–8.

National Heart Attack Alert Program (1994). Emergency department: rapid identification and treatment of patients with acute myocardial infarction. National Heart Attack Alert Program Coordinating Committee, 60 Minutes to Treatment Working Group. *Annals of Emergency Medicine*, **23**:31.

Nicholson, C. (2004). A systematic review of the effectiveness of oxygen in reducing acute myocardial ischaemia. *Journal of Clinical Nursing*, **13**:996–1007 (Comment in *Journal of Clinical Nursing*, **15**:121–2).

Norris, R. (1998). Fatality outside hospital from acute coronary events in three British health districts, 1994–5. United Kingdom Heart Attack Study Collaborative Group. *British Medical Journal* 316:1065–70.

Pinto, D.S., Kirtane, A.J., Nallomothu, B.K., et al. (2006). Hospital delays in reperfusion for ST elevation myocardial infarction. Implications when selecting a reperfusion strategy. *Circulation*, **114**:2019–25.

Purim-Shev-Tov, Y.A., Rumoro, D.P., Veloso, J. & Zettinger, K. (2007). Emergency department greeters reduce door-to-ECG time. *Critical Pathways in Cardiology*, **6**:165–8.

Quinn, T. & Thompson, D.R. (1995). Administration of thrombolytic therapy to patients with acute myocardial infarction. *Accident and Emergency Nursing*, **3**:208–14.

Quinn, T., MacDermott, A.F.N. & Caunt, J. (1998). Determining patients' suitability for thrombolysis: coronary care nurses' agreement with an expert cardiological 'gold standard' as assessed by clinical and electrocardiographic 'vignettes'. *Intensive and Critical Care Nursing*, **14**:219–24.

Quinn, T., Allan, T.F., Birkhead, J., et al. (2003). Impact of a region-wide approach to improving systems for heart attack care: the West Midlands Thrombolysis Project. *European Journal of Cardiovascular Nursing*, **2**:131–9.

Quinn, T., Weston, C., Birkhead, J., et al. (2005). Redefining the coronary care unit: an observational study of patients admitted to hospitals in England and Wales in 2003. *Quarterly Journal of Medicine*, **98**:797–802.

Rawles, J. (1997). Quantification of the benefit of earlier thrombolytic therapy: five-year results of the grampian region early anistreplase trial (GREAT). *Journal of the American College of Cardiology*, **30**:1181–6.

Reimer, K.A. & Jennings, R.B. (1979). The "wavefront phenomenon" of myocardial ischaemic cell death, II: transmural progression of necrosis within the framework of ischaemic bed size (myocardium at risk) and collateral flow. *Laboratory Investigations*, **40**:633–44.

Roberts, W.T. & Timmis, A.D. (2007). Patients with cardiac chest pain should call emergency services. *British Medical Journal*, **335**:669.

Stanley, A.G., Fletcher, S., Tan, A. & Barnett, D.B. (2006). Is warfarin a contradiction to thrombolysis in acute ST segment elevation myocardial infarction? *Heart*, **92**:1145–6.

Van 't Hof, A.W., Rasoul, S., van de Wetering, H., et al. (2006). Feasibility and benefit of prehospital diagnosis, triage, and therapy by paramedics only in patients who are candidates for primary angioplasty for acute myocardial infarction. *American Heart Journal*, **151**:1255e1–5.

Van de Werf, F., Ardissino, D., Betriu, A., et al. (2003). Management of acute myocardial infarction in patients presenting with ST-segment elevation. *European Heart Journal*, **24**:28–66.

Vaught, C., Young, D.R., Bell, S.J., et al. (2006). The failure of years of experience with electrocardiographic transmission from paramedics to the hospital emergency department to reduce the delay from door to primary coronary intervention below the 90 minute threshold during acute myocardial infarction. *Journal of Electrocardiology*, **39**:136–41.

Wilkinson, J., Foo, K., Sekhri, N., et al. (2002). Interaction between arrival time and thrombolytic treatment in determining early outcome of acute myocardial infarction. *Heart*, **88**:583–6.

Wilmshurst, P., Purchase, A., Webb, C., et al. (2000). Reducing 'door-to-needle' time by nurse-initiated thrombolysis. *Heart*, **84**:262–6.

Zijlstra, F., Ernst, N., de Boer, M.-J., et al. (2002). Influence of pre-hospital administration of aspirin and heparin on initial patency of the infarct-related artery in patients with acute ST elevation myocardial infarction. *Journal of the American College of Cardiology*, **39**:1733–7.

Useful Websites and Further Reading

Myocardial Ischaemia National Audit Project (MINAP): http://www.rcplondon.ac.uk/college/ceeu/ceeu_ami_home.htm

D2B Alliance – A nationwide US network of hospitals, physician champions and strategic partners committed to improving door-to-balloon times: http://www.d2balliance.org/WhatisD2B/CampaignHistory/tabid/146/Default.aspx

National Heart Attack Alert Program: http://www.nhlbi.nih.gov/about/nhaap/index.htm

NHS Cardiovascular Diseases Specialist Library: www.library.nhs.uk/cardiovascular

NHS Heart Improvement Programme – 'Top 10 Tips' for reducing door-to-needle time for hospital thrombolysis: http://www.heart.nhs.uk/Heart/Portals/0/docs_2004/Call%20to%20Needle%20final.pdf

21 Reperfusion Strategies

C.J. Zeitz & T. Quinn

Overview

Acute ST-elevation myocardial infarction (STEMI) occurs when an intracoronary plaque ruptures, with subsequent thrombus formation causing complete vessel occlusion. Within 15 min, myocyte death begins in an exponential fashion such that 50% of the myocardium at risk has died within 3h and 80% of the myocardium at risk is permanently damaged by 12h. Optimal management of STEMI requires the prompt recognition by patients of symptoms and immediate access to appropriate health care. From first medical contact, a prompt diagnosis must be made and an appropriate and timely reperfusion strategy chosen. Once a reperfusion strategy has been delivered, patients should be closely monitored to detect any evidence of re-occlusion or other complications. Nurses have important roles to play across the whole patient pathway. This chapter will examine in detail the rationale for choice of reperfusion strategy and the keys to maintaining an efficient reperfusion service.

Learning objectives

After reading this chapter, you should be able to:

- Identify the options for reperfusion therapy following acute coronary occlusion.

- Discuss the relative advantages and disadvantages of potential reperfusion therapies for acute coronary occlusion.
- Recognise the importance of time to treatment for reperfusion therapies.
- Recognise signs of re-occlusion following reperfusion therapy and discuss strategies for management should this occur.
- Discuss the significance of failed reperfusion.

Key concepts

Thrombolysis; fibrinolysis; primary percutaneous angioplasty; re-occlusion; failed reperfusion

Pathogenesis of STEMI

The earliest signs of coronary atheromatous plaque are present from teenage years. While the overall burden of coronary plaque is a determinant of events, the key measure of risk is the extent of vulnerable plaques. Vulnerable plaques have thin caps that are more prone to rupture. Rupture of an intracoronary plaque leads to formation of a platelet-rich thrombus, and the process also stimulates a variable degree of vascular spasm.

The development of plaque vulnerability is a generalised, rather than discrete, event with the potential for multiple acute events to occur (Goldstein et al. 2000). Indeed, one of the strategies for managing acute vascular presentations is to pacify generalised plaque inflammation to prevent further events.

Many episodes of plaque rupture are relatively minor and involve little or no thrombus formation or vasospasm, with rapid healing ensuing. Occasionally, plaque rupture is a substantial event with formation of a large thrombus load and associated vasospasm causing complete vessel occlusion. This occurrence in a coronary artery causes acute transmural myocardial ischaemia, represented by regional ST-segment elevation on the 12-lead electrocardiogram. Within 15 min of vessel occlusion, myocardial cell death begins to occur. Within 3 h, 50% of the myocardium supplied by the occluded vessel will have died (Reimer et al. 1993). Cell death can be prevented or reduced by restoring blood flow down the infarct-related artery. The extent of myocardial cell death is largely determined by the interval between vessel occlusion and reperfusion with shorter intervals being associated with maximal myocardial salvage and intervals of longer than 12 h providing negligible myocardial salvage.

The point of coronary vessel occlusion is generally estimated by the time of onset of ischaemic (usually chest) pain. However, while on a population basis this provides a reasonable estimate of duration of vessel occlusion, there is a large degree of heterogeneity in practice. The size of the myocardial infarction and degree of myocardial salvage are often only determined in retrospect. Treatment guidelines, however, are frequently written on the basis of duration of pain prior to presentation, a measure that at best is only a loose correlate of vessel occlusion.

Principles of reperfusion strategies

The key goal of any reperfusion strategy is to restore normal myocardial tissue perfusion as rapidly as possible with the aims of preventing further myocyte loss and restoring normal myocyte function. The reperfusion strategy used should seek to address, where possible, the three components of pathophysiology involved: plaque rupture, thrombus formation and vasospasm. While the dominant feature acutely is thrombus formation, plaque vulnerability and vasospasm are particularly strong determinants of early adverse events. Therapies should therefore seek to address all three aspects. Finally, the strategy needs to be available and effective in a very short time frame. Patients most frequently present within 2 h of symptom onset, a time when more than 50% of the threatened myocardium can still be salvaged by rapid reperfusion. Hence the concept, time is muscle. It is worth reinforcing the fact that only about two-thirds of patients presenting with acute STEMI receive a reperfusion strategy. The diagnosis must be suspected before it can be made.

Options for reperfusion

Reperfusion strategies include pharmacological and mechanical options, and a single strategy will not suit all patients. In making the choice of reperfusion strategy, time of onset of symptoms, availability of skilled percutaneous coronary intervention (PCI), risk of bleeding and contraindications to the procedure/pharmacotherapy must be considered.

Non-thrombolytic pharmacotherapy

It has long been recognised that restoration of patency of the infarct-related artery may occur spontaneously in a small group of patients with some pharmacological interventions increasing the potential for this to occur. With the introduction of primary PCI to reperfuse the infarct-related artery, it was recognised that a proportion of vessels were patent prior to the intervention proceeding with a small percentage having normal flow. Indeed, around 20% of patients having primary PCI have TIMI-2 or TIMI-3 flow in the infarct-related artery prior to any intervention being performed (Zijlstra et al. 2002). Such flow is probably sufficient to prevent ongoing myocardial cell death. Simple pharmacological strategies to increase the likelihood of TIMI-2 or TIMI-3 flow while waiting for primary PCI to be delivered therefore have the capacity to reduce final myocardial infarct size.

A study performed in the pre-PCI era examined the ability of simple pharmacological measures to improve patency of the infarct-related artery (Beltrame et al. 2002). Patients with STEMI considered eligible for thrombolytic therapy were given a combination of sublingual glyceryl trinitrate, intravenous glyceryl trinitrate and intravenous verapamil with or without intravenous heparin. This therapy was targeted at both reducing vascular spasm and having significant anti-platelet aggregation effects. Of the 101 patients studied, 36 showed resolution of ST-segment elevation on 12-lead electrocardiography, thus indicating reperfusion of the infarct-related artery. The advantage of such therapy is that it is widely available, cheap and able to be administered easily with a rapid onset of action. This therapy is currently being evaluated in a multi-centre study in patients undergoing primary PCI with a primary end point of vessel patency of the infarct-related artery at first coronary injection, prior to PCI.

Fibrinolysis/Thrombolysis

A major feature of vessel occlusion in acute STEMI is platelet-rich thrombus. The strategy of using various thrombolytic or fibrinolytic agents to break down freshly formed thrombus and thus restore flow in the infarct-related artery has been investigated for nearly 50 years. In 1988, the landmark ISIS-2 study demonstrated that thrombolysis with streptokinase resulted in a significant reduction in 30-day mortality for patients presenting with acute STEMI (Second International Study of Infarct Survival (ISIS-2) Collaborative Group 1988). This strategy rapidly became the major therapy for STEMI, with gradual adjustment over time to include agents that were more effective and easier to administer.

The major benefit of lysis therapy is that it can be delivered very easily and rapidly. For patients presenting to hospital where the major treatment of STEMI is lysis, the target interval from arrival (door) to administration of drug (needle) is 30 min. However, less than 50% of patients receiving lytic therapy achieve this goal (Eagle et al. 2008), although in England this is substantially higher at 84% (Walker et al. 2008), in part due to the widespread introduction of specially trained

nurses authorised to make treatment decisions and initiate thrombolysis without waiting for a physician (Quinn 1995; Heath et al. 2003), a strategy also under investigation in Australia (Kremser and Lyneham 2007). Improved outcomes have been demonstrated if drug administration can be performed in the pre-hospital setting (Rosenberg et al. 2002). Morrison et al. (2000) performed a meta-analysis of randomised controlled trials of pre-hospital verses in-hospital thrombolysis and reported significantly decreased all-cause hospital mortality among patients treated with pre-hospital thrombolysis compared with in-hospital thrombolysis. Results were similar regardless of trial quality or training and experience of the provider (physician or paramedic). The findings of this study informed policy developments in England, with a commitment in the National Health Service (NHS) Plan (Department of Health 2000) to introduce pre-hospital thrombolysis, delivered by paramedics, across the NHS. To date, more than 10,000 patients have received pre-hospital thrombolysis in England, and in 2007–08 about a fifth of all thrombolysis was given before hospital arrival (Walker et al. 2008). A range of models to assist paramedic decision-making have been described, including collaborative working with cardiac care nurses via telemedicine link (McLean et al. 2008).

There are a number of limitations to the benefits of lytic therapy. Firstly, there is hysteresis between drug administration and effect. There is a lag of 60–90 min between drug administration and evidence of restoration of coronary blood flow, as judged by resolution of ST-segment elevation and pain, or by direct visualisation of the infarct-related artery using coronary angiography. For individual patients, the length of this lag time is unknown and, therefore, the point at which lytic therapy is deemed to have failed is uncertain. Secondly, the overall success rate of lytic therapy, in terms of restoring and maintaining flow in the infarct-related artery, is only about two-thirds of cases (GUSTO Angiographic Investigators 1993). Patients with a short duration of vessel occlusion seem to have a better rate of response to lytic therapy than those with a longer duration of vessel occlusion, suggesting that as the thrombus becomes more organised with time, it becomes more resistant to the actions of lytic therapy. Lastly, lytic therapy is associated with risk as well as benefit.

The main risk of lytic therapy relates to bleeding, in particular intracranial bleeding. Because of this risk of bleeding, therapy is restricted to those patients with larger regions of myocardium at risk. Patients with small myocardial infarctions are generally not considered eligible for lytic therapy; this judgment being based on the extent of ST elevation observed on the 12-lead electrocardiogram. Generally, patients with less than 1 mm of ST elevation in two contiguous limb leads or less than 2 mm of ST elevation in two or more contiguous chest leads would not be considered eligible for lytic therapy in view of the risk/benefit ratio. Moreover, around a third of patients have a contraindication to hospital thrombolysis and around half to pre-hospital thrombolysis based on UK national ambulance guidelines (Castle et al. 2006). Such cases should be discussed with a cardiologist as a matter of urgency.

Nursing considerations for patients receiving lytic therapy, based on Australian practice, are shown in Box 21.1.

Box 21.1 Nursing considerations in the care of patients receiving thrombolytic/fibrinolytic therapy

Patients with STEMI need rapid reperfusion by the best means available. Institutions that utilise thrombolytics/fibrinolytics generally have established protocols to facilitate patient selection and reduce delay to treatment. These protocols should:

- Establish patient selection/exclusion criteria
- Identify which medical staff are responsible for the decision to administer the thrombolytic/fibrinolytic agent
- Determine which agents will be available in the institution and where they will be stored
- Delineate responsibility and method of mixing, delivering and administering the drug
- Establish the parameters of monitoring and intervention during and after thrombolytic administration (Del Bene and Vaughan, 2005)

The role of the nurse in caring for the patient with STEMI and thrombolytic therapy may vary according to institutional practice and the workplace location (e.g. ED, CCU and rural health). Nurses are usually responsible for mixing and delivering thrombolytic therapy, and monitoring patients during and after thrombolytic delivery, as well as emergency management of complications.

Patients with STEMI in whom thrombolytic therapy is planned should have:

- Continuous arrhythmia monitoring (and continuous 12-lead ST-segment monitoring if available)
- Frequent blood pressure checks – hypo- or hypertension should be reported to responsible medical officer prior to commencing thrombolytic agent
- Two IV accesses – one for taking blood (to avoid recurrent punctures) and one for drug administration
- Administered adjunct pharmacotherapies as ordered or as per unit protocol

Prior to thrombolytic administration:

- Ensure that the patient has no contraindications to thrombolytic therapy
- Explain the proposed therapy to the patient, including benefit versus risk (bleeding, stroke and allergic reaction) – warn the patient that they may feel dizzy for a few minutes due to transient hypotension during the therapy
- Obtain a 12-lead ECG to confirm the presence of ST-segment elevation
- Obtain blood for cardiac enzymes, complete blood picture, group and save (in case of need for transfusion), electrolytes, creatine, urea and lipid screen
- Administer hydrocortisone (100 mg IV) or diphenhydramine (Benadryl) (25 mg IV or 50 mg PO) as ordered to minimise the risk of allergic reaction if streptokinase is the thrombolytic of choice

During thrombolytic administration:

- A nurse should be present with the patient throughout infusion administration
- Blood pressure should be checked every 5 min, or more frequently if unstable, but bear in mind that the patient with thrombolysis will bruise

easily, and automated blood pressure cuffs exert pressure that often results in extensive bruising
- Observe for allergic reaction (breathing difficulties, angioedema and rash)
- Observe for bleeding
- Manage transient hypotension if it occurs: pause the infusion until BP recovers; fluid loading may be required (in the absence of pulmonary oedema) and/or require dopamine (if pulmonary oedema is present or if hypotension is unresponsive to fluid loading)

Following thrombolytic administration

- Obtain blood for serial CK and activated partial thromboplastin time (APPT) checks as per protocol
- Serial ECGs as per protocol or continuous 12-lead ST-segment monitoring for 24 h
- Continue to observe for signs of bleeding (including changed neurological state)
- Administer adjunct pharmacotherapies as ordered
- Assess reperfusion status (continuous ST-segment monitoring or frequent 12-lead ECG)

Non-reperfusion within 90 min of infusion commencement may necessitate rescue percutaneous intervention:

- Notify most available cardiologist with angioplasty skills
- Notify cardiac catheter laboratory staff of need for urgent transfer of patient for procedure

Mechanical reperfusion

Early studies of lytic therapy involved coronary angiography at 90 min to assess patency of the infarct-related artery. It not only became apparent that some vessels remained occluded but that PCI could safely be performed at this point. Around the same time, attempts were being made to use PCI as the first-line strategy and early results were at least encouraging (O'Neill et al. 1994). Advancement of PCI as the primary strategy for treating acute STEMI was assisted by the development of more effective and reliable anti-platelet drugs and the availability of coronary stents.

The use of PCI as the primary treatment strategy for treating acute STEMI has now become established as the ideal therapy for managing acute STEMI with lower rates of death, non-fatal reinfarction and stroke, as compared to fibrinolytic therapy (Keeley et al. 2003). The advantages of PCI are that it restores patency in the infarct-related artery in more than 95% of cases and reduces the need for repeat intervention following the acute presentation. The disadvantages are that it is only available in specialised centres and there is a time lag in the availability of the technique, due to assembly of the treatment team and preparation of the patient.

Primary PCI is performed in the setting of abundant thrombus, having implications for associated therapy, particularly when a foreign object such as a stent is inserted into the milieu. Management of patients in the peri-PCI time window involves striking a balance between aggressive prevention of platelet aggregation and the avoidance of significant bleeding. A number of individual patient factors will impact on the choice and dose of agents but can be expected to include a selection of aspirin, ADP-receptor antagonists such as clopidogrel, heparin either standard or low molecular weight, and glycoprotein IIb-IIIa inhibitors such as abciximab, integrilin or tirofiban. It should always be remembered that other commonly used drugs can also have significant anti-platelet effects, such as organic nitrates and non-dihydropyridine calcium antagonists such as verapamil and diltiazem.

Choosing the appropriate reperfusion strategy

The primary goal of therapy for acute STEMI is to minimise the time interval from vessel occlusion to reperfusion, thus limiting the extent of myocardial death and maximising salvage. The dilemma facing clinicians when patients present with acute STEMI is the need to balance the time taken to deliver a particular therapy with the likelihood of success of therapy. For example, if a patient presents with acute STEMI and the decision is made to use primary PCI as the reperfusion strategy, the expectation must be that mechanical reperfusion of the artery can be performed more rapidly than if a thrombolytic agent were administered at the decision point to use PCI, bearing in mind the lag time between administration of thrombolytic agent and ultimate reperfusion of the vessel. In general terms, thrombolysis is most effective for recently formed thrombus and least effective for vessels occluded for 12h or more. As such, patients presenting early after symptom onset are more likely to have successful and rapid reperfusion of the infarct-related artery with thrombolysis. However, for patients presenting more than 3h after symptom onset, thrombolysis is less likely to be successful and may take longer to be achieved. In the light of this, the more reliable outcome of PCI therapy is preferred, even where a moderate delay in delivering PCI therapy exists.

Learning activity

Review the last 20 patients who were admitted to your hospital with STEMI. How many of them met the criteria for thrombolysis based on local guidelines?

If your system uses primary PCI as the preferred reperfusion strategy, review the last 20 patients and determine (a) how far they had to travel and (b) the time from symptom onset to balloon inflation.

With the above factors in mind, current guidelines for the management of acute STEMI are structured according to symptom duration prior to presentation (Van de Werf et al. 2003; Antman et al. 2004; National Heart Foundation of Australia, Cardiac Society of Australia and New Zealand 2006). For centres where primary PCI facilities are available on site, it is generally recommended that all patients receive primary PCI, provided such therapy can be delivered within 60 min of the decision being made, although time to treatment is most important for those with a short duration of symptoms prior to presentation.

Key point

If PCI cannot be delivered within the specified time frame, the mortality advantage of PCI over thrombolysis may be lost, and thrombolytic therapy should be considered as an alternative strategy.

Most patients with acute STEMI present to centres that do not have primary PCI facilities available on site. Traditionally, such patients have been managed with thrombolysis. However, a number of studies have now demonstrated benefit from transfer of such patients to centres where PCI is available, the transportation time being utilised to assemble the PCI team and prepare the patient so that the overall time to treatment is only marginally greater than the transportation time (Andersen et al. 2003). Increasingly, consideration is being given to make this decision in the pre-hospital setting, with ambulances bypassing non-PCI-equipped hospitals to transport patients directly to PCI-equipped hospitals (Le May et al. 2006). In hospitals without PCI capability, it is generally considered advisable to treat patients who present <1h from onset with thrombolysis, but local arrangements will differ. For patients with up to 3h of symptoms, transfer for PCI should be considered as primary therapy provided transportation to a PCI centre can occur within 90min. For patients with >3h of symptoms, the delivery of PCI within 2h still confers an advantage over thrombolysis. The guidelines are, of necessity, somewhat complicated and require a detailed knowledge of the performance of individual health systems with respect to time-to-balloon inflation, so that a well-informed choice can be made for each patient.

It is relevant at this point to consider the concept of the difference in minutes between door-to-balloon and door-to-needle (DB-DN) time intervals. This concept seeks to quantify the incremental time penalty that can safely be employed in order to deliver PCI, before the mortality advantage of this therapy over thrombolysis is lost. Initial estimates suggested that 1h was the limit for this difference. More recently, a review of 192,509 patients at 645 hospitals contributing to the US National Registry of Myocardial Infarction (NRMI) database has shown that PCI can be delivered up to 114 min later than thrombolysis before the mortality advantage is lost (Pinto et al. 2006). However, there is substantial heterogeneity for this figure dependent not only on duration of symptoms prior to presentation but also on the age of the patient and the location of the infarct (anterior versus non-anterior). Indeed, for young patients with anterior infarction, the mortality advantage of PCI is lost within 45min. Systems therefore need to be structured such that all patients have a DB-DN within 114 min and ensure that no subgroup of patients is put at risk by a strategy of PCI over thrombolysis.

Strategies for reducing treatment time delays

> ### Key point
>
> Minutes mean myocardium! Irrespective of the reperfusion strategy, every effort must be made to reduce delay at all points of the patient pathway, to maximise the benefits of treatment.

The importance of reducing delays across the patient pathway in acute STEMI care is covered in detail in Chapter 20. There are three critical time periods to be considered when seeking to reduce the time taken to reperfuse the infarct-related artery in acute STEMI cases. The first is the time interval between symptom onset (the surrogate for vessel occlusion) and presentation to medical care. Attempts to reduce this time interval have been universally unsuccessful. Numerous public health campaigns in various settings have been used to encourage people with chest pain to seek early medical attention. Evidence shows that there is some improvement in time to presentation during the campaign but this quickly returns to background levels once the campaign ends. Furthermore, only half of the patients presenting with acute STEMI arrive by ambulance. Now that ambulances frequently have the ability to perform 12-lead electrocardiographs, failure to use an ambulance has a multiplying affect on delays in time to treatment.

The second critical time interval determining the efficiency of management of STEMI is the time from presentation to diagnosis. Unfortunately, this time period is poorly recognised as an issue, yet is a major determinant of delay. Guidelines assume that an electrocardiograph performed within 10 min of hospital arrival is the equivalent of a diagnosis of STEMI. This is not the case. Delays in the diagnosis of STEMI in the emergency department are common and can be caused by such factors as an inappropriate triage category, subtle rather than obvious electrocardiographic changes, and failure to appreciate the potential diagnosis and perform an electrocardiograph due to atypical symptoms.

The final critical time interval is from diagnosis to the delivery of a reperfusion strategy, either administration of a thrombolytic agent or the first balloon inflation. It is standard practice to monitor either door-to-needle (for thrombolysis) or door-to-balloon (for PCI) times with targets of 30 and 90 min respectively. Despite the fact that the evidence base determining the choice between thrombolysis and primary PCI is based on DB-DN, this time interval is not routinely measured. In short, the time from door to diagnosis is not routinely measured despite being the major source of variation in treatment (door-to-needle or door-to-balloon) times. Nevertheless, it is true that a number of system changes can be made which reproducibly reduce treatment times. The system changes largely result from devolving the responsibility for making the diagnosis of STEMI to earlier points in the health care chain. For example, there is good evidence supporting ambulance paramedics diagnosing acute STEMI in the ambulance and administering thrombolysis prior to hospital arrival. Furthermore, a recent, detailed analysis of factors associated with reduced door-to-balloon times included six key recommendations (Bradley et al. 2006). These are the performance of 12-lead electrocardiography in the field with activation of the catheterisation laboratory team while the patient is en route, having emergency physicians activate the catheterisation laboratory, having a single call to a central pager operator activate the laboratory, expecting staff to arrive in the catheterisation laboratory within 20 min after being paged, having an attending cardiologist always on site, and having staff in the emergency department and the catheterisation laboratory use real-time data feedback. Using any four of these strategies reduced the median door-to-balloon time by 30 min.

Detecting and managing failed reperfusion

Failed thrombolysis

Thrombolysis remains the most commonly delivered reperfusion strategy, largely due to the limited availability of PCI. The success or failure of thrombolysis is judged at around 90 min post-administration, due to the time taken for clot lysis and subsequent reperfusion of the infarct-related artery to occur. It is estimated that about one-third of arteries remain occluded 90 min following the administration of thrombolytic therapy. A number of strategies have been tried over time to improve this patency rate, including more advanced lytic agents and associated anti-platelet therapy. Nevertheless, a significant proportion of patients have failed reperfusion.

The determination of success of thrombolysis is dependent upon changes in the 12-lead electrocardiograph. Reperfusion is generally considered to have occurred if the extent of ST elevation, in the lead where this is maximal, is reduced by more than 50% by 90 min. The certainty of reperfusion is greatest when the reduction of ST elevation is greatest, particularly when associated with a dramatic improvement in symptoms. There is now reasonable evidence to support the use of PCI as a rescue strategy for patients where thrombolysis has failed (Testa et al. 2008). There are certainly advantages of rescue PCI over repeat thrombolysis or a conservative strategy. The time window during which rescue PCI may be effective extends at least 4 h beyond the dose of thrombolysis. Given that the success of thrombolysis can only be judged at 90 or more minutes post-dose, this only leaves little more than a 2-h window for the delivery of a rescue PCI strategy. Given that up to one-third of patients receiving thrombolysis will have no evidence of success at 90 min, it is therefore suggested that all patients having thrombolysis be considered for rescue PCI from the outset. This means moving patients at an early time point to a PCI facility so that, in the event that reperfusion from thrombolysis does not occur, rescue PCI can proceed within an acceptable time frame. This is particularly important for patients in a rural setting where transportation times can be quite extended. In these situations, transportation should be arranged at the same time that thrombolysis is being administered. Delaying transportation until the success or otherwise of thrombolysis is judged will delay rescue PCI to the point where any benefit is probably lost.

Patients receiving thrombolysis who are subsequently moved to a PCI facility should not receive an intervention automatically. For those patients with clear evidence of reperfusion, there is no benefit from undergoing acute angiography and PCI. Data from facilitated PCI studies have demonstrated that patients receiving thrombolysis followed by routine PCI have a worse outcome (ASSENT-4 PCI Investigators 2006; Ellis et al. 2008). However, for patients arriving at a PCI facility, who have received thrombolysis within the last few hours and where there is electrocardiographic evidence of failed reperfusion, acute angiography is indicated with rescue PCI performed as required. A French registry (FAST-MI) has recently reported 1-year survival of 94% for thrombolysis followed by routine angiography, compared with 93% for primary PCI (Danchin et al. 2008). These data suggest that a 'pharmaco-invasive' approach may have merit, and randomised clinical trials are underway.

Failed PCI – what next?

Primary PCI is regarded as the optimal management for acute STEMI. However, occasionally the procedure will be unsuccessful due to an inability to mechanically open the infarct-related artery. While this situation is uncommon (<5% of cases), it is nevertheless important to have a strategy for dealing with this eventuality. If procedural difficulties are apparent at an early stage, a second operator, if not immediately available, should be contacted to attend. In the event that mechanical reperfusion is not possible, there are a range of possibilities that need to be considered. One option is the administration of intracoronary thrombolysis. Alternatively, if the vascular territory is judged to be relatively small, a conservative approach may be selected. Finally, if the vascular territory is particularly large, acute coronary grafting may be considered if this facility is immediately available.

Preventing and detecting re-occlusion

Following successful reperfusion of the infarct-related artery, patients should be monitored closely for potential re-occlusion. Acute STEMI involves active thrombus formation in a setting where there is ongoing significant stimulus for thrombus formation, even after intervention. A range of therapies are used to balance the risk of recurrent thrombus formation against the risk of bleeding. Registry data from the UK report re-infarction rates approaching

10% following pre-hospital treatment (Horne et al. 2009). Re-occlusion of the infarct-related artery remains a significant risk for at least 24h after a reperfusion strategy has been applied. During this time, careful attention to the optimal use of anti-platelet therapies needs to occur, in concert with vigilance for any signs of overt or concealed bleeding.

Patient symptoms, although useful, are not always a reliable guide to vessel patency with some re-occlusion being relatively clinically silent. Detection of re-occlusion relies upon ongoing monitoring of the electrocardiograph. Ideally, this should involve continuous monitoring of the ST segments, particularly in the lead where ST elevation was maximal. Commercial systems are now available that will not only provide this level of monitoring but alarm when ST segments rise. The management of re-occlusion may involve any of the three major strategies outlined earlier in this chapter for therapy of acute STEMI but there is certainly a major bias towards PCI as the therapy of choice for this event. This is yet another reason why the early transfer of all patients with acute STEMI, regardless of treatment modality used, to a PCI facility should be considered.

Learning activity

- Locate and review your hospital/health system STEMI guidelines.
- Identify the preferred reperfusion strategy locally – PCI or thrombolysis? Is thrombolysis given in the ambulance?
- If ECG telemedicine is available in your practice setting, review the guidelines on decision-making: who has authority to make treatment decisions? Is there robust documentation/governance?
- Review local data on call-to-balloon and/or call-to-needle times: does your local system meet national/international standards of care?
- If thrombolysis is the preferred treatment locally, locate and review the policy on identifying patients who may have failed thrombolysis and require rescue PCI.
- Review your local protocol for alerting the catheter laboratory or arranging interhospital transfer for rescue PCI.

Conclusion

The primary goal of treatment of acute STEMI is restoration of early, complete and sustained myocardial reperfusion. For the past two decades at least, the most widely available treatment has been with intravenous thrombolysis, usually administered in hospital but increasingly available in the ambulance. In recent years, significant evidence has accumulated of the benefits of PCI. Individual patient and health system characteristics (including availability of PCI facilities) will determine the appropriate approach. Nurses have played a key role in care of patients receiving thrombolysis over past decades, and are likely to be a key to meeting the challenges of rapidly evolving reperfusion strategies in the PCI era.

References

Andersen, H.R., Nielsen, T.T., Rasmussen, K., et al. for the DANAMI-2 Investigators (2003). A comparison of coronary angioplasty with fibrinolytic therapy in acute myocardial infarction. *New England Journal of Medicine*, **349**:733–42.

Antman, E.M., Anbe, D.T., Armstrong, P.W., et al. (2004). ACC/AHA guidelines for the management of patients with ST-elevation myocardial infarction – executive summary: a report of the American College of Cardiology/American Heart Association Task Force on Practice Guidelines (Writing Committee to Revise the 1999 Guidelines for the Management of Patients with Acute Myocardial Infarction). *Circulation*, **110**:588–636.

ASSENT-4 PCI Investigators (2006). Assessment of the safety and efficacy of a new treatment strategy with percutaneous coronary intervention primary versus tenecteplase-facilitated percutaneous coronary intervention in patients with ST-segment elevation acute myocardial infarction (ASSENT-4 PCI): randomised trial. *Lancet*, **367**:569–78.

Beltrame, J.F., Stewart, S., Leslie, S., et al. (2002). Resolution of ST-segment elevation following intravenous administration of nitroglycerin and verapamil. *American Journal of Cardiology*, **89**:452–55.

Bradley, E.H., Herrin, J., Wang, Y., et al. (2006). Strategies for reducing the door-to-balloon time in acute myocardial infarction. *New England Journal of Medicine*, **355**:2308–20.

Castle, N., Owen, R., Vincent, R., et al. (2006). What percentages of patients are suitable for prehospital thrombolysis? *Emergency Medicine Journal*, **23**:444–5.

Danchin, N., Coste, P., Ferrieres, J., et al. (2008). Comparison of thrombolysis followed by broad use of percutaneous coronary intervention with primary percutaneous coronary intervention for ST-segment-elevation acute myocardial infarction: data from the French registry on acute ST-elevation myocardial infarction (FAST-MI). *Circulation*, **118**:268–76.

Del Bene, S. & Vaughan, A. (2005). Acute Coronary Syndromes In: S.L. Woods, E.S.S. Froelicher, S.U. Motzer & E.J. Bridges, (eds), *Cardiac Nursing*, 5th edn. Lippincott Williams and Wilkins, Philadelphia, pp. 572–5.

Department of Health (2000). *The NHS Plan: Investment and Reform*. Department of Health, London.

Eagle, K.A., Nallamothu, B.K., Mehta, R.H., et al. (2008). Global Registry of Acute Coronary Events (GRACE) Investigators. Trends in acute reperfusion therapy for ST-segment elevation myocardial infarction from 1999 to 2006: we are getting better but we have got a long way to go. *European Heart Journal*, **29**:609–17.

Ellis, S.G., Tendera, M., de Belder, M.A., et al. (2008). FINESSE Investigators. Facilitated PCI in patients with ST-elevation myocardial infarction. *New England Journal of Medicine*, **358**:2205–17.

Goldstein, J.A., Demetriou, D., Grines, C.L., et al. (2000). Multiple complex coronary plaques in patients with acute myocardial infarction. *New England Journal of Medicine*, **343**:915–22.

GUSTO Angiographic Investigators (1993). The effects of tissue plasminogen activator, streptokinase, or both on coronary-artery patency, ventricular function, and survival after acute myocardial infarction. *New England Journal of Medicine*, **329**:1615–22.

Heath, S.M., Baine, R.J. & Andrews, A. (2003). Nurse initiated thrombolysis in the accident and emergency department: safe, accurate, and faster than fast track. *Emergency Medicine Journal*, **20**:418–20.

Horne, S., Weston, C., Quinn, T., et al. (2009). The impact of prehospital thrombolytic treatment on reinfarction rates: analysis of the Myocardial Infarction National Audit Project (MINAP). *Heart*, **95**:559–63.

ISIS-2 (Second International Study of Infarct Survival) Collaborative Group (1988). Randomized trial of intravenous streptokinase, oral aspirin, both, or neither among 17,187 cases of suspected acute myocardial infarction: ISIS-2. *Lancet*, **2**:349–60.

Keeley, E.C., Boura, J.A. & Grines, C.L. (2003). Primary angioplasty versus intravenous thrombolytic therapy for acute myocardial infarction: a quantitative review of 23 randomised trials. *Lancet*, **361**:13–20.

Kremser, A.K. & Lyneham, J. (2007). Can Australian nurses safely assess for thrombolysis on EKG criteria? *Journal of Emergency Nursing*, **33**:102–9

Le May, M.R., Davies, R.F., Dionne, R., et al. (2006). Comparison of early mortality of paramedic-diagnosed ST-segment elevation myocardial infarction with immediate transport to a designated primary percutaneous coronary intervention center to that of similar patients transported to the nearest hospital. *American Journal of Cardiology*, **98**:1329–33.

McLean, S., Egan, G., Connor, P., et al. (2008). Collaborative decision-making between paramedics and CCU nurses based on 12-lead ECG telemetry expedites the delivery of thrombolysis in ST elevation myocardial infarction. *Emergency Medicine Journal*, **25**:370–4.

Morrison, L.J., Verbeek, P.R., McDonald, A.C., et al. (2000). Mortality and prehospital thrombolysis for acute myocardial infarction: A meta-analysis. *Journal of the American Medical Association*, **31**:2686–92.

National Heart Foundation of Australia, Cardiac Society of Australia and New Zealand (2006). Guidelines for management of acute coronary syndromes. *Medical Journal of Australia*, **184**:S1–32.

O'Neill, W.W., Brodie, B.R., Ivanhoe, R., et al. (1994). Primary coronary angioplasty for acute myocardial infarction (the Primary Angioplasty Registry). *American Journal of Cardiology*, **73**:627–34.

Pinto, D.S., Kirtane, A.J., Nallamothu, B.K., et al. (2006). Hospital delays in reperfusion for ST-elevation myocardial infarction: implications when selecting a reperfusion strategy. *Circulation*, **114**:2019–25.

Quinn, T. (1995). Can nurses safely assess suitability for thrombolytic therapy? A pilot study. *Intensive and Critical Care Nursing*, **11**:126–9.

Reimer, K.A., Vander Heide, R.S. & Richard, V.J. (1993). Reperfusion in acute myocardial infarction: effect of timing and modulating factors in experimental models. *American Journal of Cardiology*, **72**:13G–21G.

Rosenberg, D.G., Levin, E., Lausell, A., et al. (2002). Feasibility and timing of prehospital administration of reteplase in patients with acute myocardial infarction. *Journal of Thrombosis and Thrombolysis*, **13**:147–53.

Testa, L., van Gaal, W.J., Biondi-Zoccai, G.G., et al. (2008). Repeat thrombolysis or conservative therapy vs. rescue percutaneous coronary intervention for failed thrombolysis: systematic review and meta-analysis. *Quarterly Journal of Medicine*, **101**:387–95.

Van de Werf, F., Ardissino, D., Betriu, A. et al. (2003). Management of acute myocardial infarction in patients presenting with ST-segment elevation. *European Heart Journal*, **24**:28–66.

Walker, L., Birkhead, J., Weston, C., et al. (2008). *How the NHS Manages Heart Attacks*. Myocardial Ischaemia National Audit Programme Seventh Public Report. Royal College of Physicians of London and Healthcare Quality Improvement Partnership, University College London.

Zijlstra, F., Ernst, N., de Boer, M.J., et al. (2002). Influence of prehospital administration of aspirin and heparin on initial patency of the infarct-related artery in patients with acute ST elevation myocardial infarction. *Journal of the American College of Cardiology*, **39**:1733–7.

Useful Websites and Further Reading

D2B Alliance – Guidelines Applied in Practice (GAP) program launched by the American College of Cardiology (ACC) to save time and save lives by reducing the door-to-balloon times: http://www.d2balliance.org/

European Society of Cardiology 2008 STEMI guidelines: http://www.escardio.org/guidelines-surveys/esc-guideliness//Pages/act-st-segment-elevation.aspx

Get with the guidelines – American Heart Association quality improvement programme: http://www.americanheart.org/getwiththeguidelines

Myocardial Ischaemia National Audit Project (MINAP): http://www.rcplondon.ac.uk/clinical-standards/organisation/partnership/Pages/MINAP-.aspx

22 Adjunct Pharmacological Agents in Acute Coronary Syndromes

A.M. Kucia & J.D. Horowitz

Overview

Acute coronary syndromes (ACS) are a spectrum of clinical conditions associated with abrupt onset of myocardial ischaemia and/or infarction, reflecting, in most cases, the presence of an underlying intracoronary thrombus. ACS includes unstable angina pectoris, non-ST-elevation and ST-elevation myocardial infarction (MI). The management of patients with ACS encompasses a variety of interventional and pharmacological strategies. Substantial progress has been made in the understanding of the pathophysiological basis of ACS in the past two decades, and this has resulted in a large number of randomised controlled trials to guide the introduction of new therapies to treat ACS and the resulting complications.

New evidence in the knowledge of disease processes and emerging therapies with demonstrated improved outcomes has provided a stimulus for changes to medical and nursing practice. Change in prescribing practices for new pharmacological agents in the management of ACS often mandates significant change to nursing practice. This may involve change in resource requirements including equipment or more nursing hours, and formal education of all staff may be needed. An understanding of the evidence and guidelines supporting use of pharmacological agents, issues related to the administration and delivery of the agent, assessment of benefit, contraindications, side effects and management of adverse events, and any other issues related to nursing care of the patient need to be understood. It is useful to develop unit protocols for pharmacological therapies used in ACS addressing these issues.

This chapter discusses current pharmacological agents in the management of ACS and its complications and current evidence-based guidelines supporting the use of these therapies.

Learning objectives

After reading this chapter, you should be able to:

- List the adjunct pharmacological agents that are commonly used in management of ACS.
- Discuss the indications and contraindications for use of these agents.
- Evaluate and synthesise the current best evidence for management of ACS and associated cardiac conditions.
- Describe the nursing management for patients receiving these pharmacological agents.
- Demonstrate an awareness of potential side effects and hazards of these pharmacological agents.

Key concepts

Antiplatelet agents; anti-ischaemic therapies; anticoagulation; clinical trials; evidence-based guidelines

Anti-ischaemic therapies

A number of anti-ischaemic drugs are used in the treatment of ACS.

Nitrates

Nitroglycerin (NTG), also known as glyceryl trinitrate (GTN), and long-acting nitrates have been used in cardiovascular medicine for over 100 years, and have beneficial effects in stable angina, ACS and congestive heart failure (CHF). The beneficial effects of nitrates in ACS have multiple mechanisms. Atherosclerosis results in vascular endothelial dysfunction, one manifestation of which is decreased nitric oxide (NO) availability. NO is needed to stimulate vasodilation and prevent platelet aggregation. Administration of exogenous NO (released from organic nitrates) results in vasodilation in the setting of endothelial dysfunction (Abrams 1996). Nitrates increase coronary blood flow by mechanisms such as epicardial coronary artery dilation and enhanced collateral size and flow, irrespective of endothelial dysfunction. Nitrates also prevent and/or reverse coronary artery vasoconstriction, which helps to increase nutrient coronary blood flow to zones of myocardial ischaemia (Conti et al. 1985). Nitrates decrease platelet activation, aggregation and thrombosis formation (Chirkov et al. 1992). Nitrates also cause venous dilation which results in a redistribution of the circulating blood volume away from the heart to the venous capacitance system, with a resultant fall in venous return to the heart (preload) and thereby a decrease in myocardial workload (Abrams 1996). Additionally, the afterload or arterial effects of nitrates are also useful in decreasing myocardial oxygen consumption.

Nitrate tolerance

The beneficial effects of nitrates may be limited by the development of nitrate tolerance, a phenomenon that may occur even with short-term intravenous (IV) nitrate infusion. IV NTG should be converted to a non-parenteral alternative within 24 h of medical stabilisation (AHA/ACC 2007). The main mechanism of nitrate tolerance is probably decreased NO release due to a decrease in enzymatic nitrate bioconversion. This results in a need for continually increasing doses of nitrates to maintain a therapeutic effect.

Key point

It has been suggested that co-infusion of N-acetylcysteine (NAC) may be useful in ameliorating nitrate tolerance by increasing nitrate bioconversion and potentiating the vasodilatory and antiplatelet aggregatory effects of NTG (Horowitz et al. 1983, 1988; Loscalzo 1985; Winniford et al. 1986; Packer et al. 1987, Horowitz et al. 1988). NAC should only be used with low-dose IV nitrates, and the patient should be observed closely for hypotension during the first hour or with subsequent changes in nitrate dose.

Evidence for nitrate use in ACS

The evidence for the clinical utility of IV nitrate use in ACS has been limited to a number of small studies, and evidence in terms of a large prospective trial is lacking, particularly in the post-thrombolytic era. There is observational clinical evidence which documents the effect of nitrates in reducing infarct size and preservation of left ventricular (LV) function (Jugdutt & Warnica 1988), and a meta-analysis of the results of randomised clinical trials in the pre-thrombolytic era which suggests a significant reduction in mortality (Yusuf et al. 1988).

Current guidelines suggest that IV NTG be used for persistent or recurrent ischaemia and in patients with CHF. It is common clinical practice to continue IV nitrate therapy for 24–48 h and then convert to a non-parental, non-tolerance producing regimen within 24 h of medical stabilisation. It has been suggested that IV NTG should be commenced at 10 mcg/min with an increase of 10 mcg/min every 3–5 min, until relief of symptoms (dyspnoea, angina) or adverse symptoms (hypotension/headache) appear with a ceiling infusion rate of 200 mcg/min (AHA/ACC 2007).

Key point

NTG infusion rates of 10 mcg/min and above have been shown to induce nitrate tolerance within 24 h (Sage et al. 2000). It is common practice to limit infusion rates to 2.5–10 mcg/min.

Considerations in the nursing management of patients with nitrate therapy are represented in Table 22.1.

Beta-adrenoceptor antagonists

The response of the cardiovascular system to catecholamines is mediated by specific cell membrane receptors. Stimulation of beta $(\beta)_1$ receptors (primarily located in the myocardium) results in increased contractility, increased sinus discharge rate, increased atrioventricular (AV) node conduction velocity and increased AV node refractoriness. β_2-receptors (predominantly found in vascular and bronchial tissue) mediate arteriolar and bronchial smooth muscle dilation. β-adrenoceptor agonists, commonly referred to as 'beta blockers', block these responses.

Beta blockers have been used for some years in the treatment of cardiovascular diseases. The antihypertensive effects of beta blockers are due to a decrease in cardiac output. This is mediated by inhibition of the release of renin and angiotensin II, blockade of presynaptic α-adrenoceptors that increase the release of norepinephrine from sympathetic nerve terminals and decrease of central vasomotor activity. Anti-ischaemic effects of beta blockers are due to decreased myocardial oxygen demand during sympathetic stimulation due to reducing heart rate, cardiac contractility and systolic blood pressure. Increased myocardial perfusion resulting from the reduced heart rate and subsequent prolongation of diastole probably also plays a part. Beta blockers contribute to improved LV structure and function by decreasing ventricular size and increasing ejection fraction. An important action of beta blockers is suppression of arrhythmias (decreased spontaneous firing of ectopic pacemakers, slowed conduction and increased refractory period of AV node) and

reduction of sympathetic drive and associated myocardial ischaemia, and catecholamine-induced hypokalaemia (Lopez-Sendo et al. 2004).

Evidence for the use of β-adrenergic antagonists in ACS

About half of all deaths after MI are sudden cardiac deaths, and it is likely that most of these are due to ventricular fibrillation (VF) (Hjalmarson 1997). Associated reductions in total mortality and sudden cardiac death for patients with acute myocardial infarction (AMI) and beta blockers were first reported in 1981, but it should be noted that these studies were undertaken before thrombolytics and primary percutaneous transluminal coronary angioplasty (PTCA) were routinely available. Infarctions in the pre-reperfusion era were larger with a higher incidence of LV failure and ventricular fibrillation; hence the observed reduced mortality benefits in the beta-blocker groups. In the reperfusion era, the COMMIT study suggests that early aggressive beta blockade increases the risk of cardiogenic shock in haemodynamically unstable patients, and should be avoided in the setting of heart failure and haemodynamic instability (Chen et al. 2005).

The evidence for use of beta blockers in unstable angina pectoris (UAP) and non-ST-elevation MI (non-STEMI) is limited to small studies. The largest study of beta blockers in UAP was the Holland Interuniversity Nifedipine/metoprolol Trial (HINT) which produced only equivocal evidence of benefit (HINT Research Group 1986). There is good evidence for utility of beta blockers in secondary prevention after moderate to large MI (but not after small MI).

Key points

Current guidelines advise that early aggressive beta blockade should be avoided. If used, beta blockers are recommended to be initiated orally, in the absence of contraindications such as hypotension and heart failure, within the first 24 h. However, oral beta blockade is strongly recommended for secondary prevention before hospital discharge in those with compensated heart failure or LV systolic dysfunction (AHA/ACC 2007).

Table 22.1 Anti-ischaemic therapy: considerations in nursing management.

Nitrates	Beta blockers	Calcium channel blockers
Nitrates come in a variety of preparations including IV, transdermal, sublingual spray, sublingual tablets and oral tablets.	Beta blockers come in oral and some in IV preparations.	Calcium channel blockers come in oral and some in IV preparations.
Nitrates should not be administered to patients with hypotension (systolic blood pressure ≤90 mmHg or ≥30 mmHg below baseline) or severe bradycardia (<50 bpm) or tachycardia (AHA/ACC 2007).	Beta blockers are contraindicated in patients with pulmonary oedema, severe LV systolic dysfunction, cardiogenic shock, peripheral vascular disease, depression, known or suspected coronary artery spasm and heart failure (except for those specifically indicated for use in heart failure). Non-selective beta blockers are contraindicated in patients with asthma or chronic obstructive pulmonary disease because of the risk of bronchoconstriction. Sympathetic nerves innervating the bronchioles normally activate β₂-receptors that promote bronchodilation, and blockade of these receptors can lead to bronchoconstriction (Klabunde 2007).	Dihydropyridine calcium antagonists can cause flushing, headache, hypotension, peripheral oedema and reflex tachycardia.
Nitrates should not be administered to patients who have received a phosphodiesterase inhibitor for erectile dysfunction within the last 24 h (48 h for tadalafil) (Antman et al. 2004).		Cardiac selective, non-dihydropyridine calcium antagonists can cause extreme bradycardia, impaired electrical conduction (e.g. AV nodal block), depressed contractility and constipation.
Intravenous NTG should be prepared in a glass bottle and delivered via non-PVC tubing to ensure that the amount ordered is the amount delivered (PVC tubing absorbs NTG making less available to the patient).	Relative contraindications to beta-blocker therapy include heart rate <60 bpm, systolic blood pressure <100 mmHg, signs of peripheral hypoperfusion and heart block (Antman et al. 2004).	Calcium antagonists must not be used in the setting of pulmonary oedema, severe LV dysfunction, bradycardia or AV block.
Observe for hypotension on commencement of an IV NTG infusion and with upward rate adjustment.	Beta blockers should be used very cautiously in patients with diabetes. β₂-adrenoceptors normally stimulate hepatic glycogen breakdown and pancreatic release of glucagon, which work together to increase plasma glucose. Blocking the β₂-adrenoceptors lower plasma glucose and can thus precipitate hypoglycaemia. Although β₁-blocˋers have fewer metabolic side effects in diabetic patients, the effect on heart reduction means that tachycardia, which may be a sign of hypoglycaemia, may be masked (Klabunde 2007).	Calcium antagonists are contraindicated in the presence of significant LV dysfunction (ejection fraction <40%), bradycardia, conduction defects and heart failure. It is potentially dangerous to co-administer non-dihydropyridine calcium antagonists together with beta blockers in ACS patients.
Nitrates can cause severe headaches and analgesia may be required.		In addition to observing the contraindications and adverse reactions listed above, nurses should closely monitor patients on initiation of calcium antagonist therapy for hypotension, bradycardia and heart block. IV administration requires continuous ECG monitoring. The elderly are more susceptible to adverse reactions and may experience weakness, dizziness or fainting spells that may lead to falls.
Intravenous preparations of NTG should be withdrawn 24–48 h after clinical stability is achieved to minimise nitrate tolerance.		Verapamil can result in severe constipation – the patient needs education about this possibility and ways to avoid it.
Nitrates should be used with extreme caution in patients with right ventricular infarction because it may exacerbate a red\uced LV preload situation with associated reduction in cardiac output (Gardner & Altman 2005).	Continuous arrhythmia monitoring should be used for IV administration of beta blockers with a target heart rate of 50–60 bpm. Observe for bradycardia, heart block and hypotension.	

Table 22.1   *(cont'd)*

Nitrates	Beta blockers	Calcium channel blockers
For patients taking oral or transdermal nitrates, a 12-h interval between the last nitrate dose and first dose of the following day (usually between 1800 and 0600) is needed. Thus, education of patients in timing of nitrate medications is critical. Alcohol enhances the effect of NTG and puts patients at increased risk of hypotension. Ensure that patients are discharged with a short-acting nitrate and that they are educated on issues related to use and storage.	Patients should be educated about the side effects of beta blockers, including bradycardia, reduced exercise capacity, heart failure, hypotension, bronchospasm, fatigue, mood changes and nightmares.	

Calcium antagonists

Calcium antagonists (also known as calcium channel blockers) act on L-type calcium channels located on the vascular smooth muscle, cardiac myocytes and cardiac nodal tissue (sinoatrial and AV nodes). These channels are responsible for regulating the influx of calcium into muscle cells, which in turn stimulates smooth muscle contraction and cardiac myocyte contraction (Klabunde 2005). By blocking calcium entry into the cell, calcium antagonists cause vascular smooth muscle relaxation (vasodilation), decrease the force of myocardial contraction (negative inotropy), decrease heart rate (negative chronotropy) by decreasing auromaticity in the sinoatrial node and decreasing conduction in the AV junction (negative dromotropy).

Calcium antagonists have a number of therapeutic effects. The antihypertensive action of calcium antagonists is due to smooth muscle relaxation, which has the effect of decreasing systemic vascular resistance and reducing arterial blood pressure. These drugs primarily affect arterial resistance vessels, with only minimal effects on venous capacitance vessels (Klabunde 2005). Calcium antagonists also have anti-anginal actions. They cause systemic vasodilation and reduced arterial blood pressure that result in decreased ventricular afterload and decreased myocardial oxygen demand. Calcium antagonists decrease heart rate and contractility, which also leads to a reduction in myocardial oxygen demand. The more cardioselective the calcium antagonist, the greater the heart rate reduction. Calcium antagonists can also dilate coronary arteries and prevent or reverse coronary vasospasm (as occurs in Printzmetal's variant angina), thereby increasing oxygen supply to the myocardium. Calcium channel blockers have Class 4 anti-arrhythmic properties which decrease the firing rate of aberrant pacemaker sites. They also decrease conduction velocity and prolong repolarisation, especially at the AV node which helps to block re-entry mechanisms, which can cause supraventricular tachycardia (Klabunde, 2005).

Calcium antagonists can be subclassified into the *dihydropyridine* (nifedipine, amlodipine) and *non-dihydropyridine* (diltiazem, verapamil) groups, which vary in action, and subsequently, in safety, efficacy and clinical outcomes for patients with ACS. The dihydropyridines, for instance, have a greater selectivity for the vasculature rather than the heart, and consequently may produce reflex tachycardia through sympathetic nervous stimulation when blood pressure is lowered due to vasodilation. In contrast, the non-dihydropyridine group of calcium antagonists has heart-rate-lowering effects, which has been shown to tend to decrease the rate of cardiac events after AMI.

Evidence for calcium antagonist use in ACS

A meta-analysis of 16 randomised secondary-prevention trials of nifedipine concluded that in patients with coronary disease, the use of short-acting nifedipine in moderate to high doses causes an increase in total mortality (Furberg et al. 1995). There is some evidence to suggest that non-dihydropyridine calcium antagonists (verapamil, diltiazem) may be beneficial in ACS in decreasing myocardial oxygen demand and improving myocardial blood flow, and result in a reduced incidence of further ischaemic events (Gibson et al. 1986; Hansen et al. 1997). Calcium antagonists should only be used in the absence of acute pulmonary oedema or severe LV systolic dysfunction (AHA/ACC 2007).

Key points

Current guidelines suggest that calcium antagonists may be used to control ischaemia-related symptoms in patients unresponsive or intolerant to nitrates and beta blockers (AHA/ACC 2007). Calcium antagonists are particularly useful in the management of angina due to coronary artery spasm such as variant (Printzmetal's) angina. Rapid release, short-acting dihydropyridines should not be used without concomitant beta blockade. Caution should be used with this combination as the act synergistically depresses LV function and sinus and AV node conduction (AHA/ACC 2007).

Antiplatelet and anticoagulant therapy

The pathogenesis of ACS includes partial or total occlusion of a coronary artery due to thrombus formation. There have been a number of studies, in the past two decades in particular, that have focused on pharmacological agents that target the mechanisms of thrombus formation. A combination of aspirin, an anticoagulant and an additional antiplatelet therapy represents the most effective treatment for ACS (AHA/ACC 2007). Refer to Table 22.2.

Antiplatelet therapy

Coronary occlusion is complex and multifactorial, but the role of platelets in this process is well established. Platelet activation may occur in response to exposure to the subendothelial connective matrix of a plaque in plaque erosion, or as a result of sudden exposure of the plaque lipid core to the bloodstream in plaque rupture, triggering the clotting cascade. A number of mediators are associated with platelet activation, including von Willebrand factor, collagen, thromboxane A_2, thrombin and adenosine diphosphate (ADP). Activated platelets are associated with the formation of vasoconstricting and platelet-aggregating substances, including the potent thromboxane A_2.

Antiplatelet agents are medications that inhibit platelet aggregation. There are three common

Table 22.2 Antiplatelet therapies inhibitors: considerations in nursing management.

Aspirin	Clopidogrel
Aspirin is contraindicated in patients who are allergic to aspirin, active peptic ulcer disease (PUD), history of recent gastrointestinal (GI) bleeding; history of recent intracranial bleeding and bleeding disorders including haemophilia, von Willebrand's disease, thrombocytopaenia and severe liver disease.	The use of clopidogrel is contraindicated in the presence of any active bleeding and in anyone who has previously demonstrated a hypersensitivity to the drug or its components. Clopidogrel is associated with an increased risk of bleeding, particularly in the GI tract. Intracranial bleeding is also a risk. Vascular access sites should be monitored carefully for occurrence of bleeding. Signs of retroperitoneal bleed (back pain, groin discomfort, lower abdominal tenderness ipsilateral to the puncture site, femoral neuropathy and hypotension) should be promptly investigated. Monitor platelet count in patients taking clopidogrel.
Aspirin must be used with caution in people with asthma. Cautions with aspirin include asthma, uncontrolled hypertension and previous PUD.	
Proton pump inhibitors or H2-receptor antagonists may be considered for prophylaxis in people with past PUD. Enteric-coated aspirin is usually used in patients with GI symptoms, but there is no evidence to suggest that enteric-coated aspirin reduces the incidence of major GI bleed (Kelly et al. 1996).	A rare side effect of clopidogrel is thrombotic thrombocytopaenic purpura (TTP). TTP causes abnormal blood clotting causing available platelets to be consumed. Because there are no available platelets, blood cannot clot normally and bleeding occurs. TTP is a serious condition that can be fatal and requires urgent treatment including plasmapheresis (plasma exchange). Another thienopyridine, ticlodipine, is significantly more likely to cause TTP and thus is not commonly used in the setting of ACS.
The most common adverse reactions associated with aspirin are related to the GI system. Aspirin can cause ulcers in the stomach and duodenum, abdominal pain, nausea and gastritis. There is a dose-dependent relationship in upper GI bleeding.	
Intracranial haemorrhage is a rare but serious consequence of aspirin which again tends to be dose dependant.	
Allergy to aspirin is a rare but potentially lethal side effect. Sensitive individuals can develop angio-oedema, bronchospasm and anaphylaxis.	
Other side effects include renal and hepatic impairment, particularly in patients who already have renal or hepatic disease, vertigo and tinnitus.	
Observe for excessive bruising or abnormal bleeding. Keep venous and arterial punctures to a minimum. Avoid excessive inflations of automated blood pressure cuffs.	

types of antiplatelet agents used in the management of ACS: (1) aspirin, (2) thienopyridines
(clopidogrel and ticlodipine) and (3) the glycoprotein (GP) IIb/IIIa inhibitors (abciximab, eptifibatide and tirofiban). These agents differ in
mechanism of action, time to therapeutic efficacy,
potency and cost.

Aspirin

Platelet activity is increased in the setting of ACS,
and represents one of the core components of
thrombus formation. Aspirin irreversibly inhibits
the enzyme cyclo-oxygenase (COX) that produces
thromboxane A_2, a potent vasoconstrictor, and
stimulates platelet aggregation. After cessation
of aspirin, restoration of platelet function takes
around 7 days, as new platelets are released into
the circulation.

Evidence for aspirin use in ACS
Aspirin has been an accepted therapy in ACS,
since it was shown to reduce mortality and recurrent ischaemic events (The ISIS-2 Collaborative
Group 1988; Antiplatelet Trialists' Collaboration
1994). It has been shown to be beneficial in preventing rebound ischaemia following heparin cessation for patients with UAP (Theroux et al. 1988,
1992; Wallentin et al. 1991) and in long-term reduction of recurrent ischaemia (Wallentin et al. 1991).

Aspirin forms part of the early management of
all patients with suspected ACS, and in the absence
of contraindications should be given as soon as
is practicable. Given that higher doses of aspirin
are associated with an increased incidence of gastrointestinal side effects, an initial dose between
162 and 325 mg is recommended, followed by a
daily dose between 75 and 162 mg (Antithrombotic
Trialists' Collaboration 2002). For the initial aspirin
dose, there is evidence to suggest that the aspirin
is absorbed more quickly if chewed (particularly
following opiate therapy), and more rapid buc-
cal absorption takes place with non-enteric coated
preparations (Sagar & Smyth 1999).

Clopidogrel

Clopidogrel belongs to a class of drug known as
the thienopyridines. Clopidogrel blocks the ADP
receptor P2Y12 on platelet cell membranes. The
anti-aggregatory effects of clopidogrel take several

days to achieve maximal effect in the absence of a
loading dose (AHA/ACC 2007).

Evidence for clopidogrel use in ACS
Clopidogrel has demonstrated efficacy in addition
to aspirin versus aspirin alone in ACS (Yusuf et al.
2001) and is recommended for all patients after
stent implantation (Peters et al. 2003). In the acute
setting, a loading dose of clopidogrel is typically
used to achieve rapid platelet inhibition. Some
small to moderate size studies have demonstrated
benefits with a 600 mg loading dose of clopidogrel
rather than the traditional 300 mg dose, but larger
studies are required to establish the optimal dose
(AHA/ACC 2007). Optimal timing for loading
with clopidogrel in the setting of percutaneous
intervention (PCI) has not been established. There
is an association between onset of therapeutic benefit of clopidogrel and time of administration prior
to PCI (Mehta et al. 2001), but clopidogrel loading increases the risk of bleeding should coronary
artery bypass grafting (CABG) be necessary.

Evidence suggests that clopidogrel is at least
as effective as aspirin alone in secondary prevention (CAPRIE Investigators 2002), but the benefit
of clopidogrel over aspirin is probably not enough
to justify the cost of routine clopidogrel use for
this purpose alone. Clopidogrel is however a useful alternative antiplatelet therapy for individuals
who cannot tolerate aspirin.

Clopidogrel should in general be used with
aspirin in patients with STEMI, whether they receive
fibrinolysis or PTCA, or no reperfusion therapy.
Clopidogrel should continue for at least 28 days
(AHA/ACC 2007) following fibrinolytic reperfusion,
and for 12 months PTCA and stent implantation
(Aroney et al. 2006). There appears to be an increased
risk of moderate bleeding in long-term use of clopidogrel and aspirin combinations (Bhatt et al. 2007),
and thus the risk-benefit profile must be assessed in
individual patients. It is now accepted that long-term
($\geq$1 year) clopidogrel is indicated after implantation
of drug-eluting stents to reduce the risk of late-stent
thrombosis.

Prasugrel, a new generation thienopyridine,
appears to have more rapid, potent and consistent
inhibition of platelet function than the approved
300 mg clopidogrel loading dose when administered to healthy individuals. The TRITON-
TIMI 38 study (Wiviott et al. 2007) suggests some

advantages of prasugrel over clopidogrel with ACS undergoing PCI, but at the risk of a higher incidence of major bleeding. The loading dose of clopidogrel was probably suboptimal in this study (300 mg rather than 600 mg) and the results should be interpreted with this in mind.

Considerations in the nursing management of patients with antiplatelet therapy are shown in Table 22.2.

Anticoagulants

A variety of anticoagulants are available for the management of ACS. Evidence to support the use of a clearly superior agent is lacking due to differences in clinical study designs and study populations (AHA/ACC 2007), and thus anticoagulation regimes vary between institutions.

Heparin is used to prevent thrombosis or extension of an existing thrombus. Heparin is commonly available in two forms: (1) unfractionated heparin (UFH) and (2) low-molecular-weight heparin (LMWH).

Unfractionated heparin

UFH exerts its effects through potentiation of antithrombin III, resulting in indirect thrombin inhibition (Brouwer et al. 2004). It prevents coagulation by interfering with the formation of thrombin from prothrombin, and preventing thrombin from supporting the conversion of fibrinogen to fibrin. The disadvantages of UFH are that it binds to a number of plasma proteins, has a variable anticoagulant response which requires frequent monitoring of the activated partial thromboplastin time (aPPT) and it is associated with heparin-induced thrombocytopaenia in 1–3% of patients (Oler et al. 1996). An advantage of UFH is that it is easier to control anticoagulation in the case of planned percutaneous/surgical interventions compared to LMWH.

Evidence for UHF use in ACS

UHF has been in use since the pre-thrombolytic era where it was proven to improve resolution of symptoms in patients with UAP, but the magnitude of benefit has not been re-evaluated since it came into standard use with thrombolytics and

aspirin (Brouwer et al. 2004). Newer fibrinolytic preparations have not been tested without concurrent heparin, based upon the observation of clustering of re-infarctions without 10 h of heparin cessation (Granger et al. 1996).

Intravenous UFH has been shown to limit progression of UAP to AMI in the short term (Theroux et al. 1993), but in the absence of concurrent aspirin therapy, this benefit is potentially lost on cessation of the heparin infusion with ischaemia reactivation (Theroux et al. 1992; Tano & Mazzu 1995; Stewart & Voss 1997). A combined short-term therapy of aspirin and UHF has been shown to be superior to aspirin or UHF alone in preventing ischaemic events (Theroux et al. 1988; The RISC Study Group 1990; Oler et al. 1996), although there is probably an increased risk of bleeding complications with this option (Theroux et al. 1988). A meta-analysis of six randomised short-term trials involving 1353 patients to assess the value of combined UHF and aspirin therapy for UAP showed a 33% lower incidence of death and AMI in the patients receiving a combination of UHF and aspirin, when compared to aspirin alone (Oler et al. 1996), but only four of these studies reported results to 12 weeks when much of the trend in benefit was attenuated. Current practice guidelines support the combined use of aspirin and UHF in UAP (Yeghiazarians et al. 2000), but the variability of the dose–response curve for UFH limits its efficacy in some situations. There is a wide variation in antithrombotic response between patients, and it is necessary to reach target activated partial prothrombin times (aPPTs) and maintain therapeutic levels via IV infusion.

Low-molecular-weight heparins

LMWHs exert their effect primarily through inhibition of factor Xa and less by inhibition of thrombin activity (Brouwer et al. 2004). In comparison to UFH, LMWH is less likely to be inhibited by platelet factor VI and does not readily bind to plasma proteins and macrophages, which leads to a more predictable antithrombotic dose–response relationship, with a half-life of 4 hours. However, LMWH preparations do vary somewhat in their pharmacological effects (Antman & Handin, 1998), including rates of clearance, amount of non-specific binding and effects on von Willebrand factor (Montalescot et al. 1998). Ease of administration is an advantage of LMWH over UFH: LMWH can be given by subcutaneous (SC) injection. LMWH has greater bioavailability than UFH and therefore does not require constant monitoring of aPPTs and subsequent dosage titration (Fox & Antman 1998). It has a reduced rate of heparin-induced thrombocytopaenia when compared with UFH (Chong 1995) but has a higher incidence of minor bleeding (Ibbotson & Goa 2002).

Evidence for use of LMWH in ACS

A number of large-scale clinical trials have compared various preparations of LMWH with UFH in the treatment of ACS (The Fragmin During Instability in Coronary Artery Disease [FRISC] Study Group 1996; Cohen et al. 1997; Klein et al. 1997; Antman et al. 1999; Fraxiparine in Ischaemic Syndrome [FRAX.I.S.] 1999; Wallentin et al. 2001; Simoons et al. 2002; Sabatine et al. 2005). LMWH has demonstrated some therapeutic advantage over UFH which is probably related to a higher and more consistent bioavailability of LMWH leading to a more predictable anticoagulation effect without the need for laboratory monitoring (Sabatine et al. 2005). LMWH is associated with a higher rate of minor bleeding compared to UFH, but stimulates platelets less and is less likely to be associated with HIT. Enoxaparine can be used safely in ACS at a dose of 0.75 mg/kg in patients without renal impairment (Aroney et al. 2006). Where imminent PCI or CABG surgery is planned, it is reasonable to use UFH instead.

Nursing considerations in the management of patients with anticoagulant therapy are shown in Table 22.3.

Platelet GP IIb/IIIa receptor antagonists

Platelets are key contributors to the process of coron1ary thrombosis. A number of factors may stimulate platelet aggregation, but the common mechanism is the activation of the GP IIb/IIIa receptor, the platelet membrane receptor for fibrinogen (Aroney et al. 2006). GP IIb/IIIa receptor antagonists are a class of drugs that prevent platelet aggregation by preventing fibrinogen binding. They facilitate thrombolysis and reduce the rate of re-occlusion of reperfused vessels (Del Bene & Vaughan 2005).

Platelet GP IIb/IIIa receptor antagonists: evidence for use in ACS

In the past few years, a number of recent trials have evaluated the efficacy of mainly IV, and to a lesser extent, oral preparations of GPIIb/IIIa agents based on the hypothesis that interruption of this pathway of platelet aggregation with agents which block the platelet GP IIb/IIIa receptor would improve outcomes for individuals with ACS or undergoing coronary interventional procedures. Interpretation of clinical efficacy of GP IIb/IIIa inhibitor studies is made difficult because of differences between agents, but specifically differences in potential risk–benefit ratio of the various patient groups studied. Four IV GPIIb/IIIa receptor blockers have been studied extensively in ACS: abciximab (Reopro), eptifibatide, tirofiban and lamifiban (Brouwer et al. 2004). The EPIC (EPIC Investigators 1994), EPILOG (EPILOG Investigators 1997), EPISTENT (The EPISTENT Investigators 1998) and ESPRIT (The ESPRIT Investigators 2000) trials have demonstrated that compared with placebo, GPIIb/IIIa inhibitors given just prior to PCI reduce death, MI and target vessel revascularisation within 30 days of procedure. However, it should be noted that these studies were undertaken prior to routine use of clopidogrel, generally with PTCA alone, and if stents were used they were first-generation devices (Yehudai & Feit 2006).

The CAPTURE (The CAPTURE Investigators 1997), PRISM-PLUS (The PRISM-PLUS Study Investigators 1998) and PURSUIT (The PURSUIT trial investigators 1998) trials each showed a reduction in the rate of death or MI during medical management with an augmented benefit following PCI (AHA/ACC 2007).

Evidence supports the benefit of GPIIb/IIIa inhibitors in patients with unstable angina and non-ST segment elevation MI, who undergo PCI. This class of drugs is of modest benefit in patients who are not routinely scheduled to undergo PCI, and there is no strong evidence to support the use of GPIIb/IIIa inhibitors in patients who do not undergo revascularisation (AHA/ACC 2007). Further studies are required to explore the role of GPIIb/IIIa inhibitors with 'upstream' (given prior to angiography) clopidogrel.

Considerations in the nursing management of patients in whom GPIIb/IIIa inhibitors are used are shown in Table 22.4.

Table 22.3 Anticoagulant therapies: considerations in nursing management.

Unfractionated heparin	Low-molecular-weight heparin
Heparin should be used with caution in people with bleeding disorders; thrombocytopaenia; history of PUD; recent brain, spine or eye surgery and any other planned surgery that increases the potential of serious bleeding; severe hypertension; stroke; and those taking warfarin and NSAIDS. Heparin is contraindicated in patients with severe thrombocytopaenia and other bleeding disorders. It should not be used in uncontrollable active bleeding states (except when this is due to disseminated intravascular coagulation).	Many of the contraindications, cautions and nursing management issues for LMWH are similar to those for UFH.
Haemorrhage is the main potential complication of heparin therapy. GI or urinary-tract bleeding during anticoagulant therapy may indicate the presence of an underlying occult lesion. Haemorrhage can occur virtually at any site in patients receiving heparin. Adrenal, ovarian and retroperitoneal are rare sites of bleeding which are difficult to detect but can have serious consequences. An unexplained fall in haematocrit, fall in blood pressure or any other unexplained symptom should lead to serious consideration of a haemorrhagic event. Observe for excessive bruising or abnormal bleeding. Keep venous and arterial punctures to a minimum. Avoid excessive inflations of automated blood pressure cuffs.	LMWH is administered via SC injection. Injections should be given around the navel, upper thigh or buttock, and the injection site should be changed daily. Injection directly into vein or muscle should be avoided.
A serious side effect of heparin is heparin-induced thrombocytopaenia (HIT syndrome). HIT is caused by an immunological reaction that makes platelets form clots within the blood vessels, thereby using up coagulation factors. Formation of platelet clots can lead to thrombosis, while the loss of coagulation factors and platelets may result in bleeding. HIT can (rarely) occur shortly after heparin is given, but also when a person has been on heparin for a long while. Immunologic tests are available for the diagnosis of HIT.	Local irritation, bruising and pain at the site of injection are fairly common.
An overly prolonged clotting time or minor bleeding during therapy can usually be controlled by withdrawing the drug. The anticoagulant effect of UFH can be neutralised rapidly by IV protamine in a ratio of approximately 100 U UFH/mg of protamine (Hirsh et al. 2001). Protamine is not without potential adverse reactions and the risk of these should be assessed prior to administration.	The dose of LMWH may need to be reduced for those with renal or hepatic disease and adjusted for obese patients.
UFH can be administered via continuous IV or SC injection. An immediate anticoagulant effect requires an IV bolus, and thus in ACS an IV bolus dose followed by IV infusion is preferred. UFH needs to be maintained at a therapeutic level in the bloodstream and the therapeutic target needs to be reached as quickly as possible in ACS. This is achieved by maintaining aPPTs at 1.5–2.0 times the normal value. Baseline aPPT should be obtained before commencing UFH, and 6 h after therapy is started, 4–6 hourly until therapeutic target is reached, any time after a change of dose or following alterations/interruptions to infusion, then 24 hourly. To avoid variability in dosing decisions, weight-based heparin dose-adjustment nomograms should be used. In many institutions, nurses undertake the role of monitoring and adjusting heparin infusions according to nomograms. In addition to frequent monitoring of aPPT, haemoglobin, haematocrit and platelets should be monitored, and the patient should be observed for excessive bruising, bleeding or thrombocytopaenia.	LMWH may need to be changed over to UFH for individuals with planned invasive procedures that have a risk of significant bleeding.
Some patients require higher-than-average dose of heparin to prolong aPPT to the therapeutic range. Those who require more than 35,000 U in 24 h to reach therapeutic levels are known as 'heparin resistant' (Hirsh et al. 2001). Increased resistance to heparin is frequently encountered in fever, thrombosis, thrombophlebitis, infections with thrombosing tendencies, MI, cancer, and in post-surgical patients, and patients with antithrombin III deficiency (Drugs.com 2008).	Protamine sulphate should be available for reversal of heparin in the event it may be required.
Heparin should be discontinued with caution, preferably after aspirin has been commenced, to prevent episodes of rebound ischaemia. When an oral anticoagulant of the coumarin or similar type is to be begun in patients already receiving heparin sodium, baseline and subsequent tests of prothrombin activity must be determined at a time when heparin activity is too low to affect the prothrombin time. This is about 5 h after the last IV bolus and 24 h after the last SC dose.	Haemaglobin, haematocrit and platelets should be monitored and the patient should be observed for excessive bruising, bleeding or thrombocytopaenia.

For further information, visit Drugs.com at http://www.drugs.com/pro/heparin.html

Table 22.4   Platelet GP IIb/IIIa inhibitors: considerations in nursing management.

GPIIb/IIIa inhibitors are contraindicated in any conditions that involve active internal bleeding, including GI bleeds within the last 6 weeks. GPIIb/IIIa inhibitors should be avoided in people who have had an intracranial haemorrhage, intracranial neoplasms or uncontrolled hypertension within the last 2 years. There is an increased risk of bleeding at vascular access sites and a risk of thrombocytopaenia. GPIIb/IIIa inhibitors also increase the risk of stroke and may cause hypersensitivity reactions.

Vascular access sites should be monitored carefully for occurrence of bleeding. Signs of retroperitoneal bleed (back pain, groin discomfort, lower abdominal tenderness ipsilateral to the puncture site, femoral neuropathy and hypotension) should be promptly investigated.

Minimise arterial or venous punctures, intramuscular injections and inflation of automated blood pressure cuffs. Urinary catheterisation, intubation, nasogastric insertion and any other invasive procedures can trigger bleeding.

GPIIb/IIIa inhibitors should be used with aspirin and heparin for patients with ACS undergoing PCI, but the risk of bleeding is increased.

Haemaglobin, haematocrit and platelets should be monitored daily during therapy.

Inhibitors of the renin-angiotensin-aldosterone system

Angiotensin-converting enzyme inhibitors

Angiotensin-converting enzyme (ACE) inhibitors block the conversion of angiotensin I (a weak vasoconstrictor) to angiotensin II (a potent vasoconstrictor), and also prevents the enzymatic inactivation of bradykinin (a vasodilator). Their vasodilating effect helps to reduce afterload, thereby reducing the workload of the heart. They appear to inhibit inflammatory responses mediated by angiotensin II, which are central to the development of myocardial fibrosis. They play a part in ventricular remodelling and reducing the risk of congestive cardiac failure following MI (Del Bene & Vaughan 2005).

ACE inhibitors: evidence for use in ACS

There have been a number of large randomised clinical trials that have assessed the role of ACE inhibitors in early AMI, all of which demonstrated a mortality benefit (GISSI Investigators 1994; ISIS-4 Collaborative Group 1995; Chinese Cardiac Study Collaborative Group 1995). The HOPE (Yusuf et al. 2000) and EUROPA (Fox 2003) studies showed benefits of ACE inhibition in high-risk patients (those with diabetes or established vascular disease). The results of these studies seem to have been extrapolated to most patients with

atherosclerosis, diabetes mellitus, left ventricular systolic dysfunction (LVSD) or heart failure in the absence of solid evidence from placebo-controlled trials of patients with non-ST-elevation ACS (Gluckman et al. 2005). Use of ACE inhibitors in low-risk patients is not supported by evidence from the PEACE study (Braunwald et al. 2004).

ACE inhibitor use in AMI has been shown to reduce post-infarction mortality rates and reduce risk of re-infarction. The maximum benefit is demonstrated in high-risk patients, but there are short-term gains when administered to all haemodynamically stable patients in the setting of AMI.

ACE inhibitors: considerations in nursing management

Ace inhibitors should be used with extreme caution in patients with hypotension due to the marked vasodilatory effects, particularly in the setting of dehydration. Concomitant diuretic doses may need to be reduced in the first 48–72 h of initiating ACE-inhibitor therapy to avoid hypotension. Prior to commencing therapy, blood pressure should be assessed and monitored thereafter.

ACE inhibitors may not be suitable for patients with renal impairment/insufficiency and are contraindicated in patients with renal artery stenosis. Serum creatinine levels should be checked prior to initiation of therapy with ACE inhibitors and monitored thereafter (Del Bene & Vaughan 2005).

Angiotensin receptor blockers

Angiotensin II causes vasoconstriction, sodium and water retention, and activation of the sympathetic nervous system, thereby increasing blood pressure. Angiotensin receptor blockers (ARBs) prevent angiotensin II from binding to its receptor and thus inhibit the effects of angiotensin II. ACE inhibitors are often not tolerated due to their action in increasing bradykinin which causes a dry cough and angio-oedema. ARBs do not cause an increase in bradykinin and therefore are better tolerated, although it has been suggested they are not as effective in reducing blood pressure. Although ACE inhibitors appear to have clinical advantages over ARBs, ARBs are useful in post-MI and ischaemic heart failure patients who are intolerant of ACE inhibitors (Pfeffer et al. 2002, 2003). ARBs should not be administered to patients with bilateral renal artery stenosis, as it may precipitate renal failure.

Aldosterone receptor blockers

Recent studies have shown that ACE inhibitors and ARBs do not continue to effectively suppress aldosterone with chronic use (McKelvie et al. 1999). In addition to angiotensin II, other factors such as potassium, endothelin and various neurotransmitters stimulate aldosterone secretion (Coleman et al. 2002).

Spironalactone, an aldosterone receptor blocker, has been shown to decrease morbidity and death in patients with severe heart failure, including heart failure with an ischaemic cause (Pitt et al. 1999). Eplerenone, a selective aldosterone receptor blocker, has been shown to reduce morbidity and mortality when used in patients with MI complicated by LV dysfunction and either heart failure or diabetes, has been shown to reduce morbidity and mortality (Pitt et al. 2003) but has a lower binding affinity for androgenic and progestogenic receptors than spironolactone, and thus produces fewer endocrine-related adverse effects (gynaecomastia, breast tenderness and menstrual irregularities).

Statins

Statins (3-hydroxy-3-methylglutaryl coenzyme A [HMG-CoA] reductase inhibitors) have a well-

established role in secondary prevention for atherosclerotic cardiovascular disease. Recent evidence suggests that early, intensive therapy with statins has benefits including a reduction in cardiovascular death, unstable angina and revascularisation after 4 months of therapy when prescribed within 14 days of hospitalisation for ACS (Hulten et al. 2006). There is some evidence to suggest that therapy with statins may cause regression of lipid-rich lesions that are prone to rupture (Brown et al. 1993) and/or that statin therapy modulates atherosclerosis through mechanisms independent of anatomic regression (Vaughan et al. 1996). Therapy with a statin has also been associated with improvement in coronary vasomotor function (Egashira et al. 1994), decreased vasospasm (O'Driscoll 1997), reductions in platelet reactivity (Mayer et al. 1992; Lacoste et al. 1995; Notarbartolo et al. 1995) with associated improvements in myocardial perfusion (Gould et al. 1994; Eichstadt et al. 1995) and reduction in myocardial ischaemia. Statins therapy should be established during the acute admission for ACS.

Conclusion

A variety of pharmacotherapies are available for the management of ACS. Ensuring that the patient gets the best treatment available entails careful consideration of current clinical guidelines and an ability to tailor therapy to suit individual patient requirements. Education of staff and patients is an essential component in successful pharmacological management of cardiac conditions.

References

Abrams, J. (1996). Beneficial actions of nitrates in cardiovascular disease. *American Journal of Cardiology*, **77**:31C–7C.
ACC/AHA 2007 Guidelines for the management of patients with unstable Angina/Non-ST-elevation myocardial infarction: a report of the American College of Cardiology/American Heart Association Task Force on Practice Guidelines (Writing Committee to revise the 2002 Guidelines for the management of patients with unstable angina/non-ST-elevation myocardial infarction): developed in collaboration with the American College of Emergency Physicians,

the Society for Cardiovascular Angiography and Interventions, and the Society of Thoracic Surgeons: endorsed by the American Association of Cardiovascular and Pulmonary Rehabilitation and the Society for Academic Emergency Medicine (2007). *Circulation*, **116**:e148–304.

Antiplatelet Trialists' Collaboration (1994). Collaborative overview of randomised controlled trials of antiplatelet therapy – I: Prevention of death, myocardial infarction, and stroke by prolonged antiplatelet therapy in various categories of patients. *British Medical Journal*, **308**:81–106.

Antithrombotic Trialists' Collaboration (2002). Collaborative meta-analysis of randomised trials of antiplatelet therapy for prevention of death, myocardial infarction, and stroke in high risk patients. *British Medical Journal*, **324**:71–86.

Antman, E.M. & Handin, R. (1998). Low-molecular weight heparins. An intriguing new twist with profound implications. *Circulation*, **98**:294–9.

Antman, E.M., McCabe, C.H., Gurfinkel, E.P., et al. for the TIMI 11B Investigators (1999). Enoxaparin prevents death and cardiac ischemic events in unstable angina/non-Q-wave myocardial infarction: results of the thrombolysis in myocardial infarction (TIMI) 11B Trial. *Circulation*, **100**:1593–601.

Antman, E.M., Anbe, D.T., Armstrong, P.W., et al. (2004). ACC/AHA guidelines for the management of patients with ST-elevation myocardial infarction– executive summary: a report of the American College of Cardiology/American Heart Association Task Force on Practice Guidelines (writing committee to revise the 1999 guidelines for the management of patients with acute myocardial infarction). *Circulation*, **110**:588–636.

Aroney, C., Aylward, P., Allan, R.M., et al. (2006). Guidelines for the management of acute coronary syndromes 2006. *Medical Journal of Australia*, **184**:S1–32.

Bhatt, D.L., Flather, M.D., Hacke, W., et al. (2007). Patients with prior myocardial infarction, stroke, or symptomatic peripheral arterial disease in the CHARISMA trial. *Journal of the American College of Cardiology*, **49**:1982–8.

Braunwald, E., Domanski, M.J., Fowler, S.E., et al. (2004). Angiotensin-converting-enzyme inhibition in stable coronary artery disease. *New England Journal of Medicine*, **351**:2058–68.

Brouwer, M.A., Clappers, N. & Verheught, F.W.A. (2004). Adjunctive treatment in patients treated with thrombolytic therapy. *Heart*, **90**:581–8.

Brown, B.G., Zhao, X.Q., Sacco, D.E. & Albers, J.J. (1993). Lipid-lowering and plaque regression: new insights into prevention of plaque disruption and clinical events in coronary disease. *Circulation*, **87**:1781–91.

Cannon, C.P. on behalf of the CAPRIE Investigators (2002). Effectiveness of Clopidogrel Versus Aspirin in preventing acute myocardial infarction in patients with symptomatic atherothrombosis (CAPRIE Trial). *American Journal of Cardiology*, **90**:760–2.

Chen, Z.M., Pan, H.C., Chen, Y.P., et al. (2005). Early intravenous then oral metoprolol in 45 852 patients with acute myocardial infarction: randomised placebo-controlled trial. *The Lancet*, **366**:1622–32.

Chinese Cardiac Study Collaborative Group (1995). Oral captopril versus placebo among 13 634 patients with suspected acute myocardial infarction: interim report from the Chinese Cardiac Study (CCS-1). *The Lancet*, **345**:686–7.

Chirkov, Y., Chirkova, L. & Horowitz, J. (1992). Reversal of human platelet aggregation by low concentrations of nitroglycerin in vitro in normal subjects. *American Journal of Cardiology*, **70**:802–6.

Chirkov, Y., Naujalis, J., Sage, R & Horowitz, J. (1993). Antiplatelet effects of nitroglycerin in healthy subjects and in patients with unstable angina pectoris. *Journal of Cardiovascular Pharmacology*, **21**:384–9.

Chong, B.H. (1995). Heparin induced thrombocytopenia. *British Journal of Haematology*, **89**:431–9.

Cohen, M., Demers, C., Gurfinkel, E.P., et al. (1997). A comparison of low-molecular-weight heparin with unfractionated heparin for unstable coronary artery disease. Efficacy and safety of subcutaneous enoxaparin in non-Q-wave coronary events study group. *New England Journal of Medicine*, **337**:447–52.

Coleman, C.I., Reddy, P., Song, J.C. & White, M. (2002). Eplerenone: the first selective aldosterone receptor antagonist for the treatment of hypertension. *Formulary*, **37**:514–24.

Comparison of two treatment durations (6 days and 14 days) of a low molecular weight heparin with a 6-day treatment of unfractionated heparin in the initial management of unstable angina or non-Q-wave myocardial infarction: FRAX.I.S. (FRAxiparine in Ischaemic Syndrome) (1999). *European Heart Journal*, **20**:1553–62.

Conti, C.R., Feldman., R.L., Pepine, C.J., et al. (1985). Effect of glyceryl trinitrate on coronary and systemic hemodynamics in man. *American Journal of Medicine*, **74**:28–32.

Del Bene, S. & Vaughan, A. (2005). Acute coronary syndromes. In: S.L. Woods, E.S.S. Froelicher, S.U. Motzer & E.J. Bridges (eds), *Cardiac Nursing*, 5th edn. Lippincott Williams and Wilkins, Philadelphia, pp. 572–5.

Egashira, K., Hirooka, Y., Kai, H., et al. (1994). Reduction in serum cholesterol with pravastatin improves endothelium-dependent coronary vasomotion in patients with hypercholesterolemia. *Circulation*, **89**:2519–24.

Eichstadt, H.W., Eskotter, H., Hoffman, I., et al. (1995). Improvement of myocardial perfusion by short-term fluvastatin therapy in coronary artery disease. *American Journal of Cardiology*, **76**:122–5A.

Fox, K.M. (2003). Efficacy of perindopril in reduction of cardiovascular events among patients with stable coronary artery disease: randomised, double-blind, placebocontrolled, multicentre trial (the EUROPA study). *The Lancet*, **362**:782–8.

Fox, K. & Antman, E. (1998). Treatment options in unstable angina: a clinical update. *European Heart Journal*, **19**(Suppl.):K8–10.

Furberg, C.D., Psaty, B.M. & Meyer, J.V. (1995). Nifedipine: Dose-related increase in mortality in patients with coronary heart disease. *Circulation*, **92**:1326–31.

Gardner, P. & Altman, G. (2005). Pathophysiology of acute coronary syndromes. In: S.L. Woods, E.S.S. Froelicher, S.U. Motzer & E.J. Bridges (eds), *Cardiac Nursing*, 5th edn. Lippincott Williams and Wilkins, Philadelphia.

Gibson, R.S., Boden, W.E., Theroux, P., et al. (1986). Diltiazem and reinfarction in patients with non-Q-wave myocardial infarction. Results of a double-blind, randomized, multicenter trial. *New England Journal of Medicine*, **315**:423–9.

Gluckman, T.J., Sachdev, M., Schulman, S.P. & Blumenthal, R.S. (2005). A simplified approach to the management of non-ST-segment elevation acute coronary syndromes. *The Journal of the American Medical Association*, **293**:349–57.

Gould, K.L., Martucci, J.P., Goldberg, D.I., et al. (1994). Short-term cholesterol lowering decreases size and severity of perfusion abnormalities by positron emission tomography after dipyridamole in patients with coronary artery disease. *Circulation*, **89**:1530–8.

Granger, C.B., Hirsch, J., Califf, R.M., et al. (1996). Activated partial thromboplastin time and outcome after thrombolytic therapy for acute myocardial infarction: results from the GUSTO trial. *Circulation*, **93**:870–88.

Gruppo Italiano per lo Studio della Sopravvivenza nell'Infarto myocardico (GISSI) 3. (1994). GISSI-3: effect of lisinopril and transdermal glyceryl trinitrate singly and together on 6 week mortality and ventricular function after acute myocardial infarction. *The Lancet*, **343**:1115–22.

Hansen, M., Fischer, J., Hagerup, M., et al. (1997). Cardiac event rates after acute myocardial infarction in patients treated with verapamil and trandolapril versus trandolapril alone. *The American Journal of Cardiology*, **79**:738–41.

Hirsh, J., Warkentin, T.E., Shaughnessy, S.G., et al. (2001). Heparin and low-molecular-weight heparin mechanisms of action, pharmacokinetics, dosing, monitoring, efficacy, and safety. *Chest*, **119**:64S–94.

Hjalmarson, A. (1997). Effects of beta blockade on sudden cardiac death during acute myocardial infarction and the postinfarction period. *American Journal of Cardiology*, **80**:35J–9.

Holland Interuniversity Nifedipine (Metoprolol) Trial (HINT) Research Group (1986). Early treatment of unstable angina in the coronary care unit: a randomized, double blind, placebo controlled comparison of recurrent ischaemia in patients treated with nifedipine or metoprolol or both. *British Heart Journal*, **56**:400–13.

Horowitz, J., Elliott, M., Antman, E., et al. (1983). Potentiation of the cardiovascular effects of nitroglycerin by *N*-acetylcysteine. *Circulation*, **68**:1247–53.

Horowitz, J.D., Henry, C.A., Syrjanen, M.L., et al. (1988). Combined use of nitroglycerin and *N*-acetylcysteine in the management of unstable angina pectoris. *Circulation*, **77**:787–94.

Hulten, E., Jackson, J.L., Douglas, K., George, S. & Villines, T.C. (2006). The effect of early, intensive statin therapy on acute coronary syndrome. *Archives of Internal Medicine*, **166**:1814–21.

Ibbotson, T. & Goa, K.L. (2002). Enoxaparin: an update of its clinical use in the management of acute coronary syndromes. *Drugs*, **62**:1407–30.

ISIS-2 (Second International Study of Infarct Survival) Collaborative Group. (1988). Randomised trial of intravenous streptokinase, oral aspirin, both, or neither among 1787 cases of suspected acute myocardial infarction: ISIS-2. *The Lancet*, **ii**:349–60.

ISIS-4 (Fourth International Study of Infarct Survival) Collaborative Group (1995). ISIS-4: a randomised factorial trial assessing early oral captopril, oral mononitrate, and intravenous magnesium sulphate in 58,050 patients with suspected acute myocardial infarction, *The Lancet*, **345**:669–85.

Jugdutt, B.I. & Warnica, J.J. (1988). Intravenous nitroglycerin therapy to limit infarct size, expansion and complications. *Circulation*, **78**:906–19.

Kelly, J.P., Kaufman, D.W. & Jurgelon, J.M. (1996). Risk of aspirin-associated major upper-gastrointestinal bleeding with enteric-coated or buffered product. *The Lancet*, **348**:1413–6.

Klabunde, R.E. (2005). Cardiovascular Physiology Concepts. Lippincott, Williams and Wilkins, Philadelphia.

Klabunde, R.E. (2007). Beta-Adrenoceptor Antagonists (Beta-Blockers). Retrieved online 24th May 2008 from http://cvpharmacology.com/cardioinhibitory/beta-blockers.htm

Klein, W., Buchwald, A., Hillis, S.E., et al. (1997). Comparison of low molecular-weight heparin with unfractionated heparin acutely and with placebo for 6 weeks in the management of unstable coronary artery disease. Fragmin in unstable coronary artery disease study (FRIC). Circulation, 96:61–8.

Lacoste, L., Lam, J.Y.T., Hung, J., et al. (1995). Hyperlipidaemia and coronary disease: correction of the increased thrombogenic potential with cholesterol reduction. Circulation, 92:3172–7.

Lopez-Sendo, J., Swedberg, K., McMurray, J., et al. (2004). Expert consensus document on {beta}-adrenergic receptor blockers: the task force on beta-blockers of the European Society of Cardiology. European Heart Journal, 25:1341–62.

Loscalzo, J. (1985). N-acetylcysteine potentiates inhibition of platelet aggregation by nitroglycerin. Journal of Clinical Investigations, 76:703–8.

Low-molecular-weight heparin during instability in coronary artery disease, fragmin during instability in coronary artery disease (FRISC) study group (1996). The Lancet, 347:561–8.

Mayer, J., Eller, T., Brauer, P., et al. (1992). Effects of long-term treatment with lovastatin on the clotting system and blood platelets. Annals of Hematology, 64:196–201.

McKelvie, R.S., Yusuf, S., Pericak, D., et al. (1999). Comparison of candasartan, enalapril, and their combination in congestive heart failure. Randomized evaluation of the strategies for left ventricular dysfunction (RESOLVD) pilot study. Circulation, 100:1056–64.

Mehta, S.R., Yusuf, S., Peters, R.J., et al. (2001). Clopidogrel in unstable angina to prevent recurrent events trial (CURE) investigators. Effects of pretreatment with clopidogrel and aspirin followed by long-term therapy in patients undergoing percutaneous coronary intervention: the PCI-CURE study. The Lancet, 358:527–33.

Montalescot, G., Phillipe, F., Ankri, A., et al. (1998). Early increase of von Willebrand factor predicts adverse outcomes in unstable coronary disease. Beneficial effects of enoxaparin. French Investigators of the ESSENCE Trial. Circulation, 98:294–9.

Notarbartolo, A., Davi, G., Averna, M., et al. (1995). Inhibition of thromboxane biosynthesis and platelet

function by simvastatin in type IIa hypercholesterolemia. Arteriosclerosis Thrombosis and Vascular Biology, 15:247–51.

O'Driscoll, G., Green, D. & Taylor, R.R. (1997). Simvastatin, an HMG-coenzyme A reductase inhibitor, improves endothelial function within 1 month. Circulation, 95:1126–31.

Oler, A., Whooley, M.A., Oler, J. & Grady, D. (1996). Adding heparin to aspirin reduces the incidence of myocardial infarction and death in patients with unstable angina. A meta-analysis. Journal of the American Medical Association, 276:811–15.

Packer, M., Lee, W.H., Kessler, P.D., et al. (1987). Prevention and reversal of nitrate tolerance in patients with congestive heart failure. New England Journal of Medicine, 317:799–804.

Peters, R.J.G., Mehta, S.R., Fox, K.A.A., et al. (2003). Effects of aspirin dose when used alone or in combination with clopidogrel in patients with acute coronary syndromes: observations from the clopidogrel in unstable angina to prevent recurrent events (CURE) study. Circulation, 108:1682–7.

Pfeffer, M.A., McMurray, J.J., Velazquez, E.J., et al. (2002). Valsartan, captopril, or both in myocardial infarction complicated by heart failure, left ventricular dysfunction, or both. New England Journal of Medicine, 349:1893–906.

Pfeffer, M.A., Swedberg, K., Granger, C.B., et al. (2003). Effects of candesartan on mortality and morbidity in patients with chronic heart failure: the CHARM-overall programme. The Lancet, 362:759–66.

Pitt, B., Zannad, F., Remme, W.J., et al. (1999). The effect of spironolactone on morbidity and mortality in patients with severe heart failure. Randomized aldactone evaluation study investigators. New England Journal of Medicine, 341:709–17.

Pitt, B., Remme, W., Zannad, F., et al. (2003). Eplerenone, a selective aldosterone blocker, in patients with left ventricular dysfunction after myocardial infarction. New England Journal of Medicine, 348:1309–21.

Sabatine, M.S., Morrow, D.A., Montalescot, G., et al. (2005). Angiographic and clinical outcomes in patients receiving low-molecular-weight heparin versus unfractionated heparin in ST-elevation myocardial infarction treated with fibrinolytics in the CLARITY-TIMI 28 Trial. Circulation, 112:3846–54.

Sagar, K.A. & Smyth, M.R. (1999). A comparative bioavailability study of different aspirin formulations using on-line multidimensional chromatography. Journal of Pharmaceutical and Biomedical Analysis, 21:383–92.

Sage, P.R., de la Lande, I.S., Stafford, I., et al. (2000). Nitroglycerin tolerance in human vessels: Evidence for impaired nitroglycerin bioconversion. *Circulation*, **102**:2810–15.

Simoons, M.L., Krzemińska-Pakula, M., Alonso, A., et al. (2002). Improved reperfusion and clinical outcome with enoxaparin as an adjunct to streptokinase thrombolysis in acute myocardial infarction. The AMI–SK study. *European Heart Journal*, **23**:1282–90.

Stewart, S. & Voss, D. (1997). A study of planned readmissions to a coronary care unit. *Heart Lung*, **26**:196–203.

Tano, G. & Mazzu, A. (1995). Early reactivation of ischaemia after abrupt discontinuation of heparin in acute myocardial infarction. *British Heart Journal*, **74**:131–3.

The CAPTURE investigators (1997). Randomised placebo-controlled trial of abciximab before and during coronary intervention in refractory unstable angina: the CAPTURE study. *The Lancet*, **349**:1429–35.

The EPIC Investigators (1994). Use of a monoclonal antibody directed against the platelet glycoprotein IIb/IIIa receptor in high-risk coronary angioplasty. *New England Journal of Medicine*, **330**:956–61.

The EPILOG Investigators (1997). Platelet glycoprotein IIb/IIIa receptor blockade and low-dose heparin during percutaneous coronary revascularization. *New England Journal of Medicine*, **336**:1689–96.

The EPISTENT Investigators (1998). Randomised placebo-controlled coronary stenting with use of platelet glycoprotein-IIb/IIIa blockade. *The Lancet*, **352**:87–92.

The ESPRIT Investigators (2000). Novel dosing regimen of eptifibatide in planned coronary stent implantation (ESPRIT): a randomized, placebo-controlled trial. *The Lancet*, **356**:2037–44.

The PRISM-PLUS Study Investigators (1998). Inhibition of the platelet glycoprotein IIb/IIIa receptor with tirofiban in unstable angina and non-Q wave myocardial infarction. *New England Journal of Medicine*, **338**:1488–97.

The PURSUIT trial investigators (1998). Inhibition of platelet glycoprotein IIb/IIIa with eptifibatide in patients with acute coronary syndromes. *New England Journal of Medicine*, **339**:436–43.

The RISC Study Group (1990). Risk of myocardial infarction and death during treatment with low dose aspirin and intravenous heparin in men with unstable coronary disease, *Lancet* **336**:827–30.

Theroux, P., Oimet, H., McCans, J., et al. (1988). Aspirin, heparin or both to treat unstable angina. *New England Journal Medicine*, **319**:1105–11.

Theroux, P., Waters, D. & Lam, J. (1992). Reactivation of unstable angina after discontinuation of heparin. *New England Journal Medicine*, **327**:1415.

Theroux, P., Waters, D., Qiu, S., et al. (1993). Aspirin versus heparin to prevent myocardial infarction during the acute phase of unstable angina. *Circulation*, **88**:2045–8.

Vaughan, C.J., Murphy, M.B. & Buckley, B.M. (1996). Statins do more than just lower cholesterol. *The Lancet*, **348**:1079–82.

Wallentin, L.C. for the Research Group on Instability in Coronary Artery Disease in Southeast Sweden (1991). Aspirin (75 mg/day) after an episode of unstable coronary artery disease: long-term effects on the risk for myocardial infarction, occurrence of severe angina and the need for revascularization. *Journal of the American College of Cardiology*, **18**:1587–93.

Wallentin, L., Dellborg, D.M., Lindahl, B., Nilsson T., Pehrsson, K. & Swahn E. (2001). The low-molecular-weight heparin dalteparin as adjuvant therapy in acute myocardial infarction: the ASSENT PLUS study. *Clinical Cardiology*, **24**(3 Suppl):I12–4.

Winniford, M., Kennedy, P., Wells, P. & Hillis, L. (1986). Potentiation of nitroglycerin induced coronary dilation with N-acetylcysteine. *Circulation*, **73**:138–42.

Wiviott, S.D., Braunwald, E., McCabe, C.H., et al. (2007). Prasugrel versus clopidogrel in patients with acute coronary syndromes. *The New England Journal of Medicine*, **357**:2001–15.

Yeghiazarians, Y., Braunstein, J.B., Askari, A., Stone, P.H. (2000). Unstable angina pectoris. *New England Journal of Medicine*, **342**;101–14.

Yehudai, L. & Feit F. (2006). Debate of adjunctive pharmacology for percutaneous coronary intervention: thrombin inhibitors and clopidogrel are enough. *Journal of Interventional Cardiology*, **19**:464–9.

Yusuf, S., Collins, R., MacMahon, S. & Peto, R. (1988). Effect of intravenous nitrates on mortality in acute myocardial infarction: an overview of the randomised trials. *The Lancet*, **I**:1088–92.

Yusuf, S., Sleight, P. & Pogue, J., for the Heart Outcomes Prevention Evaluation Study Investigators (2000). Effects of an angiotensin converting-enzyme inhibitor, ramipril, on cardiovascular events in high-risk patients. *New England Journal of Medicine*, **342**:145–53.

Yusuf, S., Zhao, F., Mehta, S.R. et al. for the Clopidogrel in Unstable Angina to Prevent Recurrent Events Trial Investigators (2001). Effects of clopidogrel in addition to aspirin in patients with acute coronary syndromes without ST-segment elevation. *New England Journal of Medicine*, **345**:494–502.

Useful Websites and Further Reading

ACC/AHA 2007 Guidelines for the management of patients with unstable Angina/Non-ST-elevation myocardial infarction: a report of the American College of Cardiology/American Heart Association Task Force on Practice Guidelines (Writing Committee to revise the 2002 Guidelines for the management of patients with unstable angina/non-ST-elevation myocardial infarction): developed in collaboration with the American College of Emergency Physicians, the Society for Cardiovascular Angiography and Interventions, and the Society of Thoracic Surgeons: endorsed by the American Association of Cardiovascular and Pulmonary Rehabilitation and the Society for Academic Emergency Medicine (2007). *Circulation*, **116**:e148–304.

ACE Inhibitor Myocardial Infarction Collaborative Group (1998). Indications for ACE inhibitors in the early treatment of acute myocardial infarction: systematic overview of individual data from 100 000 patients in randomized trials. *Circulation*, **97**: 2202–12.

Antman, E.M., Anbe, D.T., Armstrong, P.W., et al. (2004). ACC/AHA Guidelines for the management of patients with ST-elevation myocardial infarction–executive summary. A report of the American College of Cardiology/American Heart Association Task Force on Practice Guidelines (Writing Committee to revise the 1999 Guidelines for the management of patients with acute myocardial infarction). *Circulation*, **110**:588–636.

Antman, E.M., Hand, M., Armstrong, P.W., et al. (2008). 2007 focused update of the ACC/AHA 2004 Guidelines for the management of patients with ST-elevation myocardial infarction. A report of the American College of Cardiology/American Heart Association Task Force on Practice Guidelines: developed in collaboration with the Canadian Cardiovascular Society endorsed by the American Academy of Family Physicians: 2007 Writing Group to review new evidence and update the ACC/AHA 2004 Guidelines for the management of patients with ST-elevation myocardial infarction, writing on behalf of the 2004 Writing Committee. *Circulation*, **117**:296–329.

Aroney, C., Aylward, P., Allan, R.M., Boyden, A.N. & Brieger D. (2006). Guidelines for the management of acute coronary syndromes 2006. *Medical Journal of Australia*, **184**:S1–32.

23 Arrhythmias

C. Oldroyd & A.M. Kucia

Overview

Arrhythmia is a generalised term used to indicate disturbances in heart rhythm. The majority (estimated 90%) of coronary patients will experience some sort of arrhythmia, particularly in the period immediately following a myocardial infarction (MI) (Thompson & Webster 2004). As well as coronary heart disease (CHD), arrhythmias are also associated with congenital abnormalities and cardiomyopathies, and can be induced by non-cardiac factors such as electrolyte imbalance and drugs. The interpretation of cardiac arrhythmias plays an important role in the diagnosis of cardiac disorders (Hand 2002). In England, arrhythmias are believed to be one of the most common causes for individuals to seek hospital treatment, prompting addition of a specific chapter on arrhythmias to the National Service Framework for CHD (Department of Health 2005).

In many cases, an arrhythmia may go unnoticed by the patient, or may present with a range of symptoms from palpitations to breathlessness, chest pain, heart failure or syncope. Importantly, arrhythmias are believed to be the underlying cause of sudden cardiac death syndrome (Gretton 2006). Arrhythmias producing circulatory impairment, myocardial ischaemia or risk of precipitating sudden death require prompt and effective identification and treatment. This chapter examines identification of cardiac arrhythmias, along with the principles of treatment and management.

Key concepts

Automaticity; disorders of conduction; tachycardia; bradycardia; rhythm interpretation

Learning objectives

After reading this chapter, you will be able to:

- Understand the significance of common cardiac arrhythmias.
- Use a systematic approach in arrhythmia interpretation.
- Define and identify bradyarrhythmias and understand the principles of treatment.
- Define and identify tachyarrhythmias and understand the principles of treatment.
- Identify circumstances in arrhythmia management that require expert help.

Basic electrophysiology

Electrophysiology is discussed in Chapter 3. Although cells in several areas of the atria, coronary sinus, pulmonary veins, atrioventricular (AV) junction, AV valves and Purkinje system have the property of automaticity, under normal conditions, they have slower rates than the sinus node so that they do not compete with the normal rhythm. The heart's usual rhythm is normal sinus rhythm (NSR) in which the rate is between 60 and 100 beats per minute (bpm) and all components of

the normal cardiac cycle with normal waveforms and intervals can be seen (Figure 23.1a)

Mechanisms of arrhythmia generations

Any rhythm that does not meet the criteria of NSR is by definition abnormal and termed an arrhythmia. Cardiac arrhythmias may result from:

- Abnormal impulse initiation including (1) enhanced normal automaticity, (2) abnormal automaticity and (3) triggered activity resulting from afterdepolarisations

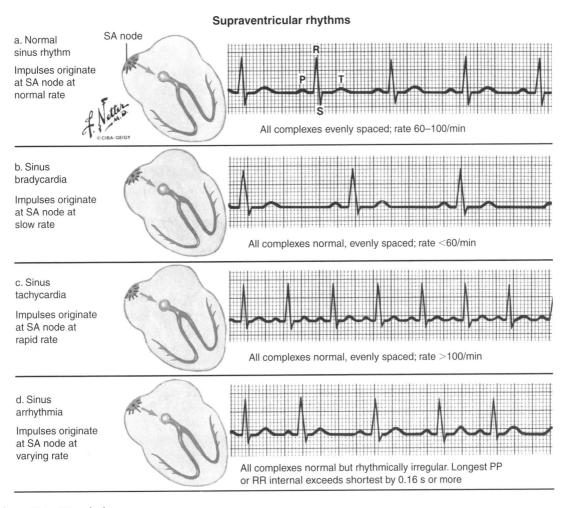

Figure 23.1 Sinus rhythms.
Source: From Scheidt (1986). Copyright Novartis A.G. Used with permission.

- Abnormal impulse conduction including (1) conduction block and (2) re-entry
- Or both of the above (Jacobsen 2005)

The site of fastest impulse initiation is referred to as the dominant pacemaker, and other cells with automaticity are known as subsidiary or latent pacemakers. This means that if the sinus rate falls below a certain level or fails altogether, these subsidiary pacemakers can take over the function of initiating the cardiac impulse and setting the heart rate. Conditions that may cause the sinus node rate to drop below that of subsidiary pacemakers include increased vagal tone, drug effects, electrolyte abnormalities and sinus node disease. Enhanced automaticity may cause sinus and atrial tachyarrhythmias and accelerated junctional and ventricular rhythms that may be due to increased sympathetic tone, some disease states and effects of drugs such as digitalis and sympathomimetics.

Abnormal automaticity may develop in myocardial cells that do not normally have this property in conditions and disease states that reduce the transmembrane resting potential, leaving the cell partially depolarised so that the time required for spontaneous diastolic depolarisation to reach threshold is reduced, thus increasing pacemaker activity and automaticity. Conditions that reduce transmembrane resting potential include ischaemia, hypoxia, acidosis, hyperkalaemia, effects of some drugs such as digitalis toxicity, metabolic abnormalities and chamber enlargement, dilation or stretch (Jacobsen 2005).

Key point

Rhythms that result from abnormal automaticity tend to occur at faster rates than rhythms that occur due to normal automaticity and include atrial and ventricular tachyarrhythmias (Jacobsen 2005).

Arrhythmias may also result from triggered activity due to afterdepolarisations, which are transient depolarisations of the cell membrane that occur during or soon after repolarisation, triggering an impulse that may sustain the activity for several beats and terminate only when the membrane finally repolarises to a high enough level to extinguish the arrhythmic activity. Afterdepolarisations occur primarily in the Purkinje fibres and ventricles and in the presence of conditions including hypoxia, acidosis, hypokalaemia, hypomagnesaemia, hypothermia, high pCO_2, high concentrations of catecholamines and in areas of stretch or mechanical injury. Afterdepolarisation activity may be triggered by slow heart rates such as bradycardia or pauses in the rhythm and is associated with genetic mutations such as congenital long QT syndrome (associated with Torsades de Pointes). Other conditions associated with arrhythmia due to afterdepolarisations are hypertrophy and heart failure (Jacobsen 2005).

Key point

Class IA and III antiarrhythmics can actually have a proarrhythmic effect because of their action in prolonging repolarisation in cardiac cells that may encourage afterdepolarisations.

Conduction may be curtailed if the propagating impulse is not strong enough to excite the tissue ahead of it, or the impulse reaches an area that is still refractory after a previous depolarisation or abnormally depolarised due to ischaemia, disease and drugs. Scar tissue from a previous MI or catheter ablation may prevent conduction. These abnormalities may result in bradyarrhythmias or aberrancy (Jacobsen 2005). Re-entrant conduction abnormalities may lead to premature beats or sustained tachycardias in any part of the heart where conduction velocity is abnormally slow. The impulse can travel through an area of myocardium, depolarise it, and then re-enter that same area to depolarise it again. Ischaemia, electrolyte abnormalities, some drugs and disease processes can facilitate this type of conduction abnormality (Jacobsen 2005).

Key points

When an impulse travels the re-entry loop only once, a single premature beat results.

If conduction velocity is slow enough and the refractory period of normal tissue is short enough, a single impulse could travel the loop numerous times, resulting in a run of premature beats or in a sustained tachycardia (Jacobsen 2005).

Cardiac monitoring

Cardiac monitoring is suitable for rhythm recognition but insufficient for diagnosis of MI or more sophisticated ECG interpretation. Wherever possible, a 12-lead ECG should be recorded, since this provides additional information not present on a single rhythm strip. However, a 12-lead ECG recording is not always possible and a cardiac monitor may be the only aid to identifying the patient's rhythm. Precise identification of many rhythm abnormalities requires experience and

expertise, but in most cases an accurate description of the rhythm is sufficient to allow effective management.

Rhythm interpretation

Deviations from the norm are not always clinically significant and manifestation of an arrhythmia is dependent on a number of factors including the ventricular rate, myocardial conduction and the patient's physiological and psychological response. Arrhythmia identification can be approached in a variety of ways, but a systematic approach to interpretation of the electrocardiographic waveforms and intervals gives the best result. Having first ensured that the ECG rhythm recording/monitor is clearly identified for a particular patient (to ensure safety), follow the steps and answer the questions in Table 23.1.

Table 23.1   Systematic interpretation of rhythm.

Is the *rhythm* regular or irregular?
Normal sinus rhythm is regular.

What is the *heart rate*?
The normal heart rate is between 60 and 100bpm.

* A heart rate ≤ 60bpm is termed 'bradycardia'.
* A heart rate ≥ 100bpm is termed 'tachycardia'.

To calculate heart rate:

One large box represents 0.2s; thus there are five large boxes in a second.

Count how many complexes there are in a second and multiply by 60 to obtain the heart rate.

This method is only reliable for regular heart rates.

Is the *P wave* normal?
Does a normal P wave precede each QRS complex?

* Normal sinus rhythm should have an upright P wave in Lead II.
* Normal P-wave width is <0.11s (3 small squares).

Is the *PR interval* normal?
Is the PR interval (measured from the beginning of P to the beginning of QRS complex) the same in each complex?

* The normal PR interval is 0.12–0.20s (3–5 small squares).

Is the *QRS* normal?
Is the QRS narrow or wide?

* The QRS is measured from the first upward/downward deflection from baseline until return to baseline.
* Normal QRS width is 0.06–0.10s (1.5–2.5 small squares).

1. Is the rhythm regular or irregular?

This is not always as easy to determine as it seems. In most cases, it is possible to see if a rhythm is regular or not merely by looking at it on the monitor screen, but as the heart rate increases, beat-to-beat variation becomes more difficult to detect. In cases of doubt, placing a piece of paper along a rhythm strip printout and marking three consecutive R waves will provide additional information: where the rhythm is regular the marks should correspond to R waves anywhere along the strip; if not, then the rhythm is irregular.

The most common reasons for irregular heart rhythms are atrial fibrillation (AF), ectopic beats and heart block. In AF, the rhythm is often described as 'irregularly irregular', meaning that it does not follow any discernable pattern. AF is very common, particularly in the elderly, and the effect on the patient is often related to the ventricular rate (Navas 2003). Heart blocks may follow a cyclical pattern, and careful analysis of the relationship between the P wave and QRS complex is required. Both atrial ectopic (atrial premature contraction) and ventricular ectopic (ventricular premature contraction) beats can make an essentially regular rhythm appear irregular. Ectopic beats are often benign, but investigation of possible underlying causes should be considered.

2. What is the ventricular rate?

Provided that discernable QRS complexes are present, the next step is to determine the ventricular rate or beats per minute. There are a number of different ways of doing this – the simplest being to read the rate shown on most modern cardiac monitors. However, this may not always be accurate, particularly in the presence of peaked T waves or an irregular rhythm such as AF, and caution is required if relying on this method. Other approaches include printing a rhythm strip and measuring the number of large squares between adjacent R waves and dividing this number into 300. For example, if there are four large squares between the R waves then the rate is 300/4 giving a rate of 75bpm. An alternative method involves counting the number of R waves in 30 large squares and multiplying by 10. Both these methods give a reasonable approximation allowing the rhythm to

be classified as regular (60–100bpm), a bradycardia (less than 60bpm) or a tachycardia (>100bpm).

3. Are there P waves present?

P waves denote atrial depolarisation and appear before the QRS complex in NSR. A normal P wave is seen as an upright, rounded deflection in Lead II on the ECG, indicating that the impulse has originated in or near the sinoatrial (SA) node. Sometimes inverted P waves are seen, indicating the impulse has originated closer to the AV node (Houghton & Gray 2003). Intermittent P waves may indicate a type of heart block, and other forms of atrial activity exist, including flutter and fibrillation waves.

4. What is the relationship between the P waves and the QRS complexes?

Having examined both atrial and ventricular activities, the final step involves analysing the relationship between them. In NSR the P wave should always be followed by a QRS complex, with a normal PR interval of 0.12–0.2s(or three to five small squares). The PR interval is measured from the beginning of the P wave to the beginning of the QRS. A distance greater than five small squares indicates some type of heart block is present. The significance of a shortened PR interval is often overlooked, but may well indicate a pre-excitation syndrome and is particularly important in patients presenting with paroxysmal tachycardias.

5. Is the QRS width broad or narrow?

Normal QRS duration is between 0.08 and 0.12s (less than three small squares on the ECG paper, using standard paper speed of 25mm/s). This interval represents the length of time the electrical impulse takes to depolarise the ventricles. A measurement of longer than three small squares indicates that there is a delay in the conduction of the impulse. This can be due to either a blockage in the conduction system (e.g. bundle branch block) or a result of the impulse being initiated from the ventricular myocardium. Widening of the QRS complex can also occur in electrolyte disturbances (e.g. hyperkalaemia) or poisoning, particularly where tricyclic antidepressants have been taken in excess (Houghton & Gray 2003).

Determining the rhythm

Having systematically used the approach described above, it should now be possible to determine the cardiac rhythm. Although it is not always possible to precisely name the rhythm, this approach should at least allow for an accurate description, which in turn will direct appropriate management, and may prove particularly useful when communicating with colleagues who do not have access to the patient or actual rhythm strip (such as in telephone consultations with off-site medical staff). In the acutely ill patient, a general 'rule of thumb' is to concentrate on the obvious and leave the details to the experts.

Arrhythmias that are usually asymptomatic

Rhythms such as sinus arrhythmia (Figure 23.1d), non-sinus atrial rhythms (including coronary sinus rhythm) (Figure 23.6a) and wandering atrial pacemaker (Figure 23.6b) usually do not cause symptoms but may be associated with underlying disease states. Likewise, atrial, junctional and ventricular ectopic beats (Figure 23.2a) are usually harmless but may cause palpitations and light-headedness if frequent, may be associated with an underlying disease state or may indicate an increased risk of other arrhythmias.

Symptom producing arrhythmias are usually those that are abnormally fast or slow.

Bradyarrhythmias

A bradyarrhythmia exists when the ventricular rate is less than 60 bpm. In many cases the patient is asymptomatic and no treatment is required. However, the bradycardia may be due to malfunction of the SA node, or a delay or blockage of AV conduction, in which case intervention may be required.

Sinus bradycardia

Sinus bradycardia occurs when the heart rate is slower than 60 bpm. This rhythm is similar to NSR, except that the RR interval is longer. Each P wave is followed by a QRS complex in a ratio of 1:1 (see Figure 23.1b).

Sinus bradycardia can occur naturally during sleep and be a normal finding in athletes, or a side effect of treatment such as beta-blockers. Other causes include hypothermia, hypothyroidism and hypoxia (Gretton 2006). A slow heart rate might be beneficial in some patients with MI by reducing the heart's oxygen demand, possibly reducing the infarct size, and thus mortality risk (Kinney & Packa 1996). It is frequently associated with inferior MI, where the right coronary artery supplies the inferior territory of the heart, including the sinus and AV nodes in many patients.

Slow heart rates are usually well tolerated and no intervention is required, but some patients may exhibit symptoms such as dyspnoea, dizziness, chest pain, syncope and hypotension. In these patients, treatment with intravenous atropine may be indicated, and if drug therapy proves ineffective, cardiac pacing may be considered (Resuscitation Council [UK] 2005).

Heart block

Atrioventricular block occurs when there is a delay or failure in impulse conduction from the atria to the ventricles. It may be transient or permanent and can be classified as first, second or third degree.

First-degree AV block

Atrial conduction is prolonged in first-degree block (Figure 23.3d). The rate is usually within normal limits, so technically first-degree block is not a bradycardia, but it is practical to consider along with other AV blocks. The impulse is delayed passing through the AV node to the ventricles, resulting in prolongation of the PR interval on the ECG. A QRS complex follows every P wave and the rhythm is regular. A prolonged conduction time is frequently found in athletes and older people. First-degree block can also present in patients on beta-blocker therapy, with digoxin toxicity, and electrolyte disturbance, such as hyperkalaemia. It is also associated with ischaemia, infarction, myocarditis and hypoxia (Hand 2002).

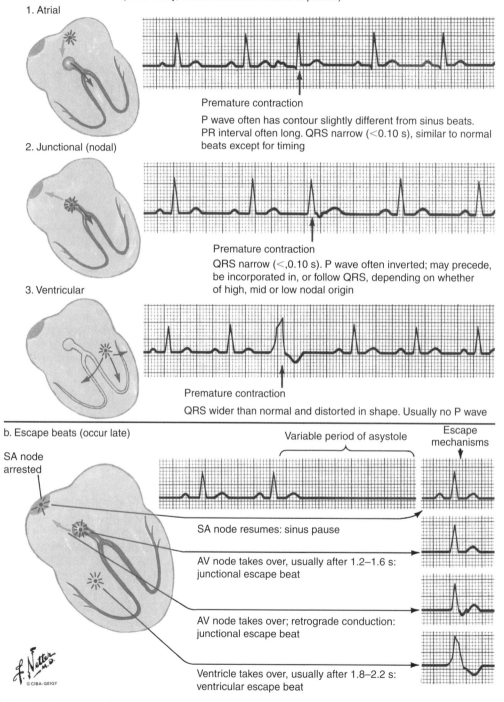

Unusual beats

a. Premature contractions (occur early, before next sinus beat is expected)

1. Atrial

Premature contraction

P wave often has contour slightly different from sinus beats. PR interval often long. QRS narrow (<0.10 s), similar to normal beats except for timing

2. Junctional (nodal)

Premature contraction

QRS narrow (<,0.10 s). P wave often inverted; may precede, be incorporated in, or follow QRS, depending on whether of high, mid or low nodal origin

3. Ventricular

Premature contraction

QRS wider than normal and distorted in shape. Usually no P wave

b. Escape beats (occur late)

SA node arrested

Variable period of asystole

Escape mechanisms

SA node resumes: sinus pause

AV node takes over, usually after 1.2–1.6 s: junctional escape beat

AV node takes over; retrograde conduction: junctional escape beat

Ventricle takes over, usually after 1.8–2.2 s: ventricular escape beat

Figure 23.2 Ectopic and escape beats.
Source: From Scheidt (1986). Copyright Novartis A.G. Used with permission.

Atrioventricular conduction variations

a. Fixed normal PR interval
   Sinus rhythm

b. Fixed but short PR interval
   1. Junctional or coronary sinus rhythm
   2. Wolff–Parkinson–White syndrome

c. P wave related to each QRS complex, but variable PR interval
   1. Wandering atrial pacemaker
   2. Multifocal atrial tachycardia

d. Fixed but prolonged PR interval
   First-degree AV block

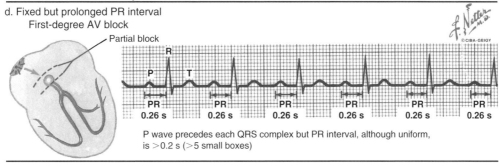

P wave precedes each QRS complex but PR interval, although uniform, is >0.2 s (>5 small boxes)

e. Progressive lengthening of PR interval with intermittent dropped beats
   Second-degree AV block: Mobitz I (Wenckebach)

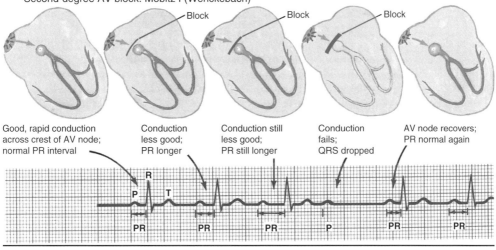

f. Sudden dropped QRS without prior PR lengthening
   Second-degree AV block: Mobitz II (non-Wenckebach)

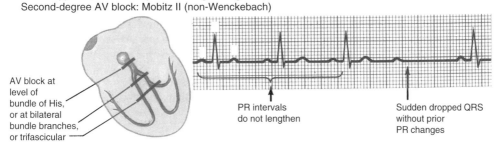

Figure 23.3   First- and second-degree heart blocks.
Source: From Scheidt (1986). Copyright Novartis A.G. Used with permission.

If the heart rate is normal and the patient is unaffected, there is no need for treatment. If, however, the block is associated with organic heart disease, such as MI, the patient might be at risk of progressing to second- or third-degree block and should be observed accordingly.

Second-degree AV block

There are two types of second-degree AV heart block known as Mobitz type I (Wenckebach) and Mobitz type II.

Mobitz type I (Wenckebach)

In Mobitz type 1 AV block, commonly referred to as Wenckebach, there is a progressive prolongation of the PR interval over several heart beats (Figure 23.3e). The phenomenon repeats itself with a gradual lengthening of the PR interval over three to six beats until an impulse is totally blocked, and the P wave occurs without a corresponding QRS complex and a pause ensues. The resulting ventricular rhythm is irregular, but follows a predictable, cyclical pattern. The rate can be normal but is often slow, varying from 75 down to 40 bpm (Gretton 2006). Second-degree heart block is usually localised to the AV node. It is characteristically periodic and of shorter duration than Mobitz type II block. It is commonly seen in digoxin overdose or following inferior MI, but does not usually cause haemodynamic compromise. Treatment involves avoidance of AV nodal blocking drugs. It does not usually require pacing unless there is evidence of haemodynamic instability.

Mobitz type II

Mobitz type II heart block is characterised by occasional non-conducted P waves without a preceding lengthening of the PR interval (Bowbrick & Borg 2006) (Figure 23.3f). The 'dropped' beat can occur irregularly or regularly every second, third or fourth beat and is referred to as 2:1, 3:1, 4:1 AV block respectively. The block in conduction occurs beneath the AV node in the bundle of His or bilaterally in the bundle branches. It is less common than type I, but is frequently associated with haemodynamic compromise when it occurs, often progressing to complete heart block (Kinney and Packa 1996).

If the block presents acutely, it is often associated with acute MI (anteroseptal or inferior), while chronic block tends to occur because of degenerative changes in the conduction system associated with ageing. In the setting of MI, Mobitz type II block is often associated with irreversible myocardial damage, and deterioration to complete AV block is common. Treatment in acute cases involves intravenous atropine, otherwise prophylactic temporary pacing is used to avert the need for pacemaker insertion in a compromised patient should complete heart block develop suddenly (Hand 2002).

Third-degree (complete) AV block

In third-degree or 'complete' heart block, there is no conduction from the atria to the ventricles. In most cases, the pacemaker function is taken over by a focus below the block acting as a 'safety net', with the heartbeat sustained by impulses from the area around the AV node, or the ventricles. The QRS complex can be either broad or narrow depending on the site where the impulses are being generated. A nodal rhythm gives a rate of around 40–60 beats with a narrow complex, whereas a ventricular rhythm gives a rate of 15–40 bpm with broad complexes (Houghton and Gray 2003) (Figure 23.4a). If an 'escape' rhythm fails to develop, ventricular standstill will occur, and the patient will require immediate resuscitation.

The atrial rate may be normal and regular, and the ventricular rate also regular, but impulse transmission between the atria and ventricles is absent. The P wave does not precede a QRS complex on the ECG. The lower down the conduction pathway an escape rhythm is generated, the slower the ventricular rate will be and less well tolerated by the patient (Hand 2002).

When associated with inferior MI, drug toxicity, acute pericarditis or myocarditis, total AV block is usually a transient phenomenon, although temporary pacing may be required if the patient is symptomatic or haemodynamically compromised (Thompson and Webster 2004). In acute anterior MI, the development of complete heart block usually indicates extensive myocardial damage and a poor prognosis, with a mortality rate as high as 75%.

Atrioventricular conduction variations
a. No relationship between P waves and QRS complexes: QRS rate *slower* than P rate
Third–degree (complete) AV block

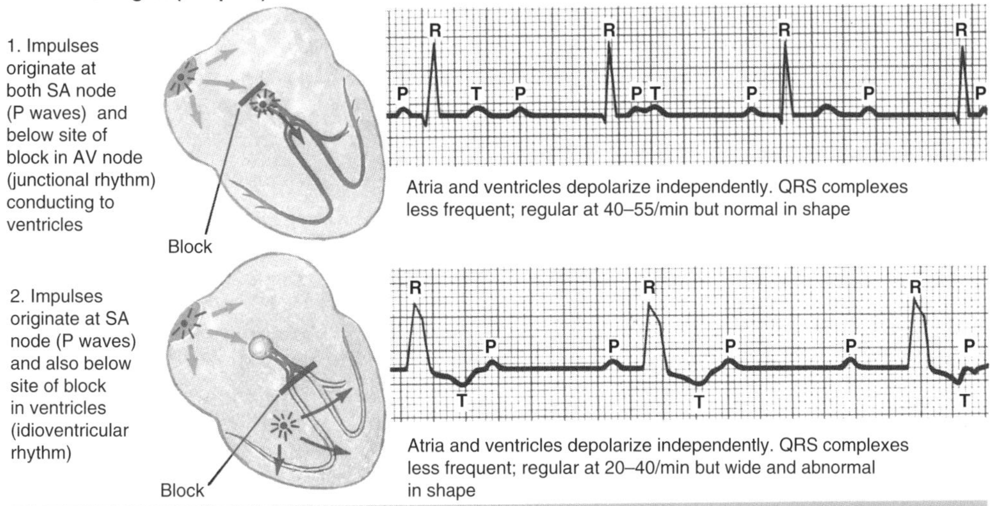

1. Impulses originate at both SA node (P waves) and below site of block in AV node (junctional rhythm) conducting to ventricles

Block

Atria and ventricles depolarize independently. QRS complexes less frequent; regular at 40–55/min but normal in shape

2. Impulses originate at SA node (P waves) and also below site of block in ventricles (idioventricular rhythm)

Block

Atria and ventricles depolarize independently. QRS complexes less frequent; regular at 20–40/min but wide and abnormal in shape

	'High'	'Low'
Features of two types of atrioventricular block		
Site of block	Crest of AV node	Bundle of His, bilateral bundle branch, or trifascicular
Type of escape rhythm	Junctional escape rhythm Narrow QRS Adequate rate (40–55)	Ventricular escape rhythm Wide QRS Inadequate rate (20–40) Danger of asystole or ventricular tachycardia
Underlying pathology	Right coronary artery disease, diaphragmatic infarction, oedema around AV node	Left anterior descending coronary artery disease, large anteroseptal infarction, or chronic degeneration of conduction system
Rhythm before complete block	Preceded by Mobitz I (Wenckebach) second-degree AV block	Preceded by Mobitz II second-degree AV block

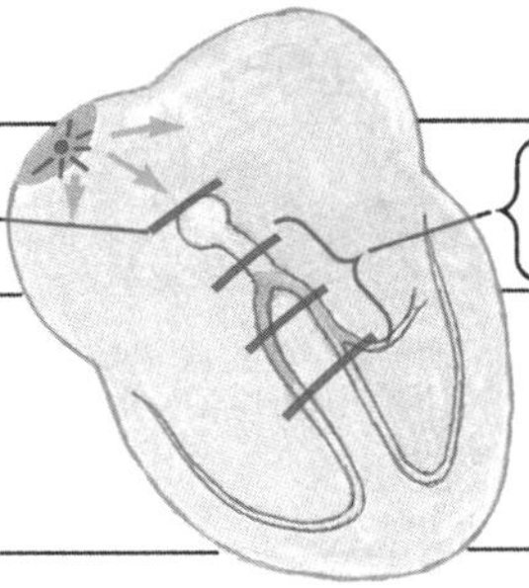

b. No relationship between P waves and QRS complexes: QRS rate *faster* than P rate
AV dissociation

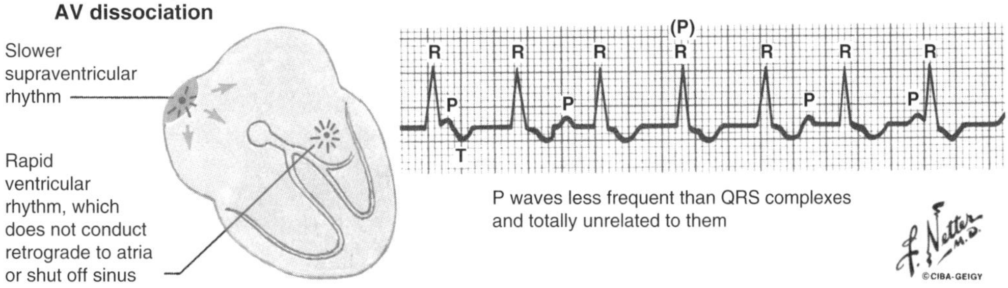

Slower supraventricular rhythm

Rapid ventricular rhythm, which does not conduct retrograde to atria or shut off sinus

P waves less frequent than QRS complexes and totally unrelated to them

Figure 23.4 Complete heart block and AV dissociation.
Source: From Scheidt (1986). Copyright Novartis A.G. Used with permission.

Atrioventricular dissociation

Atrioventricular dissociation may occur when P waves and QRS complexes occur independently, with the ventricular rate being higher than the atrial rate (Figure 23.4h). The ventricular rhythm fails to conduct retrograde and thus does not supersede the slower atrial rhythm. AV dissociation is usually a benign phenomenon that can result from (1) slowing of the dominant pacemaker (sinus node), which allows an escape junctional or ventricular rhythm or (2) acceleration of a normally slower (subsidiary) pacemaker, such as a junctional site or a ventricular site that activates the ventricles without retrograde atrial capture (Sandesara & Olschansky 2006).

Key point

Complete heart block may be described as a type of AV dissociation as the atria and ventricles operate independently, but a rhythm is usually labelled AV dissociation when the ventricular rate is faster than the atrial rate.

Escape beats

Should the SA node fail, an automatic cell must take over to maintain beating of the heart. This is known as an escape beat (Figure 23.2b). Escape beats may be asymptomatic or associated with underlying pathology eventually leading to symptomatic bradycardia requiring treatment.

Junctional rhythm

If the SA node fails, automatic cells in the AV node may take over the function of maintaining the heart's rhythm. This is known as a junctional rhythm. Rhythms originating in the junction have both retrograde (back to the atria) and antegrade (continuing down the bundle branches) conduction. Inverted P waves may be seen immediately after the QRS or may be obscured by the QRS complex (Figure 23.6k). The intrinsic rate of the junction is about 50 bpm, and this rate will signify that the rhythm is an escape rhythm. Occasionally,

the junctional rate will be faster due to causes such as ischaemia, and in this case it would be known as junctional tachycardia.

Idioventricular rhythm

Idioventricular rhythm (IVR) is an escape rhythm resulting from a slow pacemaker in the ventricle taking over when SA node and AV junctional pacemakers fail to function. The rate usually is less than 40 bpm and the rhythm is usually transient (Figure 23.5a). As with escape beats, the underlying pathology and symptoms will dictate whether treatment is required. IVR and accelerated IVR (IVR at a rate between 45 and 120 bpm) (Figure 23.5b) is common in the first 24 h of MI and generally benign.

Tachyarrhythmias

Tachycardias are defined as a heart rate greater than 100 bpm and can be supraventricular or ventricular in origin. Tachycardias can result in hypotension and reduced tissue perfusion. Because the heart is beating faster, the amount of time between cardiac contractions is reduced, thus the ventricles do not have time to fill adequately before contraction and cardiac output decreases. Heart rate is a major determinant of oxygen requirement: the harder the heart has to work, the greater its demand for oxygen. Persistent or prolonged tachycardia will, therefore, increase the amount of oxygen required by the myocardium, resulting in increased ischaemia in patients who cannot meet the increased demand (Hand 2002). Sudden cardiac death is discussed in Chapter 14.

Sinus tachycardia

Sinus tachycardia is classified as a sinus rhythm greater than 100 bpm. All the other ECG characteristics are the same as for sinus rhythm (Figure 23.1c). Sinus tachycardia is not therefore a 'true' arrhythmia but represents a response to some other physiological or pathological state. It is a normal response to stressors such as fever, pain, anxiety, exercise, hypovolaemia, shock and

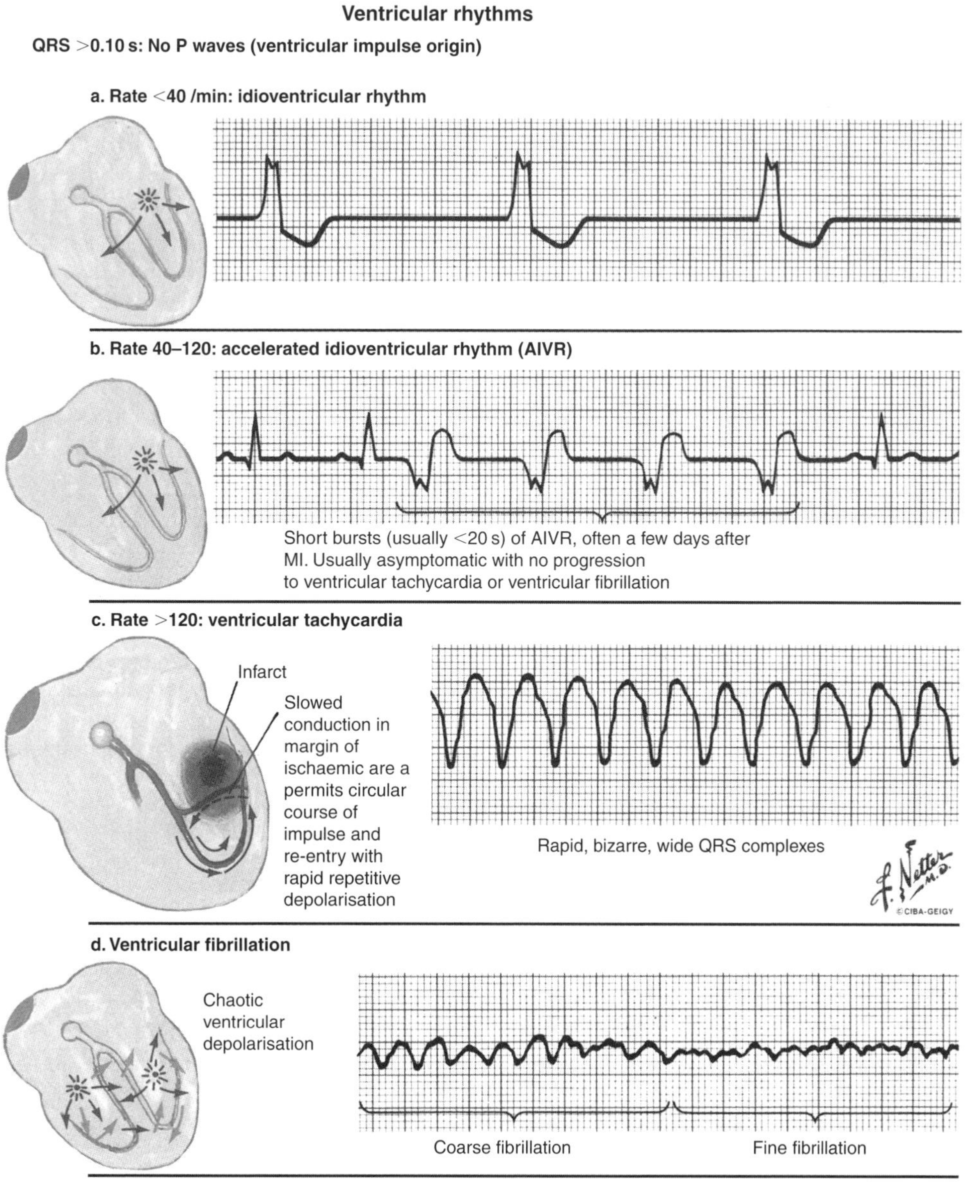

Ventricular rhythms

QRS >0.10 s: No P waves (ventricular impulse origin)

a. Rate <40 /min: idioventricular rhythm

b. Rate 40–120: accelerated idioventricular rhythm (AIVR)

Short bursts (usually <20 s) of AIVR, often a few days after MI. Usually asymptomatic with no progression to ventricular tachycardia or ventricular fibrillation

c. Rate >120: ventricular tachycardia

Infarct

Slowed conduction in margin of ischaemic are a permits circular course of impulse and re-entry with rapid repetitive depolarisation

Rapid, bizarre, wide QRS complexes

d. Ventricular fibrillation

Chaotic ventricular depolarisation

Coarse fibrillation   Fine fibrillation

Figure 23.5 Ventricular rhythms.
Source: From Scheidt (1986). Copyright Novartis A.G. Used with permission.

cardiac failure. It can also be caused by stimulants such as caffeine and alcohol, or drugs that cause sympathetic stimulation. The cause of the tachycardia and underlying condition of the myocardium will determine the prognosis (Hand 2002). Management focuses on detecting and correcting any underlying causes.

Supraventricular tachycardia

Supraventricular tachycardia (SVT), sometimes referred to as narrow complex tachycardia (NCT), is a convenient way of grouping together those tachyarrhythmias that originate above the ventricles and appear as a narrow QRS complex on the ECG (Gretton 2006). Although the impulse is not originating from the SA node, ventricular depolarisation occurs normally and results in a narrow QRS complex. The rhythm is often regular but may be irregular in the presence of AF or variably conducted atrial flutter.

Multifocal atrial tachycardia

As in wandering atrial pacemaker, the contour of the P wave and PR, PP and RR intervals may vary, but in multifocal atrial tachycardia (MAT), the rate is above 100 bpm (Figure 23.6f). MAT is almost always associated with underlying severe pulmonary disease or congestive heart failure (CHF).

Paroxysmal atrial tachycardia

Paroxysmal atrial tachycardia (PAT) is often a re-entry arrhythmia that usually occurs at a rate between 160 and 220 bpm with P waves that are regular, identical, frequently inverted in Lead II (Figure 23.6h). PAT may be associated with rheumatic heart disease, pulmonary disease, cardiac decompensation, Wolff–Parkinson–White syndrome, mitral valve prolapse or digitalis intoxication, but can also occur in people with no structural heart disease (Scheidt 1986).

Atrial fibrillation

Atrial fibrillation is one of the most commonly occurring arrhythmias in clinical practice, complicating 15–20% of MIs (Thompson & Webster 2004), and affecting 5–10% of older people (Houghton & Gray 2003). The prevalence of AF increases exponentially with age and it may be permanent, persistent or paroxysmal (Navas 2003). In MI, it is frequently associated with severe left ventricular damage and heart failure (Thompson & Webster 2004), and persistent AF following MI usually indicates extensive myocardial damage and carries a poor long-term prognosis (Davies 2001). Long-standing hypertension, hyperthyroidism and pulmonary embolus are other potential causes. Precipitating factors for AF include hydration status, recent infections, alcohol use, sympathomimetic drugs and electrolyte imbalance. It is believed that inflammation plays a part in the development of AF but the role has not yet been clearly elucidated (Lazar & Clark 2007).

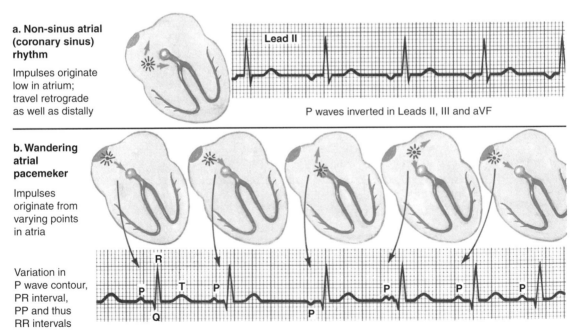

a. Non-sinus atrial (coronary sinus) rhythm

Impulses originate low in atrium; travel retrograde as well as distally

Lead II

P waves inverted in Leads II, III and aVF

b. Wandering atrial pacemeker

Impulses originate from varying points in atria

Variation in P wave contour, PR interval, PP and thus RR intervals

Figure 23.6 Supraventricular rhythms.
Source: From Scheidt (1986). Copyright Novartis A.G. Used with permission.

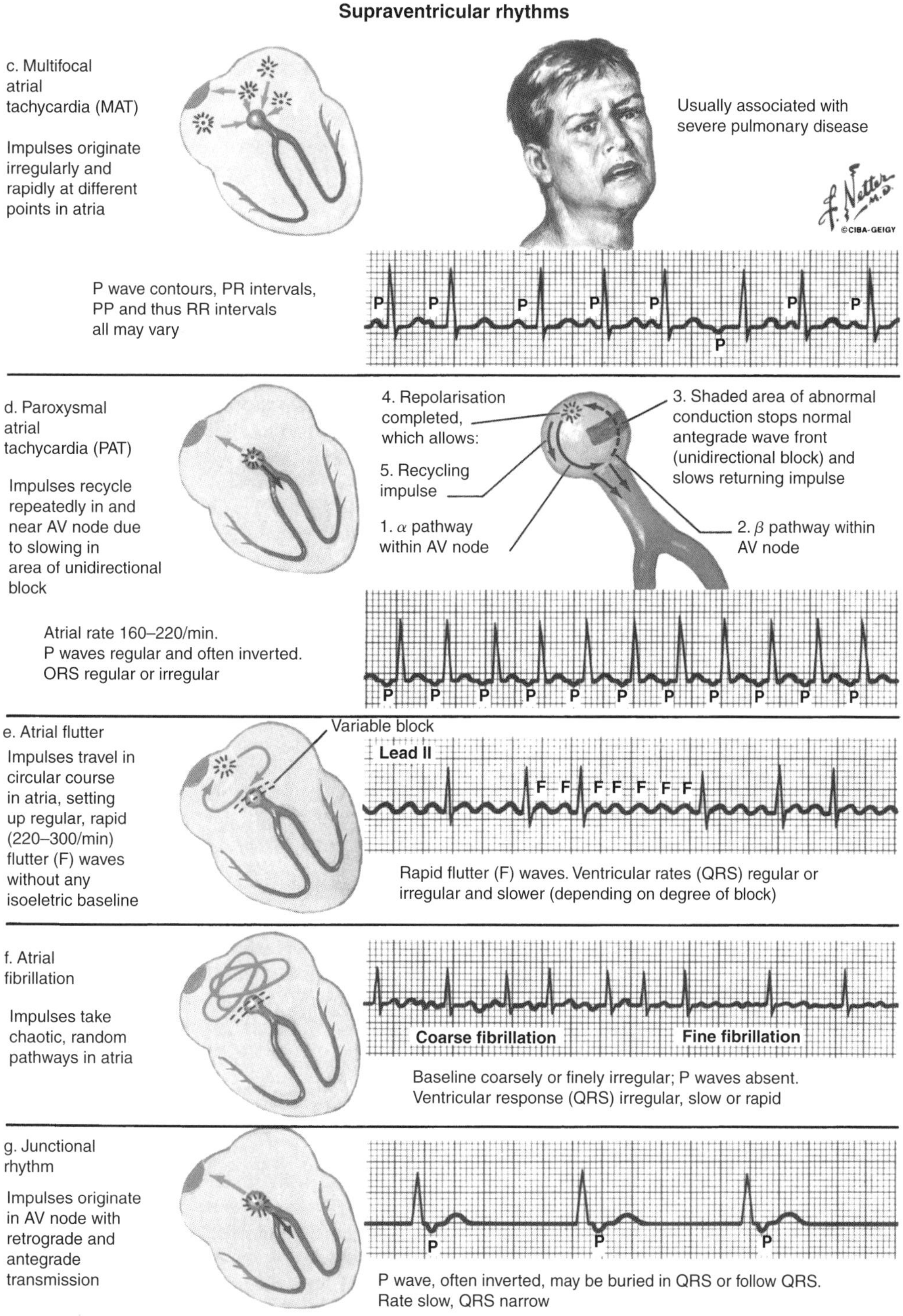

Supraventricular rhythms
c. Multifocal atrial tachycardia (MAT)
Impulses originate irregularly and rapidly at different points in atria
Usually associated with severe pulmonary disease
©CIBA-GEIGY
P wave contours, PR intervals, PP and thus RR intervals all may vary
P P P P P P P P
d. Paroxysmal atrial tachycardia (PAT)
Impulses recycle repeatedly in and near AV node due to slowing in area of unidirectional block
4. Repolarisation completed, which allows:
5. Recycling impulse
1. α pathway within AV node
3. Shaded area of abnormal conduction stops normal antegrade wave front (unidirectional block) and slows returning impulse
2. β pathway within AV node
Atrial rate 160–220/min.
P waves regular and often inverted.
QRS regular or irregular
P P P P P P P P P P P
e. Atrial flutter
Impulses travel in circular course in atria, setting up regular, rapid (220–300/min) flutter (F) waves without any isoeletric baseline
Variable block
Lead II
F F F F F F F
Rapid flutter (F) waves. Ventricular rates (QRS) regular or irregular and slower (depending on degree of block)
f. Atrial fibrillation
Impulses take chaotic, random pathways in atria
Coarse fibrillation
Fine fibrillation
Baseline coarsely or finely irregular; P waves absent.
Ventricular response (QRS) irregular, slow or rapid
g. Junctional rhythm
Impulses originate in AV node with retrograde and antegrade transmission
P P P
P wave, often inverted, may be buried in QRS or follow QRS.
Rate slow, QRS narrow

Figure 23.6 *(cont'd)*

Key point

Atrial fibrillation is described as acute or chronic, and chronic AF may be sub-classified as follows:

Paroxysmal AF: duration less than 7 days, with spontaneous termination (more common in young people)

Persistent AF: duration greater than 7 days that would last indefinitely without intervention (cardioversion)

Permanent AF: duration greater than 7 days without a possibility of reversion to sinus rhythm

Lone AF: used to describe AF in individuals (usually younger than 60 years of age) without structural or cardiac or pulmonary disease and with low risk for thromboembolism (Lazar & Clark 2007).

Atrial fibrillation results from multiple re-entrant electrical wavelets that move randomly around the atria (Lazar & Clark 2007) resulting from multiple ectopic foci in the atria discharging at up to 600 times per minute. There are no discernable P waves, but small undulating waves (known as fibrillation or fibrillatory waves) appear on the ECG. The AV node is bombarded by electrical impulses from the atria and becomes relatively refractive to conduction, resulting in erratic transmission of impulses through the AV node and subsequently, an irregular ventricular rhythm. This rhythm is frequently referred to as an 'irregularly irregular' rhythm, meaning there is no discernable pattern to its irregularity (Bowbick & Borg 2006) (Figure 23.6j). Three mechanisms that have been shown to play a role in the initiation and maintenance of AF are as follows:

- Enhanced automaticity in the left atrium extending to the proximal portions of the pulmonary veins
- Electrical remodelling of the atria which shortens the atrial refractory period and increases the duration and stability of AF (often described as 'atrial fibrillation begets atrial fibrillation')
- Areas of functional conduction block which further divide and maintain a persistently chaotic electrical state in chronic AF (Lazar & Clark 2007)

Atrial fibrillation reduces cardiac output due to (1) loss of atrial kick (synchronized atrial mechanical activity), (2) irregularity of ventricular response and (3) inappropriately rapid heart rate (Lazar & Clark 2007). The rapid rate at which the atria depolarise causes a quivering motion rather than effective contraction. This in turn leads to inadequate filling of the ventricles, which results in a 10–15% fall in cardiac output (Houghton & Gray 2003).

In patients who present with haemodynamic instability (symptomatic hypotension, altered mental status or loss of consciousness, acute myocardial ischaemia, or hypoxia) due to AF, emergency cardioversion may be indicated, but this is rarely required. AF in the presence of congestive cardiac failure will contribute to haemodynamic instability (Lazar & Clark 2007). In patients experiencing AF for more than 48 h, stasis of blood in the fibrillating atrial appendage may lead to blood clot formation and systemic embolism to the brain or lungs, which is particularly likely to happen when AF reverts to sinus rhythm (Thompson & Webster 2004). AF is the single most significant cause of ischaemic stroke in patients over 75 years of age (Hart & Halpern 2001).

Pharmacological management of AF may be aimed at (1) rate control and (2) restoring/maintaining sinus rhythm; and there may be overlap with these. In patients with an acute episode, digoxin is ineffective in controlling ventricular rate during acute episodes and digoxin or amiodarone should be used in patients with CHF. In the absence of contraindications, rate is controlled most effectively with intravenous verapamil, diltiazem, or beta-adrenergic blockers. Antiarrhythmic drugs that can terminate AF include procainamide, disopyramide, propafenone, sotalol, flecainide, amiodarone and ibutilide (Lazar & Clarke 2007).

Atrial flutter

Atrial flutter is a macro-reentrant arrhythmia characterised by atrial rates between 240 and 400 bpm. It is best defined by the presence of uniform atrial activation known as 'flutter waves' that appear in a characteristic 'saw-tooth' pattern on the ECG (Figure 23.6i), with P waves best visualised in

Leads II, III, aVF or V1. The atrial rate is faster that the ventricular rate. Commonly, there is a 2:1 conduction ratio, although the block can be 4:1, or less commonly 3:1 or 5:1. The conduction rate may vary, known as 'variable block' (Lazar & Parwani 2006).

Atrial flutter is divided into two types.

- Type 1 atrial flutter is the most common and involves a counterclockwise re-entrant circuit that encircles the tricuspid annulus of the right atrium, with a depolarising stimulus travelling up the atrial septum and then back down the atrial free wall (although a clockwise version of this has also been described). The atrial rate is typically 240–340 bpm.

Key point

Flutter waves for typical (type 1) atrial flutter are inverted (negative) in Leads II, III, aVF and V1 because of a counterclockwise re-entrant pathway, but may be upright (positive) when the re-entrant loop is clockwise (Lazar & Parwani 2006).

- Type 2 atrial flutter is less common and poorly characterised, but probably results from an intra-atrial circuit that operates at a faster rate than type 1 atrial flutter, with atrial rates greater than 340 bpm (Lazar & Parwani 2006).

Atrial flutter is commonly found in patients with heart failure, valvular disease, chronic obstructive pulmonary disease, hyperthyroidism, pericarditis, pulmonary embolism, a history of open heart surgery and, occasionally, in digoxin toxicity. Men are affected more often than women in a 2:1 ratio, and prevalence increases with age. Like AF, and depending on the ventricular rate, atrial flutter can impede cardiac output and lead to atrial thrombus formation, with risk of systemic embolisation (Lazar & Parwani 2006).

If it is not clear that the arrhythmia is atrial flutter, adenosine can be used to produce transient AV block which unmasks the flutter waves. Adenosine does not generally revert atrial flutter to NSR and is primarily used diagnostically.

Unstable presentations of atrial flutter will most likely require DC cardioversion. Generally, cardioversion of atrial flutter requires low energy (50 joule) or less. Occasionally, the DC shock results in AF, and higher energies will be required to revert AF to NSR (Lazar & Parwani 2006). When using DC cardioversion in rate-controlled patients with atrial flutter, be prepared for potential bradycardia and hypotension following reversion to sinus rhythm. The issue of anticoagulation for prevention of embolic stroke in atrial flutter has been controversial because, unlike AF, the atria are still contracting. There is evidence to show that patients with atrial flutter are still at risk of embolic stroke and so there is a case for anticoagulation (Seidl et al. 1999). If atrial flutter is resistant to DC cardioversion, atrial pacing, radiofrequency catheter ablation or drug therapy may be tried.

If medical therapy is used, the goal is usually rate control. Digoxin (after ascertaining that the arrhythmia is not due to digoxin toxicity), calcium antagonists, beta-blockers or amiodarone are drugs that may be used, but are effective in only 50–60% of patients (Lazar & Parwani 2006).

Ventricular tachycardia

Ventricular tachycardia (VT) is present when five or more ventricular extra systoles occur in rapid succession (Figure 23.5c). VT may be monomorphic (originating from a single focus with identical QRS complexes) or polymorphic (may appear as an irregular rhythm, with varying QRS complexes) (Ernoehazy 2006). The duration may vary from a few beats to many hours, and VT is 'sustained' if of more than 30-s duration. VT is often preceded by ectopic beats and evolves from a ventricular focus in the right or left ventricle that depolarises with a rate of 120–250 bpm (Thompson and Webster 2004). There are no absolute criteria for establishing that a tachyarrhythmia is VT, but the following criteria are very suggestive that the rhythm is VT:

- Rate greater than 100 bpm (usually 150–200)
- Wide QRS complex (>1q20 ms)
- Presence of AV dissociation
- Fusion beats (Ernoehazy 2006)

Atrial tachyarrhythmias with aberration may also present with a broad complex (Bowbick & Borg

2006) but it is prudent for the non-expert to consider VT the 'default' diagnosis and seek specialist advice.

Ventricular tachycardia is always serious, and the rate may be so fast that adequate ventricular filling is not possible. Because coronary blood flow occurs predominantly during diastole, high heart rates reduce filling time, resulting in poor coronary blood flow and myocardial ischaemia. Sudden reduction in cardiac output is sufficient to cause cardiac arrest (so called 'pulseless VT') (Gretton 2006). Even when cardiac output is sufficient to produce a pulse, VT can lead quickly to heart failure and shock with pulmonary oedema and requires urgent treatment. There is a high risk of VT deteriorating to ventricular fibrillation (VF) and cardiac arrest. VT is usually a consequence of structural heart disease that causes a breakdown of normal conduction patterns, increased automaticity (favouring ectopic foci) and activation of re-entrant pathways in the ventricular conduction system (Ernoehazy 2006). It is often caused by ischaemic heart disease and occurs most frequently in the first few hours following MI. Other common causes of VT include electrolyte imbalance, cardiomyopathy and congenital long QT syndromes.

Variants of VT include:

- Torsades de Pointes (twisting of the points): a distinctive pattern of VT in which the QRS axis shifts, giving a spindle-shaped pattern. Usually associated with a prolonged QT interval (congenital or acquired) and may occur with myocardial ischaemia or infarction).
- Accelerated ventricular rhythm (AVR): sometimes called 'slow VT', presents at a rate between 60 and 100 bpm and typically occurs with underlying ischaemic or structural heart disease. Often seen as a 'reperfusion arrhythmia'. Treatment is not usually required unless the AVR is prolonged with haemodynamic compromise.
- Catecholaminergic polymorphic VT: Recently described VT that appears to be congenital, exercise or stress induced, most commonly found in paediatric cases and can result in syncope or sudden death (Ernoehazy 2006).

Occasionally, VT will occur for periods where there is no haemodynamic decompensation, but

VT tends to deteriorate into unstable states and more malignant arrhythmias and thus should be treated with antiarrhythmic therapy such as amiodarone or lignocaine. Synchronised cardioversion may be necessary to stabilise the patient if medical therapy fails (Ernoehazy 2006). If VT is associated with significant haemodynamic compromise or deteriorates into VF, basic and advanced life-support guidelines are followed.

Ventricular fibrillation

Ventricular fibrillation results in cardiac arrest and if left untreated is rapidly fatal (Houghton and Gray 2003). Usually simple to recognise, VF (Figure 23.5d) occurs when portions of the ventricular myocardium depolarise independently of each other, at a fast, irregular rate. Co-ordinated ventricular activity and muscular contraction is replaced by a quivering motion, thus cardiac output is critically compromised. Irregular, chaotic and abnormal deflections of varying height and width are evident on the ECG, with no identifiable QRS complexes. VF is most commonly seen in the early phase of MI, often occurring following a ventricular ectopic beat that interferes with repolarisation (R on T ectopic). As discussed above, VF can be precipitated by an episode of VT, which can degenerate into VF.

In VF, the heart ceases to pump and after approximately 10s the blood pressure falls and unconsciousness occurs. If left untreated, death will follow within 3–5 min (Kinney & Packa 1996). VF is the most common cause of sudden cardiac death (Hudak et al. 1998). Sudden cardiac death is discussed in Chapter 14.

Asystole

Asystole (colloquially called 'flat line') refers to the absence of cardiac output and ventricular depolarisation and it eventually occurs in all dying patients. It may occur as a primary condition as a result of the failure of the heart's electrical system to generate a ventricular depolarisation due to conditions such as ischaemia or degeneration of the conducting system. Primary asystole is usually preceded by a bradyarrhythmia due to sinus node block-arrest, complete heart block or both. Secondary asystole is due to factors other than the failure of the heart's conducting system to generate an impulse. Severe tissue hypoxia with metabolic acidosis is usually the common pathway and the outcome is generally poor. Asystole is the terminal rhythm following unresolved VF (Caggiano 2008). The management of cardiac arrest due to asystole is covered in Chapter 14.

Treatment of arrhythmias

Not all arrhythmias are clinically important, and initial treatment is dictated by the effect the arrhythmia has on the individual patient. Where haemodynamic instability is identified, then this should be considered 'time critical' and effective treatment instigated promptly. Left untreated, some arrhythmias may lead to avoidable deterioration in the patient's condition, including cardiac arrest. Stable patients should undergo further assessment and referral as necessary to appropriate specialists.

The Resuscitation Council (UK) (2005), in common with other national and international organisations, publishes guidelines on the management of cardiac arrhythmias which support decision-making in clinical practice. These recommendations provide the focus for the following discussion. Clinical assessment is crucial to identify 'adverse signs' that require prompt management. The reader should note that, in this introductory text, only the 'basics' are covered and that specialist advice should be sought at the earliest opportunity.

Treatment of bradyarrhythmias

Adverse signs associated with bradycardia include a systolic blood pressure below 90 mmHg, a heart rate below 40 bpm, ventricular ectopic beats and indications of heart failure (Resuscitation Council [UK] 2005). If these features are present, cardiac monitoring should be commenced and high-flow oxygen administered without delay. Venous access should also be established at the earliest opportunity.

The drug treatment of choice for the treatment of bradycardia is atropine 500 mcg, administered intravenously and repeated every 3–5 min (depending on response) up to a maximum of 3 mg. This is often effective for sinus bradycardia, but tends to be less so for heart block. Atropine should be used cautiously in the setting of acute myocardial ischaemia or MI where there is a risk of worsening ischaemia by inducing tachycardia (Resuscitation Council [UK] 2005).

Even where atropine produces a favourable response, it is necessary to determine the potential risk of the patient developing asystole. This is most likely to occur if there has already been an episode of asystole or complete heart block, especially if the heart rate is less than 40 bpm (Gretton 2006). If such risk is identified, or there has been no improvement following atropine, cardiac pacing is indicated. The definitive treatment is transvenous pacing (Resuscitation Council [UK] 2005), involving insertion of a pacing catheter under local anaesthetic into the patient's right ventricle via a large vein. This is a specialised procedure that may not be immediately available in the emergency setting. As a 'holding' measure, transcutaneous pacing may be useful although evidence for mortality benefit is poor. External pacing devices are widely available with most modern defibrillators incorporating this facility (Jowett & Thompson 2007). Transcutaneous pacing has the advantages of being non-invasive, quickly established and can be initiated by appropriately trained personnel (although evidence for pre-hospital use remains poor). Adhesive pads applied to the patient's chest deliver an electric shock on 'demand', when the patient's heart rate drops below the rate to which the pacing device has been set. The patient may experience some discomfort, and Gretton (2006) suggests this may be one reason why some health care professionals are reluctant to initiate this procedure. Non-invasive pacing is an emergency treatment and should only be used until transvenous pacing can be instigated. For persistent bradycardia, a permanent pacemaker may need to be fitted.

In the absence of electrical pacing facilities, percussion (or fist) pacing may buy time. Repeated but firm blows are delivered to the patient's chest over the left lower sternum to produce a viable cardiac output. It is most likely to be successful in ventricular standstill where there is P-wave activity (Resuscitation Council [UK] 2005). Alternative drug therapies include intravenous infusions of adrenaline, dopamine or isoprenaline.

Treatment of tachyarrhythmias

Detection of adverse signs associated with tachycardia, such as a systolic blood pressure less than 90 mmHg, heart rate greater than 150 bpm, ischaemic chest pain, signs of heart failure or altered conscious level, should result in the immediate establishment of cardiac monitoring, high-flow oxygen and venous access.

Synchronised DC cardioversion is standard treatment for unstable/compromised patients with tachyarrhythmia, irrespective of whether broad or narrow complex. The principle of delivery is the same as that of defibrillation in cardiac arrest, but the defibrillator must be set to synchronised mode and lower energy levels may be required. It is common to start at a lower energy level than in a cardiac arrest and use increasing energy levels in accordance with manufacturers' instructions. Synchronisation enables the defibrillator to deliver the shock on the R wave of the QRS complex, thus avoiding the vulnerable part of the cardiac cycle and minimising the risk of VF. Another important difference from defibrillation in cardiac arrest is that the arrhythmia patient is often conscious and may require sedation prior to the procedure. A maximum of three shocks are recommended, and where unsuccessful in restoring NSR, drug treatment with intravenous amiodarone 300 mg over 10–20 min is advocated followed by a further synchronised shock and 24 h infusion of 900 mg of amiodarone (Resuscitation Council [UK] 2005).

In stable patients, there is time for more in-depth analysis of the ECG rhythm before proceeding with treatment – the main decision being whether the tachycardia has a broad or narrow QRS complex and whether the rhythm is essentially regular or irregular. Expert advice should be sought where time allows.

Broad-complex tachycardias

As discussed above, broad-complex tachycardia may be due to SVT with aberration, or VT. Careful examination of the 12-lead ECG recording is essential in these patients, and only rarely (e.g. in severe haemodynamic collapse) should treatment be given before this is available. For the non-expert, it is advisable to assume the rhythm is ventricular in origin since this is the more sinister rhythm and poses a greater risk to the patient (Resuscitation Council [UK] 2005). An infusion of amiodarone 300 mg over 20–60 min followed by a maintenance infusion of 900 mg over 24 h is recommended. Careful consideration should be given to possible underlying causes, with particular attention being paid to electrolyte abnormalities, especially potassium levels. Correction of hypokalaemia and associated hypomagnesaemia should be undertaken if present. Patients with broad-complex tachycardia are at high risk of deterioration and require careful monitoring (Gretton 2006).

Patients with an irregular broad-complex tachycardia may have AF with aberrant conduction. Other possibilities include AF with pre-excitation or polymorphic VT (Torsades de Pointes): if the patient is stable, it is unlikely to be the latter. Careful examination of a 12-lead ECG is required, and expert help should be sought to advise on appropriate management.

Narrow-complex tachycardias

Regular NCTs include sinus tachycardia, re-entry tachycardias and atrial flutter with regular AV conduction. As discussed above, sinus tachycardia is not a true arrhythmia but a physiological response, and it is important to determine the underlying cause. Patients with a regular NCT other than sinus tachycardia, and without adverse signs, may be treated initially by manoeuvres to stimulate the vagus nerve. The Valsalva manoeuvre (the patient is asked to force air out against a closed epiglottis, for example by blowing the plunger out of a syringe or by coughing) is simple and often effective. If this fails, carotid sinus massage may be considered by appropriately trained personnel after the presence of carotid bruits has been excluded (Richardson et al. 2000). If these measures are ineffective, adenosine is the initial drug of choice, provided the patient is not known to possess an accessory pathway such as Wolff–Parkinson–White syndrome. Adenosine has a very short half-life and must be administered rapidly to be effective. Vagal manoeuvres or adenosine will terminate most re-entry tachycardias; resistance to these measures would imply the NCT is more likely to be atrial flutter (Resuscitation Council [UK] 2005).

Irregular NCTs are likely to be AF with uncontrolled ventricular response, or possibly atrial flutter with variable block. In stable patients, treatment options include rate control drugs (e.g. beta-blockers, digoxin or magnesium) or rhythm control using either chemical or electrical cardioversion. As previously discussed, the risk of clot formation increases significantly if the arrhythmia has persisted for more than 48h, therefore full anticoagulation and expert guidance are required to help determine appropriate management (Fuster et al. 2001).

Learning activity

Locate your hospital's agreed pathway for patients with arrhythmias, particularly the pathway for AF and determine the evidence base.

Find out which ECG rhythm-interpretation tool is recommended in your hospital and use it (or the one provided in this chapter) to interpret the rhythm for the next 10 patients in your care who are undergoing continuous cardiac monitoring.

Conclusion

Cardiac arrhythmias are one of the main complications in the acute cardiac patient. Effective patient care and intervention depends on accurate assessment, observation and recognition of relevant signs and symptoms. Identification of the arrhythmia can be achieved using a systematic approach, classifying the arrhythmia as either a bradycardia or a tachycardia. Management is determined by the haemodynamic status of the patient. A haemodynamically unstable patient requires prompt intervention, whilst the stable patient allows more time for rhythm analysis. Management of arrhythmias aims to restore sinus rhythm or, if this is not possible, to control the ventricular rate and maximise cardiac output using either drugs or electrical intervention. Patients' haemodynamic tolerance varies and the focus of any intervention should always be the condition of the patient.

References

Bowbrick, S. & Borg, A.N. (2006). *ECG Complete*. Churchill Livingstone, London.

Caggiano, R.M. (2008). Asystole. *eMedicine*. Retrieved online 5th October 2008 from http://www.emedicine.com/EMERG/topic44.htm

Davies, W. (2001). The management of atrial fibrillation. *Clinical Medicine*, **1**:190–3.

Department of Health (2005). *National Service Framework for Coronary Heart Disease. Chapter 8*. HMSO, London.

Ernoehazy, W. (2006). Ventricular tachycardia. *eMedicine*. Retrieved online 5th October 2008 from http://www.emedicine.com/emerg/topic634.htm

Fuster, V., Lyden, R., Asinger, R.W., et al. (2001). American College of Cardiology/American Heart Association Task Force and the European Society of Cardiology Committee for Practice Guidelines and Policy Conferences. ACC/AHA/ESC Guidelines for the Management of Patients with Atrial Fibrillation. *European Heart Journal*, **22**:1852–923.

Gretton, M. (2006). Arrhythmias. In: D. Barrett, M. Gretton & T. Quinn (eds). *Cardiac Care: An Introduction for Healthcare Professionals*. Wiley, Chichester.

Hand, H. (2002). Common cardiac arrhythmias. *Nursing Standard*, **16**:43–53, 58.

Hart, R. & Halpern, J. (2001). Atrial fibrillation and stroke: concepts and controversies. *Stroke*, **32**:8033–8.

Houghton, A.R. & Gray, D. (2003). *Making Sense of the ECG: A Hands-On Guide*. Arnold Publishers, London.

Hudak, C., Gallo, B.M. & Gonce Morton, P. (1998). *Critical Care Nursing: A Holistic Approach*. Lippincott, Williams & Wilkins, Philadelphia.

Jacobsen, C. (2005). Arrhythmias and conduction disturbances. In S.L. Woods, E.S.S. Froelicher, S.U. Motzer & E.J. Bridges (eds). *Cardiac Nursing*, 5th edn, Lippincott, Williams & Wilkins, Philadelphia, pp. 361–424.

Jowett, N. & Thompson, D. (2007). *Comprehensive Coronary Care*. Balliere Tindall, London.

Kinney, M. & Packa, D. (1996). *Comprehensive Cardiac Care*, 8th edn. Mosby, St. Louis.

Lazar, J. & Clark, A.D. (2007). Atrial fibrillation. *eMedicine*. Retrieved online 6th October 2008 from http://www.emedicine.com/EMERG/topic46.htm

Lazar, J. & Parwani, V. (2006). Atrial flutter. *eMedicine*. Retrieved online on 5th October 2008 from http://www.emedicine.com/emerg/TOPIC47.HTM

Navas, S. (2003). Atrial fibrillation: Part 2. *Nursing Standard*, **17**:47–56.

Resuscitation Council (UK) (2005). Peri-arrest arrhythmias. Retrieved online 1st April 2009 from http://www.resus.org.uk/pages/periarst.pdf

Richardson, D., Bexton, R., Shaw, F., et al. (2000). Complications of carotid sinus massage – a prospective series of older patients. *Age and Aging*, **29**:413–17.

Sandesara, C.M. & Olschansky, B. (2006). Atrioventricular dissociation. *eMedicine*. Retrieved online 7th November 2008 from http://www.emedicine.com/Med/topic190.htm

Scheidt, S. (1986). *Basic Electrocardiography*. Ciba-Geigy Pharmaceuticals, New Jersey.

Seidl, K., Rameken, M., Siemon, G. (1999). Atrial flutter and thromboembolism risk. *Cardiology Review*, **16**:25–8.

Thompson, D. & Webster, R. (2004). *Caring for the Coronary Patient*, 2nd edn. Elsevier, London.

Useful Websites and Further Reading

Arrhythmia Alliance: http://www.arrhythmiaalliance.org.uk/

National Institute for Health and Clinical Evidence: http://www.nice.org.uk/nicemedia/pdf/word/TA095guidance.doc

National Library for Health: www.library.nhs.uk/cardiovascular

Resuscitation Council (UK): http://www.resus.org.uk/

Plummer, B. (2007). ECG challenge: how strip savvy are you? *American Journal of Nursing*, **107**:72A–C.

24 In-Hospital Resuscitation

C. Oldroyd, T. Quinn & P. Whiston

Overview

The incidence of in-hospital cardiac arrest is difficult to assess, but it is apparent that survival rates to discharge are very poor. The 'Chain of Survival' concept has formed the basis of international efforts to improve outcomes from cardiac arrest over recent decades, influencing organisation of resuscitation services within the hospital setting (Perkins & Soar 2005) and in pre-hospital care. However, despite advances in systems of care and therapeutic interventions, survival rate remains low, especially outside critical care environments (Tunstall-Pedoe et al. 1992). Most in-hospital cardiac arrests are predictable, with up to 84% of patients showing signs of deterioration prior to arrest (Kause et al. 2004). Early recognition and effective treatment may prevent cardiac arrest and also help identify individuals for whom resuscitation is not appropriate or against their wishes (Sandroni et al. 2007). To aid in early detection of critical illness, many hospitals now utilise early warning scores, and in some areas a Medical Emergency Teams (MET) have replaced the traditional cardiac arrest or 'crash' team, enabling patients to be treated as soon as a deterioration in their condition is detected, rather than waiting for cardiac arrest to occur (Lee et al. 1995; Subbe et al. 2001). Of patients resuscitated, over half die before leaving hospital, indicating the vital role

that post-resuscitation care plays in the process (Sandroni et al. 2007). The nurse, therefore, needs to be proficient in both assessment and resuscitation in order to maximise the patient's chances of a successful outcome. This chapter will address the nurses' role in in-hospital resuscitation.

Learning objectives

After reading this chapter, you should be able to:

- Understand the importance of identifying patients at-risk of cardiac arrest.
- Describe the in-hospital resuscitation process and understand how it might differ from a pre-hospital situation.
- Discuss factors contributing to outcomes of in-hospital cardiac arrest.
- Recognise the importance of post-resuscitation care.
- Discuss the need to adopt uniform reporting of outcome after cardiac arrest.

Key concepts

In-hospital cardiac arrest; medical emergency teams; advanced life support; resuscitation education; data collection and quality improvement

Introduction

Cardiac arrest can be defined as the cessation of cardiac mechanical activity, with the absence of a detectable pulse, unresponsiveness and apneoa (Cummins et al. 1997). Estimates of the annual incidence of in-hospital cardiac arrest in the United States alone vary from 370,000 to 750,000 (Sandroni et al. 2007). Reported incidence is in the range of one to five cardiac arrests per 1000 admissions, with coronary artery disease – a leading cause in most cases (Hodgetts et al. 2002).

The causes of adult cardiac arrest can be separated into two distinct categories: primary and secondary (American Association for Respiratory Care [AARC] 2004; Australian Resuscitation Council [ARC] 2006). Primary causes include acute myocardial infarction, cardiomyopathy, electrical shock, congenital heart disease and drug toxicity (AARC 2004; ARC 2006). Secondary causes include hypothermia, airway obstruction, metabolic and electrolyte imbalances, absence of breathing, major bleeding, trauma and neuromuscular disease (AARC 2004; ARC 2006). In the hospital setting, common reasons for cardiac arrest include cardiac arrhythmias, acute respiratory failure and shock (Schneider et al. 1993). Furthermore, cardiac arrest is often precipitated by a rapid deterioration in level of consciousness, arterial blood gas values, vital signs and other physiological observations (AARC 2004).

When cardiac arrest occurs, it is hypothesised that myocardial ischaemia creates ventricular irritability, which facilitates degeneration from ventricular tachycardia (VT) to ventricular fibrillation (VF) and finally asystole (Frenneaux 2003). During the onset of cardiac arrest, ischaemic injury begins to develop, and it is during this time that defibrillation and effective chest compressions are most likely to restore circulation. Prolonged cardiac arrest leads to development of toxic metabolites, depletion of phosphate stores and ischaemic cascade, with high risk of irreversible cellular injury (Dwyer 2007).

Despite technological advances, system improvements and an extensive array of therapeutic options available in the hospital setting, the mortality rate of patients suffering cardiac arrest remains high, with less than 20% of patients surviving to discharge (Tunstall-Pedoe et al. 1992; Peberdy et al. 2003).

Key point

More than two-thirds of patients who regain return of spontaneous circulation (ROSC) die within 24h or are at risk of significant adverse events as a result of resuscitation attempts (Tunstall-Pedoe et al. 1992; Skrifvars et al. 2003; Sandroni et al. 2004), including fractures, hepatic or splenic rupture and prolonged critical care stay.

Factors associated with survival can be divided into two groups: (1) those relating to the patient and (2) those pertaining to the event (Cummins et al. 1997; Sandroni et al. 2007). Factors influencing outcome from cardiac arrest include age, gender, ethnicity and clinical diagnosis (Cummins et al. 1997). Evidence suggests that older adults have a considerably poorer survival rate (Tunstall-Pedoe et al. 1992; Cooper & Cade 1997). Furthermore, a significant relationship has been reported between race and incidence of cardiovascular disease, social influences, financial status, lifestyle and the use of health care facilities contributing to critical outcomes (Ayanian 1993; Sandroni et al. 2007). Clinical diagnoses of sepsis, acute renal failure, metastatic disease and cerebrovascular accident may also be associated with increased mortality (Ebell 1992; Ballew et al. 1994; De Vos et al. 1999).

The initial monitored rhythm observed during cardiac arrest may profoundly affect the chance of survival (Sandroni et al. 2007). Higher probability of recovery is reported in patients with VT and VF (Huang et al. 2002; Peberdy et al. 2003; Resuscitation Council [UK] 2005; Sandroni et al. 2007). Most adult survivors of in-hospital cardiac arrest suffer VF caused by myocardial ischaemia and irritability (Smith 2005). VT/VF are reported as the initial arrhythmia in 20–35% of in-hospital cardiac arrests; more commonly hypoxia and hypotension are precursors to pulseless electrical activity (PEA) and asystole (Peberdy et al. 2003; Skrifvars et al. 2003). Other factors influencing survival include a witnessed arrest and presence of cardiac monitoring, duration of event, time delay and implementation of advanced life support (ALS), location of the patient and time of day (Sandroni et al. 2007). In addition, patients who suffer cardiac arrest in non-monitored (general ward) areas have particularly low survival-to-discharge rates (Smith 2005; Perkins & Soar 2005), with arrests in such circumstances often not related to underlining cardiac disease, usually predictable and following a slow period of progressive physiological deterioration (Smith 2005).

It is clear that those patients who receive prompt defibrillation require a short period of resuscitation and those who have no or minimal co-morbidities have the greatest chance of successful outcome. Meaningful neurological status (cerebral performance category of one) at discharge has been reported in around 60% of survivors (Danciu et al. 2004).

Prevention: systems for identifying patients at risk of cardiac arrest

Hospitals have experienced an increase in acuity over recent years, resulting from a larger volume of patients presenting with more complex disease states and health care needs (Boots & Lipman 2002). General wards are frequently occupied by patients who are elderly, undergoing major medical and surgical interventions or are particularly unwell. These patients require a higher level of care to reduce risk of adverse events and prevent mortality (Elliott 2006).

Acute clinical deterioration can occur at any phase of a patient's hospitalisation. However, there are specific periods in which a patient is arguably more vulnerable, such as at the onset of treatment, during therapeutic intervention and in recovery from critical illness. When deterioration occurs, patients display abnormalities directly related to their airway, breathing and circulation (McQuillan et al. 1998; Kause et al. 2004; Smith 2005), posing a significant threat to their health and increasing the risk of cardiac arrest and subsequent mortality (Smith 2005). It has also been suggested that in some instances, the deterioration of patients in general ward settings is avoidable (Robson 2002). Early recognition of deterioration is essential and should be accompanied by an appropriate response. However, Smith and Poplett (2002) argue that often members of the health care team may not have a clear plan of management for the patient, do not possess the knowledge and skills, or lack confidence in their ability to identify an acute care problem.

The monitoring of vital signs is an essential process for detection of irregularities of cardiovascular, respiratory and neurological origin (Harrison et al. 2005; Smith 2005). A typical physiology is evidenced on a regular basis in the acute care setting, but observations and key indicators of impending critical illness are often overlooked or examined infrequently (Smith 2005). Evidence suggests that cardiac arrests rarely occur in isolation, and may often be predictable, and preceded by easily recognisable changes in vital signs and physiological abnormalities (Hodgetts et al. 2002; Sandroni et al. 2007). Patients may display a period of slow progressive deterioration, that is often not recognised or adequately treated (Goldhill et al. 1999; Kause et al. 2004). Specific areas for concern include:

- Inappropriate use of oxygen therapy
- Inadequate monitoring of patients
- Failure to consult with experienced staff in the care of the acutely ill
- Failure to use a systematic approach to the assessment of critically ill patients
- Poor communication
- Lack of teamwork
- Insufficient use of treatment limitation plans (Smith & Poplett 2002; Smith 2005)

Failure to appreciate clinical urgency, lack of knowledge and organisation, and medical staff not reviewing patients in a timely fashion when nurses have raised concern are important factors in helping to prevent deterioration (McQuillan et al. 1998).

Key point

Early recognition of clinical deterioration in patients is essential to prevent the high mortality associated with cardiac arrest. A logical and organised approach is, therefore, desirable to provide timely intervention and help prevent deterioration (McQuillan et al. 1998).

Learning activity

Reflective thinking activity

Smith (2005) has outlined a number of hospital processes that have significant effects on patient outcomes. Explore the following observations and decide whether you think this applies in your workplace:

Patients who are discharged from intensive care units (ICU) to general wards at night have an increased risk of in-hospital death compared to those discharged during the day.

Patients who are discharged from ICU to general wards at night have an increased risk of in-hospital death compared to those discharged to high-dependency units.

Higher nurse–patient staffing ratios are also associated with reduction in cardiac arrest rates, as well as rates of pneumonia, shock and death.

Physiological observations of sick patients are not measured frequently enough or adequately – the respiratory rate particularly is essential, as it may predict cardiorespiratory arrest, and yet this is often overlooked.

Recommended strategies for the prevention of avoidable cardiac arrest

As described earlier, survival rates following in-hospital cardiac arrest are poor (Peberdy et al. 2003). Prevention, therefore, assumes great importance. A number of strategies to facilitate the early detection of critically ill patients and reduce the risk of cardiac arrest have been outlined in Box 24.1.

Early recognition and management of critically ill patients

The 'Chain of Survival' concept has formed the basis for the implementation of national and international efforts to prevent mortality from cardiac arrest over recent decades (Cummins et al. 1991; Cummins 1993). The foundations for this theory are based on the 'rescue chain' model for emergency medicine (Cummins et al. 1991) and the chain is comprised of four links:

(1) Early access to mobilise emergency resources and provision of prompt defibrillation
(2) Early basic life support (BLS)
(3) Early defibrillation and
(4) Early ALS (Cummins et al. 1991)

Although the Chain of Survival concept has influenced the development of in-hospital resuscitation

---

Box 24.1   Strategies to facilitate the early detection of critically ill patients

- Admit acutely ill patients (and those identified as at-risk of physiological decline) to hospital areas where high acuity care can be delivered.
- All patients at high-risk of cardiac arrest should be cared for in a monitored area, with facilities for immediate resuscitation.
- Co-ordinate the frequency and extent of observations to the acuity of the patient.
- Use a vital signs chart that encourages and facilitates regular measurement and frequent documentation of observations.
- Ensure easy access to concise guidelines that outline the specific roles of health care professionals in responding to acute deterioration of patients.
- Each hospital should have a strategic plan to deal with medical emergencies response.
- All clinical staff should be equipped with the necessary skills to enable early observation and detection of critically ill patients.
- There should be an ongoing audit on all cardiac arrests and antecedent events. Unplanned admissions/re-admissions to intensive care should also be audited for future planning, education and quality assurance activities.
- Ensure that Advanced Directives and DNR orders are in place where appropriate (Smith 2005; Sandroni et al. 2007).

---

strategies (Spearpoint et al. 2000), it appears that cardiac arrests are often not recognised promptly; nor is intervention from skilled staff always timely (Hillman et al. 2001). Traditionally, cardiac arrest teams, compromised of individuals who are competent in resuscitation, have responded to a cardiac arrest call, but it has been reported that survival-to-hospital discharge was only seen in patients who had ROSC prior to arrival of the resuscitation team (Soar & McKay 1998). It is important to consider the obstacles that potentially influence the outcome for a patient in cardiac arrest. These include:

- Members of the team come from different locations within the hospital.
- Members of the team have other responsibilities and may be occupied at the time of the call.

- Hospitals are set over a large geographical area with multiple levels and it can take a considerable amount of time to reach the location of the arrest.
- Resuscitation team members are often unaware of the patient's medical history of circumstances leading to the arrest.

A range of strategies have been suggested to improve outcomes, to address the poor outcomes from cardiac arrest. Among these are early warning scoring systems (EWS), medical emergency teams (MET), 'patient at-risk' teams (PART), intensive care liaison nurses and integrated outreach programs (Gao et al. 2007). Common elements include early recognition and detection of patients with potential or established critical illness, timely attendance by appropriately skilled staff and admission to intensive care ser-vices (Gao et al. 2007). Such systems aim to identify and manage high-risk patients through collaborative care, education, expert experience and empowerment (Bright et al. 2004).

Early warning scoring systems

EWS aim to detect early changes in patient's vital signs and identify abnormal premonitory symptoms prior to physiological decline in areas other than critical care units (Sharpley & Holden 2004). Modified EWS incorporate parameters such as oxygen requirements, urine output and neurological status (Gao et al. 2007). The aggregated score from one or more observations or the total EWS is then used as a 'trigger' to alert staff to impending patient deterioration (Subbe et al. 2003). There are, however, few robust data examining the introduction of EWS. Criticisms of EWS include a lack of sensitivity and specificity and lack of validation of their ability to identify and detect deterioration in the acutely ill patient (Naeem & Montenegro 2005; Cuthbertson & Smith 2007; Gao et al. 2007), and there is some evidence to suggest that existing EWS fail to utilise appropriate variables to detect acutely ill patients or use the wrong cut-off points (Cuthbertson & Smith 2007). Moreover, health professionals who conduct observations may not always be aware of the implications of abnormal findings; more complex systems may result in inaccurate calculation of scores (Naeem & Montenegro 2005).

Medical emergency teams/patient at-risk teams

MET and PART have been developed to replace traditional cardiac arrest teams (Lee et al. 1995; Goldhill et al. 1999). MET comprised of nursing and medical staff from critical care (or general medical officers proficient in all aspects of ALS and resuscitation) respond not only to cardiac arrests, but also to predefined situations of patient deterioration based on abnormal vital sign parameters (Lee et al. 1995; Parr et al. 2001). Many hospitals also include a 'worried' or 'concerned' category for alerting the MET for patients who do not display abnormal parameters but may be at risk of deterioration (such as those with chest pain or confusion) (Parr et al. 2001). Interventions provided by the MET include stabilisation of the airway, breathing and circulation support, ALS, transfer to critical care services and the implementation of 'Do Not Resuscitate' (DNR) orders where appropriate (Parr et al. 2001; Naeem & Montenegro 2005). It has been suggested that MET may assist in the education of general ward clinicians, provide an opportunity for the involvement of experienced medical officers in the care of the acutely ill patient and assist in development of quality improvement systems to increase overall standards of care (Kerridge 2000).

Studies of the impact of MET and PART have reported mixed results (Lee et al. 1995; Parr et al. 2001; Jaques et al. 2006). In some studies, implementation of such services appear to have reduced cardiac arrest rates, unplanned intensive care admissions, post-operative morbidity, occurrence of specific disease states and increased detection of medical errors (Bristow et al. 2000; Braithwaite et al. 2004; Jones et al. 2005), while others have reported difficulties in demonstrating such benefits. Evaluation of such systems is recognised as complex, and study findings may have been influenced by differences in implementation strategies and institutional characteristics (Kerridge 2000; Parr et al. 2001). Another reason may relate to the criteria for alerting teams (McArthur-Rouse 2001) with some considering early experience to be based upon late signs of deterioration and studies (Hillman et al. 2005; Cuthbertson & Smith 2007). Several studies have been limited by small sample size, use of historical controls and non-randomised comparisons. Further research is required to assess the utility of such systems in a variety of hospitals involving similar case mix and locations (Naeem & Montenegro 2005).

Critical care outreach and intensive care liaison nurses

Critically ill patients are increasingly managed outside of ICUs. As a result, critical care outreach teams and intensive care liaison nurse roles have emerged, and these are comprised of clinicians trained in critical care with support from experienced medical staff. The focus is on early detection and intervention for the acutely ill ward patient, in addition to taking an active role in supporting discharge from the ICU and facilitation of timely admission. The role also involves education and support of ward staff (Ball et al. 2003; Bright et al. 2004). Team composition, working patterns and activity varies, and a number of different service models have emerged to suit local needs. Some authors have questioned the value of such systems in relation to ability to simply 'troubleshoot' problems, rather than address underling causes (Riley & Falerio 2001).

In-hospital resuscitation

In the hospital setting, cardiopulmonary resuscitation involves both BLS and ALS, with the division between the two being subjective (Resuscitation Council [UK] 2005). Cardiopulmonary resuscitation is not an isolated procedure, rather a series of assessments and interventions aimed at saving life and reducing disability (American Heart Association 2005). Resuscitation should be regarded as a continual process based upon the principles incorporated in the Chain of Survival concept described earlier (AARC 2004; Perkins & Soar 2005). Interventions may vary in this process depending on the underlining cause of the arrest (American Heart Association 2005). BLS aims to maintain coronary and cerebral perfusion through support of the airway, breathing and circulation, without the use of equipment until more definitive treatment can be initiated. ALS combines BLS with the use of drugs, specialist techniques and equipment to maintain circulation and respiration

(Jowett & Thompson 2007). Adequate resuscitation attempts are extremely important in order to preserve life and prevent disability; however, the nature of the process will be influenced by site of arrest, availability and clinical expertise of staff, response time, type of equipment and implemented resuscitation system (AARC 2004; Resuscitation Council [UK] 2005; Sandroni et al. 2007).

Basic life support

Effective BLS can be implemented by both health care professionals and trained members of the community (Resuscitation Council [UK] 2005). For clinicians working in the acute care setting, knowledge of this process is essential and in many institutions accreditation is mandatory (AARC 2004). When a cardiac arrest occurs in the hospital environment, it is expected that the staff involved in the care of the patient are able to carry out a series of standard actions. These form the basis of the first three links in the chain of survival and include:

- Immediate recognition of cardiac arrest.
- Call for help (resuscitation/MET) using a predetermined emergency number.
- Commence cardiopulmonary resuscitation (using simple airway devices).
- Defibrillate within 3 min, if automated external defibrillator (AED) and trained staff are available (Cummins et al. 1991; AARC 2004; Perkins & Soar 2005; Resuscitation Council [UK] 2005).

Team activation

Hospitals have designated emergency response teams, the nature varying as described above (Resuscitation Council [UK] 2005). Many teams are devised to meet local need but regardless of the approach, a designated emergency response team should be continuously available, 24 h a day, 7 days a week (AARC 2004). All team members should be alerted simultaneously (AARC 2004; Resuscitation Council [UK] 2005). All health care workers must be familiar with local policies and procedures relating to emergency team activation (AARC 2004). In specialised areas such as the cardiac care unit, critical care and emergency departments, team activation may not be necessary as clinicians in these areas will often possess ALS skills.

Guidelines for first responders

Hospital staff are often skilled in resuscitation techniques more appropriate to the lay person in a community environment, and guidelines have been published (Nolan et al. 2005; Resuscitation Council [UK] 2005; Australian Resuscitation Council 2006) for those likely to be first responders

in the hospital setting. The Resuscitation UK algorithm for initial management of in-hospital cardiac arrest is shown in Figure 24.1.

Guidelines for BLS and ALS are reviewed and updated periodically following detailed evaluation of published evidence (Sandroni et al. 2007). A pulse check to verify cardiac arrest should generally be carried out by knowledgeable clinicians only (Resuscitation Council [UK] 2005), and the correct position for compressions should be ascertained by placing the heel of the hand on the centre of the chest (Handley 2002). BLS should be undertaken

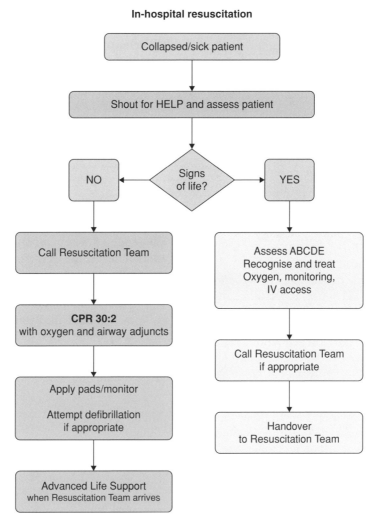

Figure 24.1   Initial management of in-hospital cardiac arrest.
Source: From Resuscitation Council UK, *2005 Resuscitation Guidelines.*

at a rate of 100 compressions per minute (a cycle of 30 compressions to two ventilatory breaths) to a depth of 4–5 cm (Nolan et al 2005). The greater emphasis on chest compressions in current guidelines is aimed at reducing interruptions to help improve the likelihood of successful outcome (Nolan et al. 2005; Sandroni et al. 2007).

Early cardiopulmonary resuscitation and defibrillation

The earlier patients receive cardiopulmonary resuscitation, the greater the chance of survival. In addition, CPR extends the 'time window' for successful resuscitation and can double the chances of survival in a witnessed cardiac arrest (Waalewijn et al. 2001). Defibrillation is performed to terminate VF or pulseless VT and restore a cardiac rhythm capable of maintaining cardiac output, tissue perfusion and oxygenation. Early defibrillation is one of the most important factors in determining survival (Resuscitation Council 2006). Evidence suggests that delay from collapse to the delivery of the first shock is the single most important factor in determining outcome, chances of successful defibrillation declining at a rate of 7–10% for every minute of delay thereafter, in the absence of BLS (Nolan et al. 2005). If BLS is commenced, mortality decreases more gradually, averaging 3–4% per minute from collapse to defibrillation (Resuscitation Council [UK] 2006). BLS helps to maintain a shockable rhythm, it is not a definitive treatment, and conversion to a perfusing rhythm is still dependant upon defibrillation (American Heart Association 2005).

Within hospital, Powers and Martin (2002) have suggested that delayed defibrillation is a fundamental weakness that may contribute to low-survival rates, especially outside emergency or critical care environments. Manual defibrillation may be performed by the resuscitation team, but introduction of AEDs has brought defibrillation within the capabilities of the first responder (American Heart Association 2005). Traditionally, hospital resuscitation has relied on initiation of BLS and summoning the cardiac arrest team, with resultant delays as described earlier. Training of more hospital personnel in ALS has the potential to further

improve chances of survival. A new 'Immediate Life Support' (ILS) course focusing on simple airway adjuncts and automated defibrillation, and requiring less intensive training (Hatfield 2006) may be more suitable (Resuscitation Council [UK] 2006).

Automated external defibrillators (AEDs) are becoming increasingly popular in the general ward environment (American Heart Association 2005). AEDs are portable and analyse the heart rhythm, prompting the user to deliver a shock if required. Use of AEDs is discussed in more detail in Chapter 15.

Working within your scope of practice

Clinicians involved in resuscitation in the hospital setting have different levels of competence and should only work within their scope of practice, utilising the skills in which they are proficient (AARC 2004). Clinicians and institutions must accept accountability for annual training, evaluation and performance monitoring of resuscitation procedures and skills. This should occur at frequent intervals in order to ensure safe and effective care (AARC 2004).

It is important for health professionals to have an understanding of their role in a resuscitation attempt. Clinicians not trained in ALS play an important role even after arrival of the resuscitation team, for example in ensuring accurate handover of details of the patient's diagnosis and events leading up to the acute event, assistance with chest compressions, attaching monitoring equipment and defibrillating under direction from the resuscitation team leader, documenting the event, moving and collecting required equipment, and liaising with family members and other staff involved in the patient's care (AARC 2004).

Advanced life support

Clinicians employed in critical care areas have often undertaken postgraduate qualifications in recognition and management of critical illness and cardiac arrest, becoming primary members of the resuscitation team and responding to calls both in and outside designated clinical areas (AARC 2004).

Clinicians with a primary role in resuscitation teams practice in line with ALS guidelines (Resuscitation Council [UK] 2004). VT and VF require prompt defibrillation; other rhythms such as asystole and PEA do not respond to defibrillation (Resuscitation Council [UK] 2005). During CPR, attempts to reduce time between compressions and shock delivery should be emphasised to increase likelihood of successful outcome (Resuscitation Council [UK] 2005). During prolonged resuscitation, attempts should be made to identify and treat potential underlying causes (Resuscitation Council [UK] 2005). Additional responsibilities include continuous monitoring, observation and assessment of the adequacy of airway, breathing (ventilation) and circulation, level of consciousness, evidence of seizure, interpretation of diagnostic data and the administration of sedatives, and/or paralysing agents (AARC 2005; Resuscitation Council [UK] 2005).

Resuscitation should continue until ROSC is achieved and signs of life restored (AARC 2004), in which case post-resuscitation care (see later) commences. If ROSC is not achieved, resuscitation attempts should continue until the appropriate senior medical officer determines that continuing interventions are futile (AARC 2004). Once resuscitation efforts have ceased, events should be carefully documented, and the process and performance of those involved reviewed and assessed (AARC 2004).

Equipment

All clinical areas must have immediate access to functioning resuscitation equipment, including defibrillators, airway adjuncts and pharmacologic agents in order to facilitate timely response and intervention (Resuscitation Council [UK] 2005). Under ideal circumstances, layout and equipment used should be consistent across the institution (AARC 2004). Regardless of scope of practice, skill level and training, all clinicians should have a thorough understanding of the location and nature of equipment available in their clinical setting to implement prompt resuscitation (Resuscitation Council [UK] 2005). Ward and resuscitation team members have a responsibility to check that equipment is in working order, with a standard checking procedure completed on a regular basis.

Post-resuscitation care

Around half of hospital patients initially resuscitated following cardiac arrest die before discharge from hospital (Peberdy et al. 2003). Post-resuscitation care forms the final link in the Chain of Survival and may be crucial in determining final outcome. The immediate post-resuscitation phase commences at the point where ROSC is achieved (Perkins & Soar 2005). In the immediate post-resuscitation phase, most patients are clinically unstable, and ongoing systematic assessment of vital functions is required using the ABCDE approach: assessment of adequacy of airway (A), breathing (B) and circulation (C) is followed by assessment of disability (D) (e.g. Glasgow Coma Scale) and the patient fully exposed (E) and examined to ensure that nothing has been overlooked that might have contributed (e.g. haemorrhage) to the arrest or occurred (such as injury) as a consequence of the arrest (Hatfield 2006).

Continuing care of the patient in the location where the cardiac arrest occurred will not always be appropriate, and transfer to a more suitable environment such as a cardiac care or critical care unit, or cardiac catheter laboratory may be required. Definitive treatment should not be delayed, but where possible the patient's condition should be stabilised prior to transfer (Resuscitation council [UK] 2004), including assessment and management of pain and distress. Appropriately trained staff should accompany patients to the destination department, fully equipped to provide ALS again should the patient deteriorate en route, and relatives should be informed. Following admission to the destination (e.g. critical care) unit, intensive therapies such as mechanical ventilation, dialysis, circulatory support and neurological monitoring may be implemented as indicated (Resuscitation Council [UK] 2005).

A 12-lead ECG is essential and may provide information on the underlying cause (for instance, ST-elevation myocardial infarction). Other interventions that should be considered in the immediate post-resuscitation phase include drawing venous blood samples and arterial blood gases. A chest X-ray will be needed to exclude possible skeletal damage that might have occurred during CPR and to confirm positioning of central lines, pacing wires or drains that may have been inserted. Other interventions such as insertion of a urinary catheter will facilitate ongoing monitoring. Recent studies have suggested that mild therapeutic hypothermia in the early post-resuscitation care phase may improve outcome in adult patients who remain unconscious after ROSC from cardiac arrest due to VT/VF (Perkins & Soar 2005). Nolan et al. (2003) recommend that patients should be cooled to 32–34°C and this temperature maintained for 12–24h. Abella et al. (2005) suggest that hypothermia is underused after resuscitation from cardiac arrest, although further research is required to fully evaluate this aspect of care.

There are currently no reliable predictors of outcome from cardiac arrest. However, there are four clinical signs that strongly predict death or poor neurological outcome within 24h of the event. These include absent corneal reflex; absent pupillary response; absent withdrawal response to pain and no motor response (Jowett & Thompson 2007).

The drama of a resuscitation attempt and its aftermath should not distract the nurse from the need to maintain the dignity and safety of the patient, nor should the fear and anxiety engendered in both patient and family members be overlooked. In the event of an initially 'successful' resuscitation attempt, both patient and relatives will require sensitive support and often questions arise relating to prognosis. Where the patient does not respond to resuscitation, often grief-stricken relatives will require considerable attention.

Advanced care directives

For many patients admitted to hospital, cardiac arrest may be a terminal event (Sandroni et al. 2007). In other circumstances, the resuscitation process may be traumatic for both the patient and loved ones, resulting in poor functional and neurological outcomes (British Medical Association, Resuscitation Council [UK] & Royal College of Nursing 2007). For those patients identified as at high-risk for cardiac arrest, early assessment of their condition may assist in identifying those for whom resuscitation measures are not considered appropriate (Sandroni et al. 2007). In patients with terminal illness, life-threatening disease or trauma where death is imminent, resuscitation attempts may not prolong life and simply extend a painful experience (British Medical Association, Resuscitation Council [UK] & Royal College of Nursing 2007). When these circumstances arise, the senior medical officer in collaboration with the patient and members of the health care team may choose to discuss the risks, benefits and likely outcomes associated with the resuscitation process (British Medical Association, the Resuscitation Council [UK] & Royal College of Nursing (2007) This may assist the patient and family with making well-informed decisions based upon their wishes. The nursing role in this process includes the clarification of information, the provision of psychological and emotional support to both the family and patient, and the implementation of palliative care if required (Elliott et al. 2006).

Advanced care planning and the implementation of DNR orders should be carried out in the early phases of the patients admission, allowing time for the patient and family members to process the facts, avoiding the making of quick decisions upon acute deterioration and critical illness (British Medical Association, Resuscitation Council [UK] & Royal College of Nursing 2007). Once a decision has been made, it must be clearly documented and members of the health care team should be updated. It is important to understand that these orders may be subject to change, and decisions regarding CPR should be reviewed at frequent intervals and viewed in the context of the patient. In circumstances where no clear, advanced directive or DNR orders exist, there should be a presumption that all health care professionals make all reasonable efforts to attempt resuscitation (British Medical Association, Resuscitation Council [UK] & Royal College of Nursing 2007).

Learning activity

Reflective thinking activity

What resources are available in your clinical setting to support patients and families after cardiac arrest, and when contemplating decisions relating to advanced care directives?

Audit and data collection

The outcome of cardiac arrest and subsequent resuscitation attempts is dependent on a number of factors, particularly early defibrillation and effective chest compressions (Jacobs et al. 2004). Survival rates from cardiac arrest vary considerably between health care systems, but most reported outcome figures are poor. In order to improve outcomes, all potential risk factors and interventions must be carefully assessed, but this process has been hindered by lack of accurate data on structure, process and outcome of care, which Jacobs et al. (2004) suggest is due, in part, to the lack of uniformity in defining and reporting results. Inconsistent reporting makes reliable comparison of results from different studies and health care systems impossible.

In 1991 and 1997, international resuscitation council task forces, now known as the International Liaison Committee on Resuscitation (ILCOR), produced guidelines for the uniform reporting of data for out-of-hospital and in-hospital cardiac arrest: the Utstein Guidelines (Cummins et al. 1991, 1997). The aim of these guidelines was to provide clear and precise definitions of interventions, intervals and outcomes, and the production of templates for reporting of resuscitation attempts. The Utstein template was used extensively and

contributed significantly to a better understanding of resuscitation practices. However, although the original had many benefits, it also had limitations; the two main ones being difficulties in capturing all required data and the focus on patients presenting in VF. A revised version was published in 2004.

The Utstein guidelines have become an important tool for quality assurance and improvement in both pre-hospital and in-hospital settings. The in-hospital version recommends a set of uniform data and 'gold standard' process indicators (such as time to defibrillation), and several outcome indicators to be assessed at regular intervals. Hospitals can incorporate these indicators into a programme for quality monitoring and improvement, which provides feedback, education and training to staff involved in resuscitation.

It is now widely acknowledged that the quality of post-resuscitation care is an important determinant of outcome following cardiac arrest, and many critical care units are involved in the collection and analysis of data on survivors of cardiac arrest. An Utstein template has recently been devised to define the way in which this data is collected, which will allow meaningful comparison. Ultimately, while registry rather than randomised data, this might assist in evaluation of emerging treatment strategies, such as therapeutic hypothermia, in the post-resuscitation phase (Resuscitation Council [UK] 2005). The science of resuscitation continues to develop and the gathering of data throughout the process is essential to improve the outcome of cardiac arrest.

Conclusion

In-hospital cardiac arrests may result from a variety of causes. However, there is evidence to suggest that these events do not occur in isolation, and they may be predictable and preceded by a period of acute deterioration (Sandroni et al. 2007). Despite technological advancements and improvements in therapeutic interventions, unexpected hospital deaths are cause for alarm: survival rate to discharge remains low (Resuscitation Council [UK] 2005). The notion that early recognition and prevention of deterioration is of paramount importance has influenced the development and implementation of a range of strategies for detecting and managing impending physiological collapse. However, the usefulness of such strategies in the clinical setting remains to be fully demonstrated. There is a need for clinicians to become proactive and proficient in their approach to patient assessment, and the implementation of resuscitation and post-resuscitation care. This may assist in the reduction of associated deaths from in-hospital cardiac arrest and provide the potential for successful patient outcomes.

References

Abella, B., Rhee, J., Huang, K. et al. (2005). Induced hypothermia is underused after resuscitation from cardiac arrest: a current practice survey. *Resuscitation*, **64**:181–6.

American Association for Respiratory Care (AARC) (2004). Resuscitation and defibrillation in the health care setting, revision and update. *Respiratory Care*, **49**:1085–9.

American Heart Association (2005). Guidelines for cardiopulmonary resuscitation and emergency cardiovascular care. Part 3: Overview of CPR. *Circulation*, **112**:IV-12–18.

Australian Resuscitation Council (2006). *Policy Statements*. ARC, Melbourne.

Ayanian, J. (1993). Heart disease in black and white. *New England Journal of Medicine*, **329**:656–8.

Ball, C., Kirkby, M. & Williams, S. (2003). Effect of the critical care outreach team on patient survival to discharge from hospital and readmission to critical care: non-randomised population based study. *British Medical Journal*, **327**:1014–22.

Ballew, K., Philbrick, J., Caven, D. & Schorling, J. (1994). Predictors of survival following in-hospital CPR: a moving target. *Archives of Internal Medicine*, **154**:2426–32.

Boots, R. & Lipman, J. (2002). High dependency units: issues to consider in their planning. *Anaesthesia and Intensive Care*, **30**:348–54.

Braithwaite, R., De Vita, M., Simmons, R., et al. (2004). Use of medical emergency team (MET) responses to detect medical errors. *Quality and Safety Health Care*, **13**:255–9.

Bright, D., Walker, W., Bion, J. et al. (2004). Clinical review: outreach – a strategy for improving the care of the acutely ill hospitalized patient. *Critical Care*, **8**:33–40.

Bristow, P., Hillman, K., Chey, T., et al. (2000). Rates of in-hospital arrests, deaths and intensive care admissions: the effect of a medical emergency team. *Medical Journal of Australia*, **173**:236–40.

British Medical Association, the Resuscitation Council (UK) & Royal College of Nursing (2007). Decisions relating to cardiopulmonary resuscitation. Retrieved online 10th October 2007 from http://www.rcn.org.uk/__data/assets/pdf_file/0004/108337/003206.pdf

Cooper, S. & Cade, J. (1997). Predicting survival, in in-hospital cardiac arrests: resuscitation survival variables and training effectiveness. *Resuscitation*, **35**:17–22.

Cummins, R. (1993). Emergency medical services and sudden cardiac arrest 'the chain of survival concept.' *Annual Review of Public Health*, **14**:313–33.

Cummins, R., Ornato, J., Thies, W. & Pepe, P. (1991). Improving survival from sudden cardiac arrest: the 'chain of survival' concept. A statement for health professionals from the Advanced Life Support Subcommittee and the Emergency Cardiac Care Committee, American Heart Association. *Circulation*, **83**:1832–47.

Cummins, R., Chamberlain, D., Hazinski, M., et al. (1997). Recommended guidelines for reviewing and conducting resuscitation on in-hospital resuscitation: the in-hospital 'Utstein Style.' *Circulation*, **95**:2213–39.

Cuthbertson, B. & Smith, G. (2007). A warning on early-warning scores! *British Journal of Anaesthesia*, **98**:704–6.

Danciu, S.C., Klein, L., Hosseini, M.M., et al. (2004). A predictive model for survival after in-hospital cardiopulmonary arrest. *Resuscitation*, **62**:35–42.

De Vos, R., Koster, R., De Haan, R., et al. (1999). In-hospital CPR: prearrest morbidity and outcome. *Archives of Internal Medicine*, **159**:845–50.

Dwyer, T. (2007). 'Resuscitation' in D. Elliott, L. Aitken, W. Chaboyer, Eds. ACCCN's Critical care Nursing. Marrickville, N.S.W.: Elsevier Australia.

Ebell, M. (1992). Prearrest predictors of survival following in-hospital CPR: a meta analysis. *Journal of Family Practice*, **34**:845–50.

Elliott, M. (2006). Readmission to intensive care: a review of the literature. *Australian Critical Care*, **19**:96–104.

Frenneaux, M. (2003). CPR: some physiological considerations. *Resuscitation*, **58**:259–65.

Gao, H., McDonnell, A., Harrison, D., et al. (2007). Systematic review and evaluation of physiological track and trigger warning systems for identifying at-risk patients on the ward. *Intensive Care Medicine*, **33**:667–79.

Goldhill, D.R., Worthington, L., Mulcahy, A., et al. (1999). The patient-at-risk team: identifying and managing seriously ill ward patients. *Anaesthesia*, **54**:853–60.

Handley, A. (2002). Teaching hand placement for chest compressions: a simpler technique. *Resuscitation*, **53**:29–36.

Harrison, G.A., Jacques, T.C., Kilborn, G. & McLaws, M.L. (2005). The prevalence of recordings of the signs of critical conditions and emergency responses in hospital wards – the SOCCER study. *Resuscitation*, **65**:149–57.

Hatfield, J. (2006). Resuscitation. In: D. Barrett, M. Gretton & T. Quinn (eds), *Cardiac Care: An Introduction for Healthcare Professionals*. Wiley, Chichester.

Hillman, K., Parr, M., Flabouris, A., et al. (2001). Redefining in-hospital resuscitation: the concept of the medical emergency team. *Resuscitation*, **48**:105–110.

Hillman, K., Chen, J., Cretikos, M., et al. (2005). Introduction of the medical emergency team (MET) system: a cluster-randomised controlled trial. *The Lancet*. **365**:2091–7.

Hodgetts, T., Kenward, G., Vlackonikolis, I., et al. (2002). Incidence, location and reasons for avoidable in-hospital cardiac arrest in a district general hospital. *Resuscitation*, **54**:115–123.

Huang, C., Chen, W., Ma, M., et al. (2002). Factors influencing the outcomes after in-hospital resuscitation in Taiwan. *Resuscitation*, **53**:265–70.

Jacobs, I., Nadkani, V., Bahr, J. et al. (2004). Cardiac arrest and cardiopulmonary resuscitation outcome reports: update and simplification of the Utstein templates for resuscitation registries. A statement for healthcare professionals from a taskforce of the International Liaison Committee on Resuscitation. *Resuscitation*, **63**:233–49.

Jaques, T., Harrison, D., McLaws, M. & Kilborn, G. (2006). Signs of critical conditions and emergency responses (SOCCER): a model for predicting adverse events in the inpatient setting. *Resuscitation*. **69**:175–183.

Jones, D., Bellomo, R., Bates, S., et al. (2005). Long term effect of a medical emergency team on cardiac arrests in a teaching hospital. *Critical Care*, **9**:808–15.

Jowett, N. & Thompson, D. (2007). *Comprehensive Coronary Care*. Balliere Tindall, London.

Kause, J., Smith, G., Prytherch, D., et al. (2004). A comparison of antecedents to cardiac arrests, deaths and emergency intensive care admissions in Australia and New Zealand, and the United Kingdom – the ACADEMIA study. *Resuscitation*, **62**:275–82.

Kerridge, R. (2000). The medical emergency team: no evidence to justify not implementing change. *Medical Journal of Australia*, **173**:228–9.

Lee, A., Bishop, G., Hillman, K. & Daffurn, K. (1995). The medical emergency team. *Anaesthesia and Intensive Care*, **23**:183–6.

McArthur-Rouse, F. (2001). Critical care outreach services and early warning scoring systems: a review of the literature. *Journal of Advanced Nursing*, **36**:696–704.

McQuillan, P., Pilkington, S., Allan, A., et al. (1998). Confidential inquiry into quality of care before admission to intensive care. *British Medical Journal*, **316**:1853–8.

Naeem, N. & Montenegro, H. (2005). Beyond the intensive care unit: a review of interventions aimed at anticipating and preventing in-hospital cardiopulmonary arrest. *Resuscitation*, **67**:13–23.

Nolan, J., Morely, P., Vanden Hoek, T., et al. and ALS task force (2003). Therapeutic hypothermia after cardiac arrest: an advisory statement by the advanced life support task force of the International Liaison Committee on Resuscitation. *Resuscitation*, **57**:221–326.

Nolan, J.P., Deakin, C.D., Soar, J., et al. (2005). European resuscitation council guidelines for resuscitation 2005. Section 4: Adult advanced life support. *Resuscitation*, **67** (Suppl. 1):S39–86.

Parr, M., Hadfield, A., Flabouris, A., et al. (2001). The medical emergency team: 12 month analysis of reasons for activation, immediate outcome and not for resuscitation orders. *Resuscitation*, **50**:39–44.

Peberdy, M.A., Kaye, W., Ornato, J.P., et al. (2003). Cardiopulmonary resuscitation of adults in the hospital: a report of 14720 cardiac arrests from the National Registry of Cardiopulmonary Resuscitation. *Resuscitation*, **58**:297–308.

Perkins, G. & Soar, J. (2005). In-hospital cardiac arrest: missing links in the chain of survival. *Resuscitation*, **66**:253–5.

Powers, C.C. & Martin, N.K. (2002). When seconds count, use an AED: in-hospital automated external defibrillators increase chances of patient survival. *American Journal of Nursing*, **102**(Suppl.):8–10.

Resuscitation Council (UK) (2004). Patient transfer and post-resuscitation care. Standards for clinical practice and training. From http://www.resus.org.uk/pages/standard.pdf

Resuscitation Council (UK) (2005). *Resuscitation Guidelines 2005*. Resuscitation Council (UK), London.

Resuscitation Council (UK) (2006). *Advanced Life Support*, 5th edn. Resuscitation Council (UK), London.

Riley, B. & Falerio, R. (2001). Critical care outreach: rationale and development. *British Journal of Anaesthesia*, **1**(15):146–9.

Robson, W.P. (2002). An evaluation of the evidence base related to critical care outreach teams–2 years on from comprehensive critical care. *Intensive Critical Care Nursing*, **18**:211–8.

Sharpley, J. & Holden, J. (2004). Introducing an early warning scoring system in a district general hospital. *Nursing in Critical Care*, **9**(3):98–103.

Sandroni, C., Ferro, G., Santangelo, S., et al. (2004). In-hospital cardiac arrest: survival depends on mainly the effectiveness of the emergency response. *Resuscitation*, **62**:291–7.

Sandroni, C., Noolan, J., Cavallaro, F. & Antonelli, M. (2007). In-hospital cardiac arrest: incidence, prognosis and possible measures to improve survival. *Intensive Care Medicine*, **33**:237–45.

Schneider, A., Nelson, D. & Brown, D. (1993). In-hospital cardiopulmonary resuscitation: a 30-year review. *Journal of American Board of Family Practice*, **6**:91–101.

Skrifvars, M., Rosenberg, P., Finne, P., et al. (2003). Evaluation of the Utstein template in CPR in secondary hospitals. *Resuscitation*, **56**:275–82.

Smith, G. (2005). Prevention of in-hospital cardiac arrest and decisions about cardiopulmonary resuscitation. In: *Resuscitation Council (UK), Resuscitation Guidelines 2005*. From http://www.resus.org.uk/pages/poihca.pdf

Smith, G.B. & Poplett, N. (2002). Knowledge of aspects of acute care in trainee doctors. *Postgraduate Medical Journal*, **78**:335–8.

Soar, J. & McKay, U. (1998). A revised role for the hospital cardiac arrest team? *Resuscitation*, **38**(3):145–9.

Spearpoint, K., McLean, C. & Ziederman, D. (2000). Early defibrillation and the chain of survival in in-hospital cardiac arrest. *Resuscitation*, **5**:297–308.

Subbe, C., Kruger, M., Rutherford, P. & Gemmel, L. (2001). Validation of a modified early warning score in medical admissions. *Quarterly Journal of Medicine*, **94**:521–6.

Subbe, C., Davies, R., Williams, E., Rutherford, P. & Gemmel, L. (2003). Effect of introducing the modified early warning score on clinical outcomes, cardiopulmonary arrests and intensive care utilisation in acute medical admissions. *Anaesthesia*, **58**:775–803.

Tunstall-Pedoe, H., Bailey, L., Chamberlain, D., Marsden, A., Ward, M., Zideman, D. (1992). Survey of 3765 cardiopulmonary resuscitations in British hospitals (The BRESUS study, methods and overall results). *British Medical Journal*, **304**:1347–51.

Waalewijn, R., De Vos, R., Tijssen, J. & Koster, R. (2001). Survival models for out-of-hospital cardiopulmonary resuscitation from the perspectives of the bystander, the first responder, and the paramedics. *Resuscitation*, **51**:113–22.

Useful Websites and Further Reading

In addition to the references listed earlier, you may find the following websites useful.

American Association for Respiratory Care: http://www.aarc.org/

American Heart Association: http://www.americanheart.org/presenter.jhtml?identifier53011764

Australian National Heart Foundation: http://www.heartfoundation.org.au/index.htm

Australian Resuscitation Council: www.resus.org.au

European Resuscitation Council: www.erc.edu

Resuscitation Council (UK): www.resus.org.uk

Royal College of Nursing (UK): http://www.rcn.org.uk/development/communities/specialisms/cardiovascular_nurses

25 Acute Heart Failure

T. Quinn

Overview

Acute heart failure (AHF) is a major health problem, accounting for 1–2% of health expenditure due mainly to the costs of acute hospital care (Berry et al. 2001). An ageing population, combined with improved survival from myocardial infarction (MI), has contributed to AHF being the single most expensive condition overall encountered in contemporary cardiological practice (European Society of Cardiology [ESC] 2005). The prognosis is poor, especially in patients where AHF complicates acute MI: almost one-third will die within 12 months (Stevenson et al. 1993). For patients with acute pulmonary oedema, mortality rates of 12% in hospital and 40% at 1 year demonstrate the gravity of this condition (Roguin et al. 2000). Of those patients admitted to hospital with AHF, almost half will be readmitted at least once in the ensuing year, and a substantial majority will undergo repeat hospitalisation.

Learning objectives

After reading this chapter, you should be able to:

- Define the syndrome of AHF.
- Identify the key causes of, and precipitating factors for, AHF.

- Describe the principal elements of clinical assessment of the patient with AHF.
- Discuss the immediate treatment goals in AHF.
- Examine the main therapeutic options and nursing challenges for AHF care.
- Discuss the role of nurses in reducing readmission to hospital by supporting patients with chronic heart failure in the community setting.

Key concepts

Acute heart failure; pulmonary oedema; cardiogenic shock; oxygenation; ventilatory support

Introduction

Acute heart failure (AHF) is defined by the ESC (2005) as the rapid onset of symptoms and signs secondary to abnormal cardiac function. AHF may occur with pre-existing cardiac disease, but also in patients who have no cardiac history. AHF is often life-threatening and requires emergency care.

Acute heart failure is a clinical syndrome with reduced cardiac output, tissue hypoperfusion, increased pulmonary capillary wedge pressure and tissue congestion. There are many causes of, or precipitating factors for, AHF, ranging from acute coronary syndromes to decompensation of chronic heart failure to septicaemia and volume overload, as shown in Table 25.1.

According to registry data, admissions for AHF are evenly split between the sexes, but women with AHF tend to be older than men and more commonly have preserved left ventricular function. Women are also reported to be less likely to have coronary disease and related risk factors but more commonly have hypertension. Treatment appears to differ: both genders receive similar intravenous diuretic regimens, but fewer women received vasoactive therapy, and evidence-based oral therapies are underused in both genders. Women consistently received less procedure-oriented therapy (e.g. percutaneous intervention and devices), and the length of stay and risk-adjusted in-hospital mortality are similar in both genders (Galvao et al. 2006).

Irrespective of the cause, AHF is associated with insufficient cardiac output to meet the needs of the peripheral circulation, establishing a 'vicious cycle' that, uncorrected, leads to chronic heart failure and death. Correction of the underlying mechanism may reverse the course of AHF, depending on the presence of a reversible cause such as myocardial ischaemia, stunning or hibernation.

Immediate goals for the care of the patient with suspected AHF focus on:

- Establishing the diagnosis
- Alleviating distress
- Providing definitive treatment to improve haemodynamics and reduce the risk of death.

Key point

The patient with AHF presents several challenges to the nurse: supporting distressed patients and carers, working with other members of the health care team to establish the diagnosis and provide increasingly complex packages of care to alleviate symptoms and achieve haemodynamic stability, and to reduce the risk of death or complications, while maintaining dignity and safety.
Immediate care needs: resuscitation and symptom relief

In the absence of a palpable pulse, resuscitation, including advanced life support, should be provided in line with standard guidelines. Where arrhythmias (e.g. atrial fibrillation) are identified as the cause of, or thought to be aggravating, AHF, then standard treatments as discussed in Chapter 23 should be considered under specialist guidance.

Key point

The patient with AHF can be extremely distressed and unwell on presentation. Care should ideally be provided by expert cardiology staff in designated areas (ESC 2005) but in the 'real world' this will not always be achievable in the first few minutes and hours, where ambulance, emergency department and general medical personnel will often play a main role in resuscitation and symptom relief. All such staff should be aware of, and practice under, locally agreed protocols and pathways derived from published evidence-based guidelines.

Establishing the diagnosis

Diagnosis is based on symptoms and clinical findings supported by investigations including 12-lead ECG, chest radiograph, echocardiography and biomarkers. These are discussed in more detail in this chapter. As with all such investigations, it is important that competent professionals, taking into account the clinical context of the individual patient, undertake the interpretation of test results appropriately.

Clinical features

The patient may often have a history of chronic heart failure or acute MI, but other causes (Table 25.1) need to be identified so that appropriate treatment can begin, or excluded.

The principal presenting features in AHF are those associated with fluid overload and reduced cardiac output (Table 25.2). Symptoms remain the most important method of diagnosing overt AHF. Pulmonary rales and peripheral oedema may be absent in a majority of patients during the chronic

Table 25.1   Causes and precipitating factors for AHF.

Cardiac	Non-cardiac
Acute coronary syndromes (e.g. cardiogenic shock, right ventricular infarction)	Anaemia
Acute valvular disease (e.g. severe aortic stenosis, ruptured chordae tendinae, deterioration of pre-existing regurgitation)	Asthma
	Infection (e.g. septicaemia)
Arrhythmias (atrial fibrillation or flutter, other narrow- and broad-complex tachycardias)	Non-concordance with prescribed medication
	Post-operative complication
Aortic dissection	Renal impairment
Cardiac tamponade	Serious brain injury
Decompensation of pre-existing chronic heart failure (including cardiomyopathy)	Substance abuse (drugs, alcohol)
	Thyroid crisis
Hypertensive crisis	Volume overload
Myocarditis	
Post-partum cardiomyopathy	

Table 25.2   Principal clinical features of AHF.

Features indicating fluid overload	Features indicating low cardiac output
Dyspnoea (difficult or laboured breathing)	Tachycardia
Orthopnoea (shortness of breath when lying flat)	Hypotension
Pulmonary inspiratory crackles on auscultation	Cool peripheries
	Slow capillary refill
	Mentally obtunded/confused/drowsy
	Oliguria

phase, but are more pronounced during episodes of decompensation. Positive hepatojugular reflux and Valsalva square-wave signs may indicate elevated filling pressures in acute presentations (Dec 2007).

Key point

It is important to remember that dyspnoea alone is insufficient to diagnose AHF. Lack of physical fitness in patients who are well otherwise often results in exertional dyspnoea, for example. Other conditions associated with dyspnoea include chronic obstructive pulmonary disease (COPD – in some studies, as many as two-fifths of patients with presumed AHF had a history of COPD), asthma, pneumonia and myocardial ischaemia. A prior history of chronic heart failure is an important predictor of a true diagnosis of AHF.

A majority of patients, typically younger and with little or no overt pulmonary congestion, present with AHF with a history of gradual worsening of symptoms, weight gain and peripheral oedema over a period of days, with normal blood pressure and less pulmonary congestion compared to a minority (10–20% of cases) of older, frequently female, patients presenting with hypertension, marked pulmonary oedema and rapid onset (Gheorghiade & Bebazaa 2005). Less than 10% of AHF patients will present with hypotension and marked haemodynamic compromise, and less than 1% with cardiogenic shock (Gheorghiade et al. 2005).

A simple '2-minute' bedside tool for clinical assessment of a patient's haemodynamic status in AHF has been described by Nohria et al. (2003). Physical assessment has been reported to correlate closely with acute haemodynamic measurements and assist in prognostication. In Nohria's paradigm, 'warm and dry' patients have normal haemodynamics and are well compensated at rest, a profile that should prompt the clinician to explore other potential causes (e.g. pulmonary embolism) of acute dyspnoea and related symptoms. Conversely, 'warm and wet' patients – accounting for around half of patients admitted with worsening heart failure – are primarily volume overloaded but with adequate end-organ perfusion. A small minority of patients fall into the 'cold and dry' profile, with impaired cardiac output, and a slightly larger minority of AHF patients will present 'cold and wet', with marked haemodynamic abnormalities on admission as described earlier.

Investigations and monitoring in AHF

Electrocardiography

The 12-lead ECG is an essential component of the initial assessment of the patient with suspected AHF, although the test performs poorly as a predictor of heart failure in the primary care setting (Khunti et al. 2004). ECG abnormalities associated with acute coronary syndromes can guide the use of reperfusion and other treatments to reduce myocardial ischaemia, particularly in the setting of acute ST-segment elevation MI (STEMI). Other ECG abnormalities, such as those associated with right or left ventricular strain, left or right ventricular hypertrophy or dilated cardiomyopathy, may be present. Arrhythmias such as atrial fibrillation, and both broad- and narrow-complex tachycardia, which may have precipitated AHF and be correctable, may also be identified.

> **Key point**
>
> During the acute phase, continuous monitoring of the ECG (alongside other variables such as blood pressure and oxygen saturation) in an appropriate clinical area with staff trained in providing high dependency/critical care is essential.

Chest radiograph – X-ray

The chest X-ray provides important information on heart size and the presence of pulmonary congestion and establishes a useful baseline on which

to assess the impact of treatment. Differential diagnoses such as pneumonia, other respiratory infections and other mediastinal abnormalities may be identified or excluded with the assistance of a carefully interpreted X-ray. Pulmonary embolism and aortic dissection can be excluded using CT scanning and/or transoesophageal echocardiography.

> **Key point**
>
> Classic chest X-ray (CXR) findings include cardiomegaly (in patients with underlying chronic heart failure), alveolar oedema with pleural effusions, fluid in the major fissure, horizontal lines in the periphery of the lower posterior lung fields (Kerley B lines), loss of sharp definition of pulmonary vasculature and the thickening of interlobular septa. However, the diagnostic use of a CXR in abrupt onset AHF may be limited as it can take up to 12 h for the development of classic CXR abnormalities.

Non-invasive monitoring

Non-invasive monitoring systems using bioimpedance (BI) technology allowing the calculation of cardiac output, systemic vascular resistance and thoracic fluid volume are under investigation and may provide a convenient and useful proxy to the collection of invasive haemodynamic measurements (Springfield et al. 2004).

Echocardiography

Echocardiography is considered essential for assessing functional and structural changes associated with AHF. Echocardiography with Doppler is used to assess both regional and global ventricular function, together with the condition and function of heart valves, to exclude pericardial effusion and mechanical complications of MI, and to measure cardiac output (ESC 2005).

Blood gases

Arterial blood gas (ABG) analysis is required in all patients with severe AHF, especially in the presence of a low-output state where the patient is in shock and vasoconstricted. For patients who are not so severely ill, pulse oximetry and end-tidal CO_2 monitoring may be more convenient than ABG analysis, although the latter provides superior evaluation of oxygenation, respiratory adequacy and acid–base balance. It is important to appreciate the limitations of monitoring systems and monitored data, and to understand that invasive monitoring is not without hazard to the patient (Andrews & Nolan 2006).

Laboratory tests

A range of laboratory tests are required routinely, including full blood count, platelet count, C-reactive protein, D-Dimer, urea and electrolytes, blood sugar, and cardiac biomarkers such as troponin T or I. Patients on oral anticoagulation (e.g. warfarin) require measurement of International Normalised Ratio (INR) (ESC 2005).

Plasma B-type natriuretic peptide (BNP), released from the ventricles in response to increased wall stretch and volume load, has good negative predictive value to exclude heart failure, and may help assess prognosis. While considered more accurate than any other single finding on history, examination or laboratory tests (Myerson et al. 2006), BNP may be normal in the early stages of 'flash' pulmonary oedema, and its role has yet to be fully clarified, particularly in older patients where it has been poorly studied. Moreover, other conditions such as septicaemia and renal impairment may affect BNP concentration.

Readily available clinical variables such as blood urea nitrogen levels, serum creatinine and systolic blood pressure have been identified as useful independent predictors of in-hospital mortality in patients with AHF, and may help focus on resource utilisation and intensity of care according to outcome (Adams et al. 2008).

Invasive investigations and monitoring

More invasive investigations such as coronary angiography may be indicated in the presence of AHF complicating STEMI, and where other tests have failed to identify a cause of AHF.

The use of invasive monitoring with pulmonary artery catheters was commonplace in cardiac care and intensive care units for several decades and was thought to be beneficial in patients with AHF (Ivanov et al. 1997), but their use had been called into question by recent findings suggesting lack of mortality benefit (Binanay et al. 2005). Central venous access will usually be required where powerful vasoactive medicines are being administered.

Management specifics

Patients should be nursed in the most comfortable position for them, often sitting upright with appropriate backrest/pillow support, or leaning across a bedside table. There is no 'hard and fast' rule, and for some patients, sitting in an armchair may be the only comfortable position. The nurse, working closely with the patient and other team members, will need to assist the patient to suit individual preferences while maintaining safety and dignity, particularly in the presence of intravenous infusions and monitoring equipment.

Oxygenation

Adequate oxygenation is essential. Maintenance of SaO_2 within the normal range (95–98%) is considered important to maximise oxygen delivery and tissue oxygenation, to reduce the risk of end-organ dysfunction and multiple organ failure. As with acute MI (Nicholson 2004; Wijesinghe et al. 2008), however, there remains uncertainty surrounding the administration of high concentration oxygen in the absence of hypoxaemia.

Non-invasive positive pressure ventilation

If the patient's blood gases fail to improve despite supplementary oxygen, or respiratory distress or exhaustion ensue, then non-invasive positive pressure ventilation (NIPPV) in the form of continuous positive airways pressure (CPAP) ventilation or bi-level positive airway pressure (BiPAP) ventilation may be required. NIPPV has been shown to be effective at improving oxygenation, reducing symptoms and the need for endotracheal intubation in patients with acute cardiogenic pulmonary oedema (Gray et al. 2008; Vital et al. 2008). NIPPV has clear benefits over intubation including:

- Ease of application: it is easy to initiate and remove, can be used intermittently and reduces the need for sedation.

- Avoidance of hazards of intubation: not associated with airway trauma that is experienced by the majority of intubated patients, doesn't bypass upper airway defence mechanisms and decreases the risk of intubation-associated pneumonia that carries a high mortality and increased length of hospital stay.
- Patient comfort: the patient is able to maintain control of breathing, coughing, speaking and swallowing.

In the few instances that NIPPV is ineffective, endotracheal intubation may be required to facilitate mechanical ventilatory support.

Key point

The key to success with NIPPV in acute pulmonary oedema is rapid recognition of the condition and early commencement of NIPPV. Mehta & Hill (2001) suggest that patients with AHF and the following criteria should be considered for NIPPV:

Dyspnoea, shortness of breath, accessory muscle use and respiratory rate > 24.

$SpO_2 < 90$.

ABG analysis results: pH < 7.35; $PaCO_2$ > 45 mmHg; $PaO_2/FIO_2 < 200$.

Pharmacotherapy

Key point

Immediate management aims to reduce preload and afterload using a combination of diuretics and vasodilators. Medicines which may have precipitated heart failure (e.g. non-steroidal anti-inflammatory agents and calcium channel blockers) should be withdrawn. Temporary withdrawal of beta blockers or ACE inhibitors (many AHF patients will be taking such medicines) may also be required while the patient stabilises. Some long-established components of recommended treatment for AHF are, however, the subject of uncertainty regarding safety and efficacy, as discussed below.

Diuretics

Historically, diuretics have been the mainstay, with opiates, of the early management of AHF

associated with fluid retention. The widespread acceptance over many years of diuretics as a means of improving symptoms means, however, that there is a paucity of clinical trial data to quantify the benefits of use in this group of patients. When compared with intravenous nitrates, high-dose furosemide has been shown to be inferior to titration to the highest (haemodynamically) tolerable dose of nitrate. Intravenous administration of loop diuretics such as furosemide or bumetanide, which have a strong and rapid effect, is preferred in the context of AHF, whether in the pre-hospital setting (for example by general practitioners or paramedics) or on hospital admission.

Diuretics decrease plasma and extracellular fluid volume by enhancing the extraction of water, sodium chloride and other ions, leading to increased urine output. This reduces total body water and sodium, and thus peripheral and pulmonary congestion, lowering filling pressures in the ventricles (Conversely, where AHF is thought to be due to low filling pressures as in, for example, right ventricular MI, then intravenous fluids may be required to boost cardiac output). When administered intravenously, loop diuretics cause vasodilation, with a fall in pulmonary resistance, capillary wedge pressure and right atrial pressure, thus adequate monitoring and clinical observation are essential for patient safety. In severe cases of AHF, the possible reduction in neurohormonal activation provided by short-term use may also be beneficial in reducing the vicious cycle of deterioration. Higher intravenous doses paradoxically risk vasoconstriction, and should therefore be avoided or used with caution in acute coronary syndromes, where nitrates may be the preferred approach.

Opiates

Opiate analgesia (morphine or diamorphine) features in international guidelines for AHF and in recent authoritative texts (Myerson et al. 2006), primarily for its vasodilator properties and to relieve acute distress. Despite being in routine use for many years, the haemodynamics effects of morphine in AHF are poorly understood. Morphine has been shown to be associated with increased adverse events, including greater frequency of mechanical ventilation, prolonged admission and increased mortality in a recent analysis of the large

($n = 147{,}362$) Acute Decompensated Heart Failure National Registry (ADHERE) (Peacock et al. 2008). As these findings are based on retrospective analysis of a registry, a prospective trial of the use of morphine (and for that matter, supplementary oxygen as discussed earlier) in AHF is required to provide a definitive answer on the safety of continuing to administer this treatment routinely in AHF patients.

Vasodilators

Vasodilators are recommended as first-line therapy for AHF, provided there is an adequate blood pressure (ESC 2005). Vasodilators are used to 'open up' the peripheral circulation and thus lower preload, and their use is associated with significantly lower in-hospital mortality than positive inotropic therapy in patients with acute decompensated heart failure (Abraham et al. 2005). Emerging vasoactive agents such as nesiritide, tolvaptan and more recently the inotropic agent levosimedan could offer improved haemodynamics and congestive relief to patients in acute pulmonary oedema, but confirmation of their safety and efficacy in further clinical trials are required prior to their international approval as first-line therapy (Gauthier et al. 2008).

Nitrates are used to relieve pulmonary congestion, particularly in patients with acute coronary syndromes. The effects are dose-dependent, and arterial (especially coronary) dilation requires higher doses to achieve than does venodilation. A balance is required between arterial and venodilation to reduce left ventricular preload and afterload, and dosages should be titrated to effect as judged by haemodynamic and clinical parameters, especially blood pressure, aiming for a reduction of 10 mmHg in mean arterial pressure. Nesiritide is another powerful vasodilator associated with immediate reduction in filling pressures and relief of dyspnoea, but has been subject to safety concerns (Sackner -Bernstein et al. 2005).

Key point

Although in common use, nitrates should be used with 'extreme caution' (ESC 2005) under careful monitoring conditions, especially in patients with aortic stenosis. Nitrate tolerance develops within a few hours of continuous infusion, limiting the effective use of this approach to around 24 h.

For patients with severe AHF, especially those with hypertensive heart failure or mitral regurgitation, and thus mainly increased afterload, intravenous infusion of sodium nitroprusside is recommended (ESC 2005), although its use has not been subjected to rigorous evaluation in controlled trials. This treatment should only be administered under close observation including invasive arterial pressure monitoring, and avoided altogether in patients with severe renal or liver impairment. Prolonged use has been associated with cyanide and related toxicity.

Positive inotropic agents

Inotropic agents are potentially life-saving in the severely decompensated AHF patient, where outcome is to a large extent dependent on haemodynamic improvement. However, as with several of the treatments for AHF discussed elsewhere in this chapter, there is a paucity of robust data from clinical trials on their effectiveness in improving symptoms or long-term outcome. These medicines must be used with caution and under specialist guidance, since increases in oxygen consumption and calcium loading associated with inotrope use are potentially harmful to patients. Inotropic drugs are indicated where peripheral hypoperfusion or pulmonary oedema refractory to optimal doses of diuretics and vasodilators are present.

The inotropic agents in common use in AHF are dopamine, dobutamine, the phosphodiesterase inhibitors (milrinone, enoximone), epinephrine, norepinephrine, the cardiac glycosides (e.g. digoxin) and levosimendan. The need for further clinical trials, as mentioned earlier, is an important consideration.

Beta-adrenergic blockers

Beta blockers inhibit excessive sympathetic neurohormonal activation in heart failure. Acute decompensation in the patient with AHF leads to increases in sympathetic neural activity, resulting in peripheral vasoconstriction, impaired renal sodium handling and arrhythmias. In AHF patients already taking a beta blocker, halving of the dose may be necessary in the early, acute phase of admission while haemodynamic and symptomatic stability is achieved using the treatments described earlier. Patients with marked haemodynamic instability should have beta blockers withdrawn until stabilised, and beta blockers should not be 'up-titrated' in the acute phase in the presence of acute volume load of haemodynamic instability. In severe heart failure patients, administration of carvedilol during hospitalisation (provided the patient was not receiving critical care or inotropic support in the preceding 4 days) has been shown to significantly reduce all-cause mortality and subsequent readmission with AHF (Packer et al. 2001).

Refractory AHF

Patients who do not respond to the treatments outlined above are described as being in 'refractory' AHF. Temporary mechanical circulatory support may be required in such patients. The key options for mechanical assistance are intra-aortic balloon counterpulsation or 'balloon pump' (IABP) and ventricular assist devices.

Intra-aortic balloon pump

The IABP has been available for several decades and is used in patients where AHF is refractory to fluid administration, vasodilators and inotropic drugs, or where there is significant mitral regurgitation or septal rupture. The aim is to provide a 'bridge' of haemodynamic stability pending definitive diagnosis and treatment or in preparation for coronary intervention or surgical revascularisation if indicated (Lewis et al. 2007; Chang et al. 2008).

The IABP necessitates the placement of a balloon catheter in the aortic arch via the femoral artery. The catheter is attached to an external device (the 'pump') which synchronises inflation of the balloon in diastole to increase aortic diastolic pressure and coronary blood flow. During systole, deflation of the balloon decreases afterload facilitating emptying of the left ventricle.

While IABP can dramatically improve the patient's condition, use tends to be reserved for those in whom spontaneous recovery or a realistic chance for correction of the underlying condition by surgery or intervention. IABP is not suitable for use in patients with aortic dissection or significant aortic insufficiency, those with severe peripheral arterial disease, or multi-organ failure (ESC 2005).

> ## Learning activity
>
> Datascope offers some helpful e-learning programmes at http://www.datascope.com/ca/elearning_programs.html – Visit the website and examine the available education material on intra-aortic balloon counterpulsation therapy.
>
> London Health Sciences Centre offers Nursing Standards of Care for the patient with IABP therapy at http://www.lhsc.on.ca/icu/protocol/iabp.htm – If you work in a unit where IABP is used, examine your own protocols for care of the patient with IABP against other available standards.

Ventricular assist devices

Ventricular assist devices can be used to temporarily replace mechanical work of the ventricle, decreasing myocardial work by unloading the ventricle and pumping blood into the arterial circulation, thus increasing blood flow to organs and the peripheral circulation. The devices tend to be expensive and are associated with a range of complications from thromboembolism, bleeding, infection to haemolysis and device malfunction. Types of devices in current use/investigation include extracorporeal pumps for short-term use and intracorporeal devices for long-term use as a bridge to transplant, and the total artificial heart.

Ventricular assist devices also give rise to important ethical challenges. Such devices can prolong survival, but in some patients the overall quality of life can be adversely affected due to infection, neurological complications and device malfunction (Rizzieri et al. 2008). End-of-life trajectories may also be modified by the presence of a device, as seen also with implantable defibrillators for example. The nurse needs, in addition, to be mindful of the impact on family members, who may experience depression, anxiety and post-traumatic stress disorder in addition to social and financial ramifications. Early consideration of a palliative care approach may be appropriate depending on a careful assessment of individual patient and family circumstances (Rizzieri et al. 2008).

Key point

The ESC (2005) considers the use of ventricular assist devices unacceptable if recovery or transplantation is not possible and recommends that these devices should be restricted to use in centres where there is a dedicated programme.

Cardiac resynchronisation therapy

A substantial proportion of patients with AHF, particularly where there is associated haemodynamics derangement, will have evidence of intraventricular mechanical dys-synchrony, independent or underlying QRS width on the ECG (Mullens et al. 2008). The implications of this for the use of cardiac resynchronisation therapy (CRT), increasingly used to benefit patients with chronic heart failure, remain unclear in the acute treatment of patients with AHF. Implantation of such devices may, however, be appropriate prior to discharge once patients have responded to the pharmaceutical treatments outlined above (Dec 2007). Use of CRT in hospitalised heart failure patients has recently been described by Piccini et al. (2008). Of almost 34,000 patients admitted to 228 hospitals, 12% were discharged alive with CRT, although only one-fifth of these were new implants. Patients with CRT were older and had poorer left ventricular function than patients not requiring CRT, and more CRT recipients had ischaemic cardiomyopathy, more atrial fibrillation and higher rates of beta blocker and aldosterone antagonist use. Ten per cent of patients discharged with a new CRT implant had left ventricular ejection fraction <35%. Important variations in CRT use were observed based on racial and geographical differences as well as the age and presence of co-morbidities (Piccini et al. 2008).

Learning activity

Visit the cardiac resynchronisation therapy page at the Medtronic website at http://www.medtronic.com/physician/hf/# It has useful information including educational resources and guidelines.

Dignity, communication and preventing complications: 'back to basics'

The patient with AHF will often be seriously ill, anxious and with limited mobility. The nurse must as a matter of priority ensure that careful attention is paid to ensuring high standards of personal care, safeguarding dignity, ensuring that the communication and spiritual needs of patients and family members receive priority and that meticulous attention is paid to personal hygiene. Patients will be at significant risk of complications such as venous thromboembolism, respiratory and urinary tract infection, constipation and pressure ulcers, and appropriate nursing measures must be instituted to reduce such risk. In the midst of the high technology aspects of treatment, it is of vital importance that the 'essence of care' remains a key priority.

Every effort must be made to maintain patient comfort, including simple measures such as providing regular ice to suck (high concentration oxygen and dyspnoea commonly give rise to a dry mouth), attention to oral hygiene and regular offers of a cool face flannel. Where powerful diuretics are being administered then, in the absence of a urinary catheter, the ready availability of appropriate equipment such as urinary bottles, bedpans or commodes, and attention to privacy, will be most welcome. Communication with, and support for, family members is another consideration, with evidence that a mismatch exists between the perceptions of nurses and relatives regarding support needs (Maxwell et al. 2007).

Attention must also be paid to the nutritional status of the patient. Heart failure has long been associated with nutritional disorders, malnutrition and cachexia being particularly frequent during the late phases of chronic heart failure. Suboptimal nutritional status is also a determinant of outcome, even after cardiac transplantation. Shifting the substrate metabolism from lipids to carbohydrates and reinforcing the antioxidant status reduces the deleterious biological and clinical consequences of acute ischaemic events which are often associated with AHF (Berger & Mustafa 2003). Expert advice from a dietician should be sought.

Managing chronic heart failure better to reduce the need for re-hospitalisation

More than 70% of unscheduled admissions to hospital with AHF are a result from deterioration in a patient with chronic heart failure (Felker et al. 2003). While a detailed discussion of the evidence is outside the scope of this chapter, in recent years, the role of multidisciplinary, and often nurse-mediated, support for patients with chronic heart failure in the community has been evaluated as a means of reducing unplanned readmission with AHF (Holland et al. 2005; Yu et al. 2006). Other strategies under evaluation include the use of home monitoring of basic parameters, including weight and blood pressure (Barlow et al. 2007), and the role of social support in influencing outcome (Luttik et al. 2005). Similarly, the important role of palliative care strategies in patients with chronic heart failure is being increasingly recognised (Selman et al. 2007).

Conclusion

Acute heart failure is common and carries significant mortality risk. Acute decompensation often occurs secondary to chronic heart failure, and improved long-term management has the potential to reduce unplanned readmission. For those patients presenting with AHF, care is increasingly complex, although several 'mainstay' treatments lack sound underpinning evidence of safety and efficacy. The nurse caring for the patient with AHF has a key role to play as part of the multidisciplinary team in ensuring that therapeutic goals are met whilst patient safety and dignity are maintained.

References

Abraham, W.T., Adams, K.F., Fonarow, G.C., et al. for the ADHERE Scientific Advisory Committee and Investigators; ADHERE Study Group (2005). In-hospital mortality in patients with acute decompensated heart failure requiring intravenous vasoactive medications: an analysis from the Acute Decompensated Heart Failure National Registry (ADHERE). *Journal of the American College of Cardiology*, **46**:57–64.

Adams, K.F., Jr., Uddin, N. & Patterson, J.H. (2008). Clinical predictors of in-hospital mortality in acutely decompensated heart failure – piecing together the outcome puzzle. *Congestive Heart Failure*, **14**:127–34.

Andrews, F.J. & Nolan, J.P. (2006). Critical care in the emergency department: monitoring the critically ill patient. *Emergency Medicine Journal*, **23**:561–4.

Barlow, J., Singh, D., Bayer, S. & Curry, R. (2007). A systematic review of the benefits of home telecare for frail elderly people and those with long-term conditions. *Journal of Telemedicine and Telecare*, **13**:172–9.

Berger, M.M. & Mustafa, I. (2003). Metabolic and nutritional support in acute cardiac failure. *Current Opinion in Clinical Nutrition and Metabolic Care*, **6**:195–201.

Berry, C., Murdoch, D.R. & McMurray, J.J.V. (2001). Economics of chronic heart failure. *European Journal of Heart Failure*, **3**:283–91.

Binanay, C., Califf, R.M., Hasselblad, V., et al. for the ESCAPE Investigators and ESCAPE Study Coordinators (2005). Evaluation study of congestive heart failure and pulmonary artery catheterization effectiveness: the ESCAPE trial. *Journal of the American Medical Association*, **294**:1625–33.

Chang, S.N., Hwang, J.J., Chen, Y.S., et al. (2008). Clinical experience with intra-aortic balloon counterpulsation over 10 years: a retrospective cohort study of 459 patients. *Resuscitation*, **77**:316–24.

Dec, G.W. (2007). Management of acute decompensated heart failure. *Current Problems in Cardiology*, **32**:321–66.

European Society of Cardiology (ESC) (2005). Executive summary of the guidelines on the diagnosis and treatment of acute heart failure. Task force on acute heart failure. *European Heart Journal*, **26**:384–416.

Felker, G.M., Adams, K.F., Jr., Konstam, M.A., et al. (2003). The problem of decompensated heart failure: nomenclature, classification, and risk stratification. *American Heart Journal*, **145**(Suppl. 2):S18–25.

Galvao, M., Kalman, J., DeMarco, T., et al. (2006). Gender differences in in-hospital management and outcomes in patients with decompensated heart failure: analysis from the Acute Decompensated Heart Failure National Registry (ADHERE). *Journal of Cardiac Failure*, **12**:100–7.

Gauthier, N., Anselm, A.H. & Haddad, H. (2008). New therapies in acute decompensated heart failure. *Current Opinion in Cardiology*, **23**:134–40.

Gheorghiade, M. & Bebazaa, A. (2005). Introduction to acute heart failure symptoms. *American Journal of Cardiology*, **96**(Suppl.):1G–4.

Gheorghiade, M., De Luca, L., Fonarow, G.C., et al. (2005). Pathophysiologic targets in the early phase of acute heart failure syndromes. *American Journal of Cardiology*, **96**(6A):11G–17.

Gray, A., Goodacre, S. & Newby, D.E. (2008). Non-invasive ventilation in acute cardiogenic pulmonary oedema. *New England Journal of Medicine*, **359**: 142–51.

Holland, R., Battersby, J., Harvey, I., et al. (2005). Systematic review of multidisciplinary interventions in heart failure. *Heart*, **91**:899–906.

Ivanov, R.I., Allen, J., Sandham, J.D. & Calvin, J.E. (1997). Pulmonary artery catheterization: a narrative and systematic critique of randomized controlled trials and recommendations for the future. *New Horizons*, **5**:268–76.

Khunti, K., Squire, I., Abrams, K.R. & Sutton, A.J. (2004). Accuracy of a 12-lead electrocardiogram in screening patients with suspected heart failure for open access echocardiography: a systematic review and meta-analysis. *European Journal of Heart Failure*, **6**:571–6.

Lewis, P.A., Mullany, D.V., Townsend, S., et al. (2007). Trends in intra-aortic balloon counterpulsation: comparison of a 669 record Australian dataset with the multinational Benchmark Counterpulsation Outcomes Registry. *Anaesthesia and Intensive Care*, **35**:13–9.

Luttik, M.L., Jaarsma, T., Moser, D., et al. (2005). The importance and impact of social support on outcomes in patients with heart failure: an overview of the literature. *Journal of Cardiovascular Nursing*, **20**:162–9.

Maxwell, K.E., Stuenkel, D. & Saylor, C. (2007). Needs of family members of critically ill patients: a comparison of nurse and family perceptions. *Heart Lung*, **36**:367–76.

Mehta, S. & Hill, N.S. (2001). Non-invasive ventilation. *American Journal of Respiratory Critical Care Medicine*, **163**:540–77.

Mullens, W., Borowski, A.G., Curtin, R., et al. (2008). *Mechanical dyssynchrony in advanced decompensated heart failure: relation to hemodynamic responses to intensive medical therapy.* Heart Rhythm; **5**:1105–10.

Myerson, S.G., Choudhury, R.P. & Mitchell, A.R. (2006). *Oxford Handbook of Emergencies in Cardiology.* Oxford University Press, Oxford.

Nicholson, C. (2004). A systematic review of the effectiveness of oxygen in reducing acute myocardial ischaemia. *Journal of Clinical Nursing*, **13**:996–1007.

Nohria, A., Tsang, S.W., Fang, J.C., et al. (2003). Clinical assessment identifies hemodynamic profiles that predict outcomes in patients admitted with heart failure. *Journal of the American College of Cardiology*, **41**:1797–1804.

Packer, M., Coats, A.J., Fowler, M.B., et al. for the Carvedilol Prospective Randomized Cumulative Survival Study Group (2001). Effect of carvedilol on survival in severe chronic heart failure. *New England Journal of Medicine*, **344**:1651–8.

Peacock, W.F., Hollander, J.R., Diercks, D.B., et al. (2008). Morphine and outcomes in acute decompensated heart failure: an ADHERE analysis. *Emergency Medicine Journal*, **25**:205–9.

Piccini, J.P., Hernandez, A.F., Dai, D., et al. for the Get With the Guidelines Steering Committee and Hospitals (2008). Use of cardiac resynchronization therapy in patients hospitalized with heart failure. *Circulation*, **118**:926–33 [Epub ahead of print, doi: 10.1161/CIRCULATIONAHA.108.773838].

Rizzieri, A.G., Verheijde, J.L., Rady, M.Y. & McGregor, J.L. (2008). Ethical challenges with the left ventricular assist device as a destination therapy. *Philosophy, Ethics, and Humanities in Medicine*, **3**:20.

Roguin, A., Behar, D., Ben Ami, H., et al. (2000). Long-term prognosis of acute pulmonary oedema – an ominous outcome. *European Journal of Heart Failure*, **2**:137–44.

Sackner-Bernstein, J.D., Kowalski, M., Fox, M. & Aaranson, K. (2005). Short-term risk of death after treatment with nesiritide for decompensated heart failure: a pooled analysis of randomised controlled trials. *Journal of the American Medical Association*, **293**:1900–5.

Selman, L., Harding, R., Beynon, T., et al. (2007). Improving end-of-life care for patients with chronic heart failure: "Let's hope it'll get better, when I know in my heart of hearts it won't". *Heart*, **93**:963–7.

Springfield, C.L., Sebat, F., Johnson, D., et al. (2004). Utility of impedance cardiography to determine cardiac vs. noncardiac cause of dyspnea in the emergency department. *Congestive Heart Failure*, **10**(Suppl. 2):14–6.

Stevenson, R., Ranjadayalan, K., Wilkinson, P., et al. (1993). Short and long term prognosis of acute myocardial infarction since introduction of thrombolysis. *British Medical Journal*, **307**:349–53.

Vital, F.M., Saconato, H., Ladeira, M.T., et al. (2008). Non-invasive positive pressure ventilation (CPAP or bilevel NPPV) for cardiogenic pulmonary edema. *Cochrane Database of Systematic Reviews*, Jul 16; **3**: CD005351.

Wijesinghe, M., Perrin, K., Ranchord, A., et al. (2009). The routine use of oxygen in the treatment of myocardial infarction: systematic review. *Heart*, **95**:198–202 [Epub ahead of print, doi:10.1136/hrt.2008.148742].

Yu, D.S., Thompson, D.R. & Lee, D.T. (2006). Disease management programmes for older people with heart failure: crucial characteristics which improve post-discharge outcomes. *European Heart Journal*, **27**:596–612.

Useful Websites and Further Reading

American Association of Heart Failure Nurses: http://aahfn.org/

British Society for Heart Failure: http://bsh.org.uk/BSH/Home/tabid/82/Default.aspx

Cardiovascular Diseases Specialist Library: http://www.library.nhs.uk/cardiovascular/

Heart Failure Association: http://www.escardio.org/communities/HFA/Pages/welcome.aspx

National Heart Foundation of Australia: http://www.heartfoundation.org.au/index.htm

Society of Chest Pain Centres Recommendations for the Evaluation and Management of the Observation Stay Acute Heart Failure Patient: http://www.scpcp.org/library/introduction_pdf.html

26 Convalescence

P. Davidson & R. Webster

Overview

Hospitalisation for an acute cardiac event can evoke a range of emotions and responses for patients and their families. Undeniably, hospitalisation for an acute cardiac event is a stressful event in the life of the individual and their loved ones and is often a time for appraising life goals and plans. Nurses play an important role in not only assisting patients in coping and adjusting to their diagnosis, but also planning for their future (Di Benedetto et al. 2007). In many instances, people are required to change their lifestyles and make considerable adjustments that can result in an impact on not only the individual, but also their family members and friends. An important issue for cardiac nurses to consider is that this situation of crisis can often cause new, and evoke latent, conflicts and stressors among family members (Moser & Dracup 2004). Associated disability and time off work mean that many families face economic loss and uncertainty. Although the illness course can seem straightforward and commonplace to the cardiac nurse, these events can be very distressing to individuals, and unless patients and their families adjust appropriately a range of physical, social and psychological disabilities can ensue.

This chapter seeks to describe the importance of appropriate assessment and identification of patient needs; discuss models of interventions; implementing strategies to facilitate convalescence and identify key nursing strategies to assist recovery and enable effective secondary prevention strategies. Additional information relating to discharge planning and secondary prevention is discussed in Chapter 27. At the conclusion of this chapter there are two case studies, which will assist you in applying critical factors in planning convalescence. It is also important to consider that planning for convalescence is not solely the responsibility of the nurse, and the nurse should look to members of the multidisciplinary team including social workers, occupational therapists and community nurses to assist in care planning.

Learning objectives

After reading this chapter, the reader will be able to:

- Discuss potential emotions and reactions experienced by patients and their families in response to an acute cardiac event.
- Describe strategies to assist the patient and their family to cope and adjust following an acute cardiac event.

- Identify models of care to assist the patient and their family in the convalescence phase.
- Distinguish the importance of strategies to promote continuity of clinical care and promote secondary prevention.
- Incorporate strategies to promote convalescence in nursing care plans.

Key concepts

Identification of patient needs; models of intervention; convalescence strategies; coping with illness

Introduction

Convalescence refers to the process of recuperation and recovery following an acute illness. As a consequence, this requires the cardiac nurse to look beyond the confines of the coronary care unit (CCU) and consider key factors impacting on the individual's life experience. The period of convalescence is a time of recuperation and adjustment and often marks a life-transition phase. Sustaining a heart attack or being diagnosed with heart failure (HF) often marks a period of transition from a perception of invincibility to adjusting to living with a chronic condition. The indicators of successful transitions are emotional well-being, role mastery and well-being of relationships (Meleis et al. 2000). Following an acute cardiac event – in contrast to other models of convalescence, such as following an acute illness or operation, the key goals are to:

- Promote physical, social, psychological and existential well-being
- Assist the individual to achieve optimal physical, social and psychological functioning
- Support the individual and their families to make the necessary adjustments to cope with a potentially life-limiting chronic illness
- Facilitate the adoption of effective secondary prevention initiatives
- Ensure communication and continuity of care across care provider settings

The Chronic Care Model, originally developed by Wagner and subsequently adapted by the World

Health Organization (Epping-Jordan et al. 2004) (Box 26.1) shows the critical elements in improving chronic care. Figure 26.1 shows key elements of this model. In particular, the Chronic Care Model recognises the importance of patient-centred care and self-management as part of a multidimensional approach to improving the management of chronic care. Also nurses play a critical role in delivering effective chronic care (Bodenheimer et al. 2005). Many patients leave hospital with

---

Box 26.1   Key elements in improving outcomes in chronic conditions

Self-management

Self-management involves providing people with information and resources to inform their choices regarding health-seeking behaviours.

Decision support

Evidence-based practice guidelines and strategies such as clinical pathways and electronic prompts and recall.

Delivery system design

This infers careful delineation of roles and responsibilities in promoting continuity of care.

Clinical information system

Information systems, ideally registries, are optimal for managing chronic illness.

Organisation of health care

Health care systems can create an environment in which organised efforts to improve the care of people with chronic illness take hold and flourish.

Community

Effective chronic care involves health care organisations developing partnerships with communities to deliver effective health messages and decreasing misinformation and prejudices.

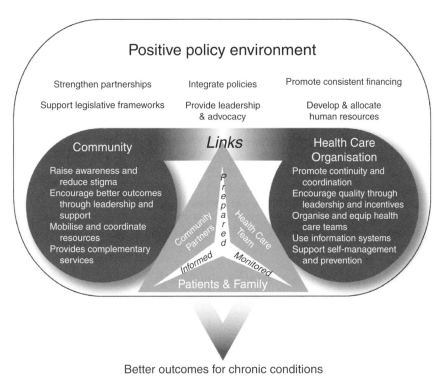

Figure 26.1   World Health Organization – Chronic Care Model.
Source: From World Health Organization, Innovative Care for Chronic Conditions Framework.

a misconception that they are 'cured'. Cardiac nurses are only too aware that heart disease is a chronic condition and our challenge is to engage our patients and their families as partners in chronic disease management strategies. Self-management strategies aim to empower individuals with the confidence, resources and strategies to be active participants in managing their condition (Bodenheimer et al. 2002). Through active participation, self-management has been shown to increase the patient's independence in their activities of daily living, improve adherence with treatment recommendations and promote optimal health outcomes. These are all important strategies in promoting a successful convalescence.

As part of the discharge process and planning for convalescence, it is vital that nurses reinforce the importance of strategies, such as medication adherence (Rolley et al. 2008). For example, stopping clopidogrel can potentially have disastrous consequences for a patient who has undergone a percutaneous coronary intervention (Rhee et al. 2008).

Often people's medication behaviours are associated with past experiences, such as taking antibiotics for an infection, and they do not understand the significance of long-term pharmacotherapy. In addition, models of nursing care are commonly configured to the needs of people with acute illnesses and, as a consequence, a range of strategies have been undertaken to introduce models related to chronic care. The individual's response to a cardiac event is dependent on prior experiences, individual psychological characteristics, level of social support and disease prognosis. The responses of patients and their families in this situation range from a flat affect relating to processing the impact of an acute cardiac event, to a debilitating depression. Adverse psychological reactions to cardiac conditions have significant implications for treatment and health-related outcomes. Clinical depression can delay the recovery process, exacerbate functional impairment and have adverse outcomes on health-related quality of life. In addition to depression, anxiety is also associated with worse prognosis, lower compliance and poorer quality of life. Beyond the psychological and social distress associated with anxiety and depression, these factors are associated with increased risk for recurrent cardiac events and mortality. An increasing body of research demonstrates the importance of psychosocial adjustment in the recovery process and underscores the importance of nurses' interventions in planning the convalescent phase (Thompson & Froelicher 2006; Moser 2007). An important goal of both planning for discharge and convalescence is supporting patients and their families to incorporate self-management strategies. If the individual appears to have an inability to self-care, either due to cognitive impairment, physical, psychological or social issues, a long-term case-management plan is recommended. This involves liaising with community-based services, general practitioners and other health providers. In countries such as the United Kingdom, New Zealand and Australia, the general practitioner is a key provider of community-based care and should be considered as an integral element of the convalescent plan (Halcomb et al. 2006).

Assessment and identification of patient needs

An integral part of planning the convalescent care for patients and their families is recognising the unique knowledge, attitudes, values and experiences that the individual brings to the experience of an acute cardiac event. These factors are influenced by the individual's cultural and socio-economic standpoint as well as physiological and psychological characteristics. Key issues emerge in the immediate post-discharge phase including: reappraisal of life circumstances; searching for a sense of control and certainty in changing circumstances; looking for continuity and coordination of care; seeking reassurance.

Many people experience psychological difficulties after a cardiac event including anxiety, depressed mood, adjustment difficulties, and feelings of grief and loss. The immediate post-discharge phase is certainly a period of vulnerability (Thompson et al. 1995). Feelings of perceived control are important for psychosocial recovery after a cardiac event. In addition to these factors Higgins and colleagues interviewed health professionals who identified trauma, guilt, and anger as emergent issues for

patients and their families (Higgins et al. 2007). Therefore, these factors should be key concerns for the nurse in facilitating the convalescent phase.

High risk groups

As the cardiac nurse approaches working with the patient and their family in preparing for the convalescence phase, it is important to consider both individuals and groups at higher risk of adverse outcomes and particularly re-hospitalisation. The ageing of the population, increasing numbers of co-morbid conditions, shortened lengths of stay and the increased complexity of treatment highlight the importance of identifying those at higher risk. Box 26.2 summarises the key signs to indicate potential poor adjustment and higher risk for adverse health outcomes.

Promoting self-management in the convalescent phase

An important strategy of preparing people for the convalescent phase is planning for self-management. Although for many decades health professionals, particularly nurses, have sought to involve patient in their own health, recent developments have extended this concept beyond purely providing information to engaging in active partnerships and empowering the individual to participate in their care plans (Marks et al. 2005). Consumer engagement involves the nurturing of collaborative and fostering mutual respect and partnerships. This occurs at both an individual level, for example, between patients,

> ### Box 26.2   High risk factors for adverse health outcomes
>
> - Prolonged and complicated hospital stay
> - Recent hospitalisation
> - Poor social support
> - Cognitive impairment
> - Socio-economic disadvantage
> - Depression, anxiety and stress
> - Low health literacy
> - Financial challenges
> - Physical disability
> - Poor prognosis

their families and health professionals, and at a systems-based level with policy makers and funding bodies. In recent times, the role of self-management in chronic care has gained significant support from clinicians, consumers and policy makers and is now widely recognised as a necessary element of effective chronic disease management, particularly heart disease. Although commonly associated with chronic care, self-management should play an important role at all entry points into the health care system, and ideally, reframe the way that health care services are delivered.

The terms 'self-care' and 'self-management' are often used interchangeably. Riegel and colleagues view these constructs as discrete entities, defining self-care as the everyday decisions people make regarding their health. Self-care involves both healthy individuals and those who experience an illness (Riegel et al. 2000, 2007). In contrast, self-management is a deliberate, active decision-making process whereby a person with an illness engages in either maintenance or management of their condition and is part of the broader construct of self-care. Self-management involves working with health professionals to assist in making informed choices and developing problem-solving skills.

The principles of self-management rely on a partnership between the health professional, patients, their families and their carers. Carers are generally family members, volunteers and friends who actively engage in supporting patients and health professionals in providing care. The role of the cardiac nurse is to facilitate the development of knowledge and skills, so that the patient may engage in self-management practices. The use of a traditional education-delivery approach, which involves didactic teaching methods with little follow-up to assess how well the patient has understood the information, are often ineffective as they fail to engage the patient in a meaningful relationship and employ principles of adult learning. Failing to provide individuals with an opportunity to make informed decisions and relate these to their lifestyle circumstances minimises information acquisition and, more importantly, decreases engagement in recommended health care behaviours. In order to improve knowledge and promote engagement in health-seeking behaviours, nurses need to adopt the role of facilitator, rather than instructor, promoting the individual's self-efficacy to manage their condition. Self-efficacy, the level of confidence an individual

has in their ability to perform a task, is an important consideration in self-management strategies.

In summary, the process of self-management, including self-care, is dynamic and includes a range of values, attitudes, behaviours and skills directed toward managing the impact of a condition(s) on daily living. Important considerations for the nurse planning convalescence following an acute cardiac event are:

- Providing the patient and their family with knowledge of their heart condition, the management plan and likely outcomes
- Participating in decision-making with health professionals, family members and/or carers
- Negotiating a self-management care plan in partnership with health professionals, family members and/or carers
- Providing the patient with strategies for monitoring and managing signs and symptoms of their heart condition
- Minimising the impact of the condition on physical, emotional, occupational and social functioning
- Adopting lifestyles that promote favourable health behaviours and minimise risk of complications, adverse events and unplanned admissions to hospital and the emergency department
- Facilitating access to support services in the community
- Empowering the patient with the confidence to participate in their care planning

Particular concerns of spouses and family members

Many spouses of patients who have undergone an acute cardiac event experience psychological distress and report stressors relating to living with a partner with heart disease. A range of factors can contribute to marital and family discord in the convalescent phase. This can range from over-vigilance and over-protectiveness to emotional distancing. Often, care-giving family members are concerned about what to do in case another event happens or if another medical emergency occurs once they have brought their family member home. For instance, wound sites or implantation of implantable cardioverter defibrillators (ICDs), may cause caregivers to be fearful of hurting the patient or themselves. In addition, many couples experience concern regarding their capacity to engage in sexual activity.

In some instances, a health crisis can bring a family or couple closer together and in others, it can erupt long-simmering conflicts and exacerbate existing difficulties. An acute cardiac event can alter the dynamics within families and also promote distress. Both the patient and their family must adjust to either temporary or longer-term changes in roles of household members. The inability to resume previous roles may cause the patient psychological distress, which may in turn affect the family members. If caregivers take on too many roles, they may suffer physical and psychological exhaustion. A loss of income is an important concern, particularly given the associated costs related to medication and health care. Marital and family concerns need to be addressed as soon as possible through referral to appropriate counselling services.

Accommodating convalescence and discharge planning following an acute cardiac event

As lengths of hospital stay following an acute cardiac event continue to decrease, traditional models of in-hospital cardiac rehabilitation (CR), traditionally referred to as Phase 1, become difficult to achieve. In spite of this challenge, the following important information should be provided to patients and their families. Where time is limited, the emphasis should be on providing:

- Initial contact and introduction
- Basic information and reassurance
- Supportive counselling
- Guidelines for increasing physical activity
- Information on pharmacotherapy and use of sub-lingual nitrates
- Appropriate discharge planning, including follow-up by the general practitioner/primary care provider and referral to a secondary prevention programme

Models of intervention to facilitate convalescence and secondary prevention

Cardiac rehabilitation (CR) has been shown to improve health outcomes for people with

cardiovascular disease. Nevertheless, despite robust evidence obtained from well-designed, controlled trials to support the benefits of CR and endorsement of peak cardiovascular bodies, such as the American Heart Association and National Heart Foundation of Australia, low participation rates continue to be a challenge internationally. The barriers to CR have been replicated in many studies. Factors associated with low participation rates include system-related factors such as lack of availability of programmes; provider factors such as physician's endorsement and individual patient-related factors such as limited access to transport, low self-efficacy for exercise and the need to return to work. In order to address the barriers to standardised models of CR, a range of innovative solutions to address promoting effective convalescence and the facilitation of chronic disease management have been implemented. A number of models that support the needs of people who cannot or do not want to attend a centre-based service are currently being evaluated. These range from web-based and home-based models to services provided by practice nurses in the general practice setting.

An interdisciplinary team is required to produce the best outcomes in the convalescence phase. Team members include the patient's physicians, both specialist and general practitioners, ideally working with a team of nurses, physiotherapists or exercise physiologists, dieticians, social workers, psychologists, occupational therapists and others depending on an individual's needs. Key models of interventions are discussed later in this chapter. Unfortunately, the choice of service provision is often dictated by availability rather than appropriateness to the patient's clinical condition. Therefore, in order to facilitate convalescence, the cardiac nurse has to be aware of services available to patients and their families in their local community. Simple strategies such as calling the patient in the early post-discharge phase can be reassuring and can also identify potential problems early. Increasingly, it is apparent that a nurse-coordinated approach is important in achieving optimal outcomes (Grady et al. 2000).

Home-based services

The evidence supporting home-based nursing care provided by HF nurse specialists is indisputable

(McAlister et al. 2004). Although the evidence is not as robust for CR, several randomised controlled trials (RCTs) have compared the effectiveness of home-based CR to traditional hospital-based CR (Dalal et al. 2007). Results from these trials demonstrate significant improvements in serum lipid levels, blood pressure and body mass index. Improvements in exercise participation and exercise capacity have also been reported as participants could incorporate physical activity in their daily routine and not have to wait for physical activity during CR. In addition, the home-based programmes also demonstrated a decrease in readmission to hospital, improved psychological well-being, anxiety levels, self-confidence, self-esteem, knowledge of angina, return to work, resumption of driving and improved quality of life (Warrington et al. 2003; Dracup et al. 2007).

Home-based CR has also been reported to promote physical activity and facilitate convalescence. Home-based programmes have been associated with lower costs. Although there have been concerns raised about the risk of sudden death in patients participating in home-based programmes, there are limited data about the safety of home-based training among higher-risk patients, such as those with exercise-induced ischaemia or advanced HF. A disadvantage of the home-based programme, however, is the lack of the psychodynamic support derived from a group-based programme.

Nurse-coordinated clinics

Increasing nurse-directed clinics are used to manage people with heart disease in a community-based setting. The emerging role of nurse practitioners has facilitated this process (Patel et al. 2003; Saxe et al. 2007). Effective implementation is largely dependent on mechanisms that facilitate reimbursement. In a systematic review of six RCTs, the majority of which were undertaken in the United Kingdom, nurse-led clinics demonstrated significant improvements in anxiety and depression, quality of life, general health and lifestyle. A reduction in the severity of angina, blood pressure and cholesterol levels, and adherence to cardiovascular risk-reduction strategies were also reported (Page et al. 2005).

Community health workers

Liaising with community health workers within the target community can be useful in gaining access to vulnerable populations. Culture influences individual's views of both illness and health, help-seeking behaviour and the capacity to adhere with health care recommendations (Webster et al. 2003). A range of cultural values and beliefs dictate an individual's view of convalescence. For example, in many cultures, bed rest is advocated which is in stark contrast to evidence-based recommendations (Webster et al. 2002). Bilingual health care workers are valuable resources who understand the cultural elements associated with particular conditions and can assist in formulating culturally competent care plans. Engaging health workers is particularly important in indigenous communities. Collaborating with these health workers is particularly useful because of not only their knowledge, resources and skill base, but also their standing within their communities (Davidson et al. 2008).

Information technology

Advances in information technology have expanded the capacity of nurses and other health professionals to engage with people with heart disease remotely (Clark et al. 2007). Examples of these interventions include the Internet, telephone and clinic-based interventions involving touch screen computers. A recent meta-analysis concluded that computer-generated interventions were effective in bringing about behaviour change (Revere & Dunbar 2001). This is a rapidly evolving area of practice with interventions evaluating remote monitoring and a range of communication strategies. However, cost and accessibility often limit these models of interventions but this is likely to change over time.

Nursing strategies to promote convalescence

As discussed above, a range of models of interventions are available to assist patients and their families in the convalescence phase. In order to achieve a seamless transition and ensure that coordination of care is optimal, communication across health care settings is critical. Therefore, strategies such as clinical pathways, discharge planning meetings and other integrated patterns of follow-up can facilitate optimal patient outcomes. In order to prepare the patient and the family for the convalescence phase, it is important that people know:

- What to expect – including a realistic view of their prognosis
- Important issues to follow-up and their timing
- Where to get information and assistance

Palliative care

Although improvements in cardiovascular care over recent decades have been remarkable, in many instances the prognosis for many individuals remains poor. This is particularly the case for those with HF. Unfortunately, a growing literature describes the limitations of acute health systems in delivering palliative and supportive care in HF (Addington-Hall & Gibbs 2000). These limitations range from failing to meet the physical, social, emotional and existential needs of patients and their families to ethical dilemmas. Professional bodies are increasingly recognising the role of palliative and supportive care in cardiovascular care and this is reflected in recent clinical practice guidelines. As part of preparing for discharge and convalescence, the notion of living with a potentially life-limiting illness needs to be considered. Effective and honest communication is an important strategy in ensuring patients and their families are well prepared for the future. Failing to address the patient's prognosis and discuss available treatment choices and the options to develop advance care plans can often lead to an unnecessary burden on patients, their family's health care systems (Davidson 2007).

Conclusion

As discussed earlier and illustrated in the case studies, preparing the patient for convalescence requires the nurse to undertake a comprehensive patient assessment and knowledge of community-based resources. As the population ages and lengths of hospital stays shorten, the significance of this planning increases in importance to optimise

health outcomes and minimise burden on health care systems as a result of unnecessary hospitalisation. Chapter 27 provides important information to plan for the patient's discharge and implement effective secondary prevention strategies.

Learning activity

Reflective case study 1

Felicity is a 64-year-old widow, living alone, who recently experienced a cardiac arrest while having dinner at a local restaurant with friends. Fortunately, she was resuscitated by bystanders and taken to her local hospital where she underwent primary angioplasty. Following the procedure, Felicity had a further cardiac arrest. Echocardiography revealed impaired systolic dysfunction and she had an automated ICD inserted. Other post-procedural complications included a urinary tract infection and pneumonia. Felicity has two children living abroad who are concerned for her well-being. Understandably, Felicity is anxious regarding her future and this anxiety is likely exacerbated by dealing with stopping smoking. Felicity also tells you that she has experienced some 'weird' feelings about the cardiac arrests she has experienced. It is Day 4 and you are being told by the discharge services that Felicity should be discharged by Day 7.

Reflect on the information provided within this chapter and the text and consider:

What are the important strategies to consider in planning Felicity's discharge and convalescent period?

What information would you consider providing to Felicity and her family to assist them in planning for the future?

How would you approach discussing the emotions and existential issues surrounding the cardiac arrest?

What services in your local area could you mobilise to support Felicity in her convalescence?

What sort of follow-up and support do you think will be appropriate to support Felicity?

Reflective case study 2

Frank is a 42-year-old man who was admitted to hospital with alcoholic cardiomyopathy that was

diagnosed when he went to see his general practitioner for investigation of impotence. Frank is a
truck driver but his shifts are being cut back as the
company he works for is in financial stress because
of rising fuel problems. Frank tells you that things
have not been going well for him and his wife
for nearly 2 years. He has two teenage sons who
have been getting into trouble at school, which has
added to the conflict in the relationship. Frank says
his real enjoyment is going to the pub and spending times with his friends. His wife does not drink
and hates the environment. Frank talks about his
impotence and the conversation becomes uncomfortable. He admits to having used Sildenafil in
the past but in an extra-marital relationship. Frank
is very embarrassed, but needs to ask your advice
about whether it is safe for him to have sexual
intercourse.

***Consider how you address Frank's need for
information, support and counselling about the
following:***

Resuming sexual activity and his erectile dysfunction

Interpersonal relationships – particularly those with
his wife and sons

Long-term work plans and his capacity to continue
in his present occupation

References

Addington-Hall, J.M. & Gibbs, J.S.R. (2000). Heart failure now on the palliative care agenda. *Palliative Care
Medicine*, **14**:361–62.

Bodenheimer, T., Lorig, K., Holman, H. & Grumbach, K.
(2002). Patient self-management of chronic disease in primary care. *Journal of the American Medical
Association*, **288**:2469–75.

Bodenheimer, T., MacGregor, K. & Stothart, N. (2005).
Nurses as leaders in chronic care. *British Medical
Journal*, **330**:612–13.

Clark, R.A., Inglis, S.C., McAlister, F.A., et al. (2007).
Telemonitoring or structured telephone support
programmes for patients with chronic heart failure:
systematic review and meta-analysis. *British Medical
Journal*, **334**:942–5.

Dalal, H.M., Evans, P., Campbell, J., et al. (2007). Home-based
versus hospital-based rehabilitation after myocardial
infarction: A randomized trial with preference arms –
Cornwall Heart Attack Rehabilitation Management

Study (CHARMS). *International Journal of Cardiology*,
119:202–11.

Davidson, P.M. (2007). Difficult conversations and chronic
heart failure: do you talk the talk or walk the walk?
Current Opinion in Supportive and Palliative Care,
1:274–8.

Davidson, P., DiGiacomo, M., Abbott, P., et al. (2008).
A partnership model in the development and implementation of a collaborative, cardiovascular education program for Aboriginal Health Care Worker.
Australian Health Review, **32**:139–46.

Di Benedetto, M., Lindner. H., Hare, D. & Kent, S. (2007).
The role of coping, anxiety, and stress in depression
post-acute coronary syndrome. *Psychology Health &
Medicine*, **12**:460–9.

Dracup, K., Evangelista, L., Hamilton, M., et al. (2007).
Effects of a home-based exercise program on clinical outcomes in heart failure. *American Heart Journal*,
154:877–83.

Epping-Jordan, J., Pruitt, S., Bengoa, R. & Wagner,
E. (2004). Improving the quality of health care for
chronic conditions. *Quality & Safety in Health Care*,
13:299–305.

Grady, K., Dracup, K., Kennedy, G., et al. (2000).
Team management of patients with heart failure:
a statement for healthcare professionals from The
Cardiovascular Nursing Council of the American
Heart Association. *Circulation*, **102**:2443–56.

Halcomb, E., Patterson, E. & Davidson, P. (2006).
Evolution of practice nursing in Australia. *Journal of
Advanced Nursing*, **55**:37688.

Higgins, R., Murphy, B., Nicholas, A., Worcester, M. &
Lindner, H. (2007). Emotional and adjustment issues
faced by cardiac patients seen in clinical practice: a
qualitative survey of experienced clinicians. *Journal of
Cardiopulmonary Rehabilitation and Prevention*, **27**:291–7.

Marks, R., Allegrante, J.P. & Lorig, K. (2005). A review
and synthesis of research evidence for self-efficacy-
enhancing interventions for reducing chronic disability: implications for health education practice (part
II). *Health Promotion Practice*, **6**:148–56.

McAlister, F.A., Stewart, S., Ferrua, S., et al. (2004).
Multidisciplinary strategies for the management of
heart failure patients at high risk for admission: a
systematic review of randomized trials. *Journal of the
American College of Cardiology*, **44**:810–19.

Meleis, A., Sawyer, L., Im, E., et al. (2000). Experiencing
transitions: an emerging middle-range theory. *Advances
in Nursing Science*, **23**:12–28.

Moser, D.K. (2007). "The rust of life": impact of anxiety
on cardiac patients. *American Journal of Critical Care*,
16:361–9.

Moser, D.K. & Dracup, K. (2004). Role of spousal anxiety and depression in patients' psychosocial recovery after a cardiac event. *Psychosomatic Medicine*, **66**:527–32.

Page, T., Lockwood, C. & Conroy-Hiller, T.I. (2005). Effectiveness of nurse-led cardiac clinics in adult patients with a diagnosis of coronary heart disease. *International Journal of Evidence-Based Healthcare*, **13**:2–26.

Patel, L., Abriam-Yago, K. & Harkins, E.A. (2003). A comparison study of the utilization of National Cholesterol Education Program (NCEP) guidelines by cardiology and internal medicine practices: implications for the advanced practice nurse. *Journal of the American Academy of Nurse Practitioners*, **15**:557–62.

Revere, D. & Dunbar, P.J. (2001). Review of computer-generated outpatient health behavior interventions: clinical encounters "in absentia". *Journal of the American Medical Informatics Association*, **8**:62–79.

Rhee, S., Yun, K., Lee, S., et al. (2008). Drug-eluting stent thrombosis during perioperative period. *International Heart Journal*, **49**:135–42.

Riegel, B., Carlson, B. & Glaser, D. (2000). Development and testing of a clinical tool measuring self-management of heart failure. *Heart & Lung*, **29**:4–15.

Riegel, B., Dickson, V.V., Goldberg, L.R. & Deatrick, J.A. (2007). Factors associated with the development of expertise in health failure self-care. *Nursing Research*, **56**:235–43.

Rolley, J., Davidson, P., Dennison, C., et al. (2008). Medication adherence self-report instruments: implications for practice and research. *Journal of Cardiovascular Nursing*. **23**:497–505.

Saxe, J., Janson, S., Stringari-Murray, S., Hirsch, J. & Waters, C. (2007). Meeting a primary care challenge in the United States: chronic illness care. *Contemporary Nurse*, **26**:94–104.

Thompson, D. & Froelicher, E. (2006). Depression in cardiac patients: what can nurses do about it? *European Journal of Cardiovascular Nursing*, **5**:251–2.

Thompson, D., Ersser, S.J. & Webster, R.A. (1995). The experiences of patients and their partners 1 month after a heart attack. *Journal of Advanced Nursing*, **22**:707–14.

Warrington, D., Cholowski, K. & Peters, D. (2003). Effectiveness of home-based cardiac rehabilitation for special needs patients. *Journal of Advanced Nursing*, **41**:121–9.

Webster, R.A., Thompson, D.R. & Mayou, R.A. (2002). The experiences and needs of Gujarati Hindu patients and partners in the first month after a myocardial infarction. *European Journal of Cardiovascular Nursing*, **1**:69–76.

Webster, R.A., Thompson, D.R. & Davidson, P.M. (2003). The first 12 weeks following discharge from hospital: the experience of Gujarati South Asian survivors of acute myocardial infarction and their families. *Contemporary Nurse*, **15**:288–99.

Useful Websites and Further Reading

In addition to the references, you may find the following useful.

Clark, A.M., Hartling, L., Vandermeer, B. & McAlister, F.A. (2005). Meta-analysis: secondary prevention programs for patients with coronary artery disease. *Annals of Internal Medicine*, **143**:659–72.

Davidson, P.M., Paull, G., Rees, D.R., et al. (2005). Narrative analysis of documentation: authentication of the home-based heart failure nurse specialist role and function. *American Journal of Critical Care*, **14**:1–8.

Grady, K.L., Dracup, K., Kennedy, G., et al. (2000). AHA scientific statement. Team management of patients with heart failure: a statement for healthcare professionals from the Cardiovascular Nursing Council of the American Heart Association. *Circulation*, **102**: 2443–56.

Inglis, S.C., Pearson, S., Treen, S., Gallasch, T., Horowitz, J.D., Stewart, S. (2006). Extending the horizon in chronic heart failure: effects of multidisciplinary, home-based intervention relative to usual care. *Circulation*, **114**:2466–73.

McAlister, F.A., Stewart, S., Ferrua, S., et al. (2004). Multidisciplinary strategies for the management of heart failure patients at high risk for admission: a systematic review of randomized trials. *Journal of the American College of Cardiology*, **44**:810–19.

The World Wide Web is a rich and lucrative resource of informatiwon to assist you in preparing the patient for recovery and convalescence. Take the time to find out the best source for community services in your local region.

American College of Cardiology: www.acc.org/
American Heart Association: http://www.americanheart.org/
American Heart Failure Nurses Association: www.aahfn.org/
Australasian Cardiovascular Nursing College: www.acnc.net.au/links.htm

British Heart Foundation: www.bhf.org.uk/
Cardiac Society of Australia and New Zealand: www.csanz.edu.au/
Carers Australia: www.carersaustralia.com.au/
Caresearch: www.caresearch.com.au/

European Society of Cardiology: www.escardio.org/
National Health Service – National Library for Health: www.library.nhs.uk/cardiovascular
National Heart Foundation: www.heartfoundation.org.au

27 Discharge Planning and Secondary Prevention

R. Webster & P. Davidson

Overview

In contemporary health environments, where patient acuity is increasing and there is an increasing pressure on hospital beds, discharge planning is increasingly becoming a critical concern for nurses working in acute cardiac care. This chapter will discuss discharge planning and the nurses' role and also outline key pharmacological and non-pharmacological strategies involved in discharge planning. Chapter 26 provides information related to convalescence, which may inform your thoughts regarding discharge planning.

- Identify key strategies to promote effective secondary prevention for people with an acute cardiac event.
- Discuss the need to identify patients at higher risk for adverse outcomes following discharge.

Key concepts

Multidisciplinary team; secondary prevention; risk factor management; reducing readmissions; counselling

Learning objectives

After reading this chapter, the reader will be able to:

- Discuss the importance of discharge planning in optimising optimal health outcomes.
- Describe the importance of the multidisciplinary team in discharge planning.
- Recognise the significance of evidence-based guidelines to inform secondary prevention plans.

Discharge planning

Discharge planning needs to start from the time of admission and be a coordinated effort by the multidisciplinary team, including physicians, nurses, dieticians, pharmacists, rehabilitation specialists, physiotherapists, occupational therapists and key members of the primary care team.

The broad goals during the hospital discharge phase are to:

- prepare the patient for as normal activities as possible

- use the acute event as an opportunity to re-evaluate the plan of care, particularly lifestyle and risk factor modification (American College of Cardiology/American Heart Association [ACC/AHA] 2007).

The decision about when to discharge a patient will depend on the patient's diagnosis, their clinical state, the risk of complications and/or other cardiac events as well as their prognosis. The discharge planning process will also be influenced by the individual's physical, social and family circumstances. It is important that patients are discharged from hospital with a clear plan of treatment that is appropriate for their condition as well as their social and psychological circumstances. For those recovering from an acute cardiac event, episodes of an acute coronary syndrome (ACS) are most likely to occur in the first 3 months after discharge. Therefore, it is important to initiate interventions in hospital that are designed to reduce this immediate risk as well as develop a strategy to reduce the longer-term adverse events and prepare the patient with realistic expectations and goals for recovery.

A clinical risk assessment prior to discharge can categorise patients into low, medium and high risk of further cardiac events and thus help guide subsequent intervention. High risk is associated with increased age, previous cardiac events, poor left ventricular function, post-infarction angina, arrhythmias, persistent ST/T wave changes on the ECG and co-existing hypertension and diabetes. High-risk patients will need post-discharge angiography and possible revascularisation. Those thought not to be at high risk may require echocardiography and a pre-discharge exercise tolerance test to confirm this, followed by medical management therapy if their low risk status is confirmed.

Key point

Hospital stays for acute coronary patients are becoming shorter and therefore there is a need to ensure strategic initiatives to prepare the patient for discharge. A typical length of stay for uncomplicated myocardial infarction (MI) patients in the United States has been reported as being 5 days (Spencer et al. 2004), and it is not unusual for uncomplicated

---

patients to be discharged 72 h after thrombolysis (Newby et al. 2000) or primary angioplasty. Nurses are in a key position to manage the patient journey and nurse-led services for admission, post-operative care and patient discharge are being successfully developed in some areas (Jesson et al. 2007).

Prior to discharge the patient and family need to receive face-to-face information that is backed up with written advice sheets that they can refer to once they are at home. This face-to-face communication is critical in ensuring that the patient and their family understand the discharge plan. Telephone follow-up, particularly in the early days after discharge, can reinforce the information that has been given in hospital and also serve as a method for answering questions, addressing concerns, monitoring progress and engaging the patient (Beckie 1989). Both the patient and family will need to know what to expect during recovery and what to do if cardiac symptoms reoccur (Dracup et al. 1997). They will also need information about lifestyle modification, exercise, drug therapy and practical advice on return to work and resuming normal activity. This period often marks the beginning of a patient's secondary prevention input and as such needs to set the tone for future intervention from health care professionals.

Secondary prevention

Secondary prevention involves identifying and managing those with established coronary heart disease (CHD) and those at very high risk of developing it. It also involves treating and rehabilitating patients who have had a cardiac event in order to reduce the risk of recurrence. The rationale for secondary prevention is based on the assumption that the progression of vascular lesions, arterial thrombosis and the occurrence of arrhythmias in those with existing CHD can be influenced by a variety of metabolic and cardiovascular factors. Secondary prevention is an evolving process designed to help people address their risk factors and thereby reduce the impact of the disease on the quality and quantity of life (American Association of Cardiovascular and Pulmonary Rehabilitation [AACVPR] 2004).

Comprehensive secondary prevention aims to:

- extend overall survival
- improve quality of life
- decrease the need for interventional procedures such as angioplasty and bypass grafting
- reduce the incidence of subsequent cardiac events

Effectiveness of secondary prevention

With an intervention that has many components it is difficult to establish which elements are the most effective or is it the combination of the whole. Evidence from clinical trials supports the merits of aggressive risk factor reduction therapies for patients with established coronary artery disease with increasing evidence that appropriate secondary intervention strategies improve survival and quality of life, limit recurrent events and reduce the need for interventional procedures (Mukherjee et al. 2004; Clarke et al. 2005; Smith et al. 2006). Exercise-based programmes for patients with CHD have been shown to be effective and reduce all-cause mortality (Joliffe et al. 2004; Taylor et al. 2004). One study (Mukherjee et al. 2005) looked at the treatment effect of combination drug therapy in ACS patients stratified according to their risk of future cardiovascular events using the thrombolysis in myocardial infarction (TIMI) risk score. This study demonstrated that when patients were given individually appropriate prescriptions of the four main prophylactic drug groups (antiplatelet drugs, lipid-lowering drugs, angiotensin-converting enzyme [ACE] inhibitors and beta blockers) for secondary prevention, the 6-month mortality was reduced. The benefits of secondary prevention were seen in the low-, intermediate- and high-risk ACS patients with the high-risk patients receiving the most benefit. In other words: the higher the risk, the greater the benefit. Risk stratification is discussed in Chapter 19.

> **Key point**
>
> Populations at highest risk of future cardiovascular events derive the greatest benefit from aggressive secondary prevention.

Target population

Effective targeting of secondary prevention is a significant challenge, particularly as the number of individuals identified as being eligible for such intervention is increasing. This is in part due to the increased numbers now living with CHD. Data from the 2003 Health Survey for England suggested that the prevalence of CHD in England was 7.4% of men and 4.5% of women. One reason for this is the demographic shift in many populations towards a higher proportion of elderly people. As populations age they take on the increased risk of cardiovascular disease with older individuals being more likely to experience a cardiac event. The elderly often have multiple pathology and complex social circumstances and therefore the potential to put increased demand on secondary prevention services.

Another reason for there being more candidates for secondary prevention is the result of improvements in treatment and more individuals now surviving an initial cardiac event. It is estimated that the incident rate for MI for those aged between 30 and 69 is between 2 and 2.5 times the mortality rate (British Heart Foundation [BHF] 2007). Those that survive are then at a higher risk of re-occurrence. It is thought that half of all incidences of MI occur in those who are already known to have cardiovascular disease (Allender et al. 2006).

> **Key point**
>
> Candidates for formal secondary prevention strategies were historically those who had recently had a MI or had undergone coronary artery bypass surgery but the scope has now widened to include those who have undergone percutaneous coronary interventions (PCI), or who have stable chronic heart failure and valvular disease (Leon et al. 2005).

Provision of secondary prevention

The health care teams that deliver secondary prevention services can be hospital, office or community based and may include chronic disease management teams as well as cardiac rehabilitation

(CR) services (ACC/AHA 2007). In fact, there is debate over what such a service should be called (Austin & Closs 2007). To be effective, secondary prevention needs to be delivered in conjunction with the patient's primary care provider and/or cardiologist (Balady et al. 2007). Since the mid-1990s, there has been a move to include secondary prevention alongside the exercise and support of conventional CR (AHA 1994; Ades et al. 2001) and it has been acknowledged that CR services are often the best forum for delivering secondary prevention initiatives (Thompson & De Bono 1999).

Commencing secondary prevention when the patient is in hospital lays a strong foundation for education and support and targets the patient when they are potentially most likely to appreciate the need for long-term treatment and lifestyle change. However, the hospital may not always be the most appropriate environment, or the best time for detailed teaching and discussion. This is often more effective when continued after discharge and in the community setting. Traditionally, it is nursing teams who coordinate CR services, and nurses have an important role in integrating hospital and community secondary prevention services and in moving the delivery of secondary prevention forward. Nurse-led secondary prevention clinics in primary care that monitor, manage and support patients and families with CHD have been shown to be an effective method of facilitating long-term structured care and optimal secondary prevention (Dalal 2003; Murchie et al. 2003). Economic analysis of these nurse-led programmes has shown that they can lead to significant improvements in life expectancy at a low cost when compared to more traditional service delivery (Raftery et al. 2005).

Components of secondary prevention

Secondary prevention programmes should build on specific core components designed to optimise cardiovascular risk reduction, foster healthy behaviours, reduce disability and promote an active lifestyle in patients with cardiovascular disease (Balady et al. 2007). Those with previous vascular events are at high risk of occurrence of the same and other vascular events, and therefore a broad menu of secondary prevention strategies, from which to select those most appropriate for an individual, is necessary

for optimal treatment. Secondary prevention strategies need to bring together medical treatment, education, exercise, sexual and vocational counselling and behaviour change (Ades et al. 2001). Box 27.1 summarises the key factors to be considered in secondary prevention.

Key point

The mnemonic ABCDE (aspirin, antianginals and ACE inhibitors; beta blockers and blood pressure; cholesterol and cigarettes, diet and diabetes; education and exercise) has been found useful in guiding treatment (Gluckman et al. 2005).

Services need to be flexible enough to accommodate the individual's clinical condition and psychological state and take into account their

---

Box 27.1   Key prevention strategies

- Assessment of fasting lipid profile to ascertain appropriate therapy. Most CHD patients will require drug therapy together with a low-saturated-fat diet.
- Assess patients for co-morbid depression, anxiety and stress and treat appropriately.
- Optimise social support.
- Engage in self-management and strategies to promote treatment adherence.
- Undertaking physical activity that can be done for 30–60 min, preferably daily, or at least 5 days per week.
- Maintaining an ideal weight through appropriate diet and an individualised exercise program.
- Limiting alcohol and sodium (salt) intake.
- Regular monitoring of blood pressure. Those who are hypertensive to be prescribed antihypertensive medication.
- Taking aspirin or other antiplatelet medication daily.
- Stopping smoking. This is likely to involve counselling, nicotine-replacement methods and formal programs.
- Regular reviews to evaluate treatment targets.

lifestyle, health beliefs, goals and expectations. It has been reported (Timms 2005) that patients mostly want information that is pertinent to survival (such as symptom management) rather than broader lifestyle issues, such as exercise and diet. Thought therefore needs to be given to presenting information on these subjects in a way that renders them both relevant and accessible. The long-term changes in behaviour and lifestyle that are recommended are not always easy for patients to accommodate unless they acknowledge the need for change and fully understand the change that is required. A regime that fosters ownership, encouragement and positive feedback and allows the patient to progress at a realistic pace is most likely to be successful. The family need to be involved at all stages and advised on how best to support the patient by encouraging changes in risk behaviour. Family members may be identified as having risk factors themselves and so a family approach to lifestyle change is a positive way forward.

In 2007, the AHA and the AACVPR (Balady et al. 2007) in a statement on the current state of secondary prevention outlined the core components of secondary prevention in terms of patient evaluation, interventions and expected outcomes. The core components are as follows:

- Baseline patient assessment
- Nutritional counselling
- Risk factor management (lipids, blood pressure, weight, diabetes mellitus and smoking)
- Psychosocial interventions
- Physical activity counselling and exercise training

The above-mentioned recommendations advocate documenting ongoing patient assessment information in order to reflect the patient's current status and to guide in developing and prioritising goals in a treatment plan. Patients need to be educated in detail regarding specific targets for risk factor modification and other appropriate lifestyle changes. It is recommended that goals should be set for the short term (weeks/months) after which follow-up plans are developed. These plans need to be communicated with the patient and appropriate family members in collaboration with the primary health care team.

Best practice for secondary prevention changes with new evidence and the results from systematic reviews. Practitioners have a responsibility to keep up to date and provide patients and families with information and advice that is contemporary and evidence based. The core components of secondary prevention presented later are based on the 2007 AHA/AACVPR 2007 guidelines.

Patient assessment

Patient assessment involves a comprehensive review incorporating a full medical history to identify cardiovascular problems, interventions, co-morbidities (including psychological) and symptoms. Physical examination incorporates a full cardiovascular assessment and resting 12-lead ECG. It also requires that wound sites are identified and orthopaedic and neuromuscular status and cognitive function assessed. Quality of life tools that allow the patient to self-assess their perceived quality of life are increasingly used (Dempster & Donally 2000; Thompson and Roebuck 2001). A review of medications including dose, frequency and compliance will help identify if the patient is taking appropriate medication (aspirin, clopidogrel, beta blockers, lipid-lowering agents and ACE inhibitors or angiotensin receptor blockers [ARBs]) (see later). Establishing the date of the most recent influenza injection can also be useful. A cardiovascular risk profile will help quantify the patient's risk for cardiovascular disease and help prioritise secondary prevention strategies. Individual risk factors should not be considered in isolation (Joint British Societies 2005).

Identifying patient characteristics such as communication difficulties, education barriers and mobility problems can help in developing individualised delivery of secondary prevention, as can identifying family networks, social support structures, work and social roles. Knowledge of health problems, health beliefs, expectations, goals, misconceptions and an appreciation of the patient's motivation and ability to engage in the process of secondary prevention are also helpful.

Nutritional counselling

A diet that is rich in saturated fat, low in fruit and vegetables and high in salt intake is associated with an increased risk of CHD (Kromhout et al. 2002).

Diets that are high in fibre and polyunsaturated fats (the typical Mediterranean diet) have been shown to have a positive impact on cardiac morbidity and mortality in MI patients (de Lorgeril et al. 1999). Eating and drinking are often embedded within social, family-centred, culturally defined behaviours that over time become established as normal routine. Changing such established behaviour is a challenge and can be difficult for patients and their families. Individuals are likely to be exposed to conflicting and ever-changing information via the media and from family and friends. They therefore need to be provided with dietary advice that is straightforward and which sets realistic targets for long-term healthy eating. Patients need to understand the basic principles of dietary content, such as calories, fat cholesterol and nutrients. A diet that contains protein, complex carbohydrates, omega-3 fatty acids, fruits, vegetables, nuts and whole grains, and is restricted in saturated fat and cholesterol, should be adopted by all patients with cardiovascular disease (Gluckman et al. 2004).

Nutritional counselling needs to include specific advice to support patients to:

- Reduce intake of saturated fat (to <7% of calories), trans-fatty acids and cholesterol (to <200 mg dietary cholesterol per day).
- Add plant stanol/sterols (2 g/day) and viscous fibre (more than 10 g/day) to further lower low-density lipoprotein cholesterol (LDL-C).
- Promote daily physical activity and weight management (see later).
- Encourage increased intake of omega-3 fatty acids in the form of fish oil in capsule form (1 g/day) for risk reduction. A higher dose is usually required for patients with elevated triglycerides.

Risk factor management

Lipid management

Guidelines classify normal triglyceride levels as less than 150 mg/dL (3.8 mmol/L) and normal high-density lipoprotein cholesterol (HDL-C) levels as 40 mg/dL (1.0 mmol/L) or greater (National Cholesterol Education Program 2001). The target level for LDL-C for those with cardiovascular

disease or diabetes mellitus is less than 100 mg/dL (2.6 mmol/L) and further titration to 70 mg/dL is reasonable in high-risk patients (Grundy 2004). Early intensive lipid lowering after ACS has been shown to reduce mortality and further cardiac events (Cannon et al. 2004) and the benefit of lowering even mildly elevated cholesterol levels in secondary prevention has been demonstrated (CARE 2002). Because guidelines are regularly reviewed by national and international bodies, the reader is encouraged to visit the links provided at the end of this chapter to access up-to-date recommendations.

There is evidence that significant numbers of patients admitted to hospital with an acute cardiac event are not being prescribed appropriate lipid-lowering therapy. (Schwiesow 2006). Thus practitioners have a responsibility to be aware of current guidelines and be advocates for appropriate implementation.

The main classes of drugs involved in lipid management are statins, fibrates and nicotinic acid.

- Statins are the most powerful drugs for lowering LDL-C, but also help raise HDL-C and lower triglyceride levels. Statins should be considered as the first-line drug for lipid lowering in cardiovascular patients and have been shown to reduce mortality (Scandinavian Simvastatin Survival Study 1994) in MI patients.
- Fibrates lower triglyceride and HDL-C levels and are appropriate first-line agents for those with hypertriglyceridemia. Combination therapy with a statin can be effective in those high-risk patients with raised LDL-C and either low HDL-C or high triglyceride levels (Gluckman et al. 2004).
- Nicotinic acid (niacin) raises HDL-C and inhibits the production of LDL-C. It can be used in combination therapy with statins and for treating hyperlipidaemia in those with normal or low HDL-C levels (Brown et al. 2001).

All patients should have a fasting lipid profile. Those admitted with an acute coronary event should have a fasting lipid profile within 24 h of hospitalisation and lipid-lowering medication initiated before discharge. Lipid profiles need to be repeated 4–6 weeks after hospitalisation and 2 months after initiation or change in lipid-lowering medication.

- The primary goal is an LDL-C of less than 100 mg/dL with further reduction of LDL-C to less than 70 mg/dL being reasonable.
- The intake of saturated fats should be less than 7% of calories. The intake of *trans*-fatty acids and cholesterol should be less than 200 mg/day. Adding plant stanol/steroids and viscous fibre will further lower LDL-C. Patients should aim for increased consumption of omega-3 fatty acids found in fish oil.
- If baseline LDL-C is 100 mg/dL or greater, LDL-lowering therapy should be initiated (typically with a statin).
- If on treatment, the LDL-C is 100 mg/dL or greater, then the LDL-lowering drug therapy needs to be increased (may require LDL-lowering drug combination [statin + ezetimibe, bile acid sequestrant, or niacin]).
- If baseline LDL-C is 70–100 mg/dL, it is reasonable to treat until the LDL-C is less than 70 mg/dL.
- If triglycerides are 200–499 mg/dL, the non-HDL-C should be less than 130 mg/dL, and further reduction of non-HDL-C to less than 100 mg/dL is reasonable.
- Therapeutic options to reduce non-HDL-C are:
  - More intense LDL-C-lowering therapy, or
  - Niacin (after LDL-C-lowering therapy), or
  - Fibrate therapy (after LDL-C-lowering therapy)
- If triglycerides are 500 mg/dL or greater, therapeutic options to prevent pancreatitis are fibrate or niacin before LDL-lowering therapy; and treating LDL-C to the target concentration after triglyceride-lowering therapy. Patients with very high triglycerides should be advised to not consume alcohol.
- Creatine kinase levels and liver function tests are recommended for patients on lipid-lowering therapy (National Cholesterol Education Program 2002).

Blood pressure control

Lowering blood pressure is likely to be one of the most effective and generalisable strategies across a variety of major vascular events including stroke and MI (Arima et al. 2006). The target goal for blood pressure is for it to be lower than 140/90 mmHg (Chobanian et al. 2003). In those patients who are diabetic or have chronic renal disease the target blood pressure is less than 130/80 mmHg (Chobanian et al. 2003). Blood pressure recordings should be taken with the patient seated and resting on at least two occasions with readings in both arms and on lying and standing at entry to the programme.

- Patients need to initiate and maintain a lifestyle that incorporates weight control, appropriate physical activity, alcohol in moderation, sodium reduction and an emphasis on increased consumption of fresh fruits, vegetables and low-fat dairy products.
- Those who are diabetic or who have chronic renal disease should be given initial treatment with beta blockers and/or ACE inhibitors, with the addition of other drugs such as thiazides as needed to achieve the target blood pressure.
- Most patients will require at least two antihypertensive medications to achieve their target blood pressure (Cushman et al. 2002).

Weight management

Achieving a normal body weight is the most important aspect of dietary modification. Being overweight is associated with raised plasma lipids, glucose intolerance and hypertension. Those with a body mass index (BMI) of 25–29.9 kg/m^2 are considered overweight, while those with a BMI of 30 kg/m^2 or greater are considered obese. The regional accumulation of body fat around the waist, known as abdominal obesity, confers an increased risk of cardiovascular disease that is age, sex and race dependent (IDF 2005) and may be an indicator of metabolic syndrome(linked to insulin resistance and hypertension). Waist circumference (measured horizontally at the iliac crest) begins to confer a risk if greater than 94 cm in European and African men and greater than 90 cm in South Asian and Chinese men (JBS-2 2005). The hip waist ratio is also useful for assessing cardiac risk (Yusuf et al. 2005) and is dependent upon age and gender.

Weight loss produces a reduction in blood pressure, triglyceride concentrations, insulin levels and increases HDL-C levels (James et al. 2000). A 10% weight reduction will reduce the risk of developing diabetes by over 50% and is associated with around a 25% reduction in total mortality.

Weight loss will also improve self-esteem and confidence. The goal is a BMI of 18.5–24.9 kg/m². Patients need to aim for a waist circumference of ≤40 inches/94 cm for men and ≤35 inches/80 cm for women. Strategies for effective weight loss include:

- Calculating the BMI and/or waist circumference on each visit and encouraging weight maintenance/reduction through an appropriate balance of physical activity, caloric intake and formal behavioural programmes as appropriate to maintain/achieve a BMI between 18.5 and 24.9 kg/m².
- Setting weight-loss targets that are realistic and achievable. The initial goal should be to reduce body weight by approximately 10% from baseline. Weight losses of around 0.5 kg/week is a realistic target and is best achieved through regular and slow eating of meals and regular physical activity.
- Initiating appropriate treatment of metabolic syndrome if a patient has a waist circumference over the target size.

Diabetes management

A fasting plasma glucose level of greater than 126 mg/dL (7.0 mmol/L) and/or 200 mg/dL (11.1 mmol/L) after loading with oral glucose defines diabetes mellitus (Alberti & Zimmet 1998). Diabetic patients with CHD have been shown to have worse risk factor management than non-diabetic patients (Pyorala et al. 2004).

Patients with cardiovascular disease who have been diagnosed with diabetes (or have impaired glucose tolerance and/or insulin deficiency) need to initiate lifestyle changes to manage their condition and reduce their cardiac risk factors. Preventing the onset of diabetes in those with predisposing factors through a weight-loss programme and regular physical activity has been shown to reduce the incidence of diabetes by 58% (Knowler et al. 2002). The goal for diabetic patients centres on the glycosylated haemoglobin (HbA1c) test which measures the average amount of sugar in the blood over the preceding 2–3 months. The United Kingdom Prospective Diabetes Study (UKPDS-35) found that for each 1% reduction in HbA1 there was a corresponding 14% reduction for non-fatal MI (Stratton et al. 2000). The target is

an HbA1c of less than 7%. Secondary prevention strategies need to include:

- A vigorous modification of risk factors (e.g. physical activity, weight management, blood pressure control and cholesterol management) as recommended above is necessary
- Reviewing medication to aim to reach the target HbA1
- Coordinating care with the patient's primary care team and endocrinologist

Smoking cessation

Smoking has been shown to be an important predictor of future cardiovascular events (Tofler et al. 1993). Men less than 60 years old with ACS who continue to smoke have been found to have a risk of death from all causes 5.4 times that of the men of the same age who stop smoking (Daly et al. 1983). Stopping smoking reduces cardiovascular risk by about 50% within 2–3 years. Secondary prevention aims to encourage the patient to stop smoking completely and involves a combination of long-term behavioural support and pharmacological therapy. Individual counselling has been shown to be an effective way of helping patients stop smoking (Lancaster & Stead 2002). Patients may also require pharmacological support, and nicotine-replacement therapy is an established method of facilitating the weaning-off process together with newer non-nicotine replacement therapies buproprion and varenicilin that have also been shown to be of benefit (Jorenby et al. 1999, 2006). An effective intervention needs to incorporate:

- Asking the patient about their tobacco use at every visit.
- Advising the patient and family members to give up alongside the patient in order to provide encouragement and support.
- Assessing the patient's willingness to quit and identify psychological factors that may inhibit success.
- Stressing the benefits of stopping smoking – healthier, improved sense of taste/smell; avoidance of nicotine-stained fingers; fresher home environment; improved lung function, easier breathing, increased self-esteem; better example to children, financial advantages,

preventing harm to others through passive smoking.

- Assist through counselling, motivational strategies and developing a stepwise plan for quitting.
- Arranging follow-up and ongoing contact, referral to special programmes and/or pharmacotherapy (including buproprion, varenicilin and/or nicotine replacement).
- Supplementary strategies if desired – for example, acupuncture, hypnosis.
- Advising against exposure to environmental tobacco smoke at work and home.

Key point

Many initiatives designed to help smokers stop smoking are being led by nurses and include smoking-cessation clinics in both secondary and primary care. Encouragement and support have been shown to be effective strategies (Van Berkel et al. 1999) with more intensive interventions being marginally more effective than less intense ones (Silagy & Stead 2001).

Psychosocial interventions

Psychological coping responses to a cardiac event, in particular anxiety and depression, can hamper recovery irrespective of the patient's physical condition. Other psychological problems include anger or hostility, social isolation, marital and family distress, sexual dysfunction and alcohol and other substance abuse. It is not known how many deaths could be avoided if psychosocial well-being were improved. However, major depression has been found to be an independent risk factor for cardiac events after MI and has been shown to occur in up to 25% of such patients (Frasure–Smith et al. 1995). Anxiety is an acceptable adaptive response to a perceived threat such as a cardiac event but it can become maladaptive and be a precursor to depression in certain circumstances. Patients often feel that stress has contributed to their condition, although its precise role as

a risk factor is unclear. Relaxation has been shown to enhance recovery from ischaemic cardiac events and has a role to play in secondary prevention.

Strategies designed to reduce stress and anxiety and improve overall psychological well-being include:

- Planned periods of rest and relaxation
- Frequent exercise
- Avoidance of polyphasic activities (not doing more than one thing at once)
- Instruction in anticipating/recognising emotions and how to manage them – encouraging self-help
- Group sessions to offer social and peer support
- Individual sessions on counselling and education on adjustment to heart disease, stress management and lifestyle change
- Including family members in the support
- Referring patients experiencing clinically significant psychosocial distress to appropriate medical health specialists for further evaluation and support

Individualised educational and behavioural support delivered by cardiac nurses in hospital has been shown to reduce psychological consequences and improve quality of life after discharge (Mayou et al. 2002).

Physical activity counselling and exercise training

Regular exercise has been shown to have the potential to regress atherosclerosis (Hambrecht et al. 1993) and reduce the rate of cardiac and all-cause mortality in those with known cardiovascular disease (Wannamethee et al. 2000; Taylor et al. 2004). The goal for exercise for all patients is 30 min, 7 days per week (minimum goal, 5 days per week). This exercise needs to be moderate-intensity aerobic activity, such as brisk walking, on most, preferably all, days of the week, supplemented by an increase in daily lifestyle activities (e.g., walking to work, gardening, house work) and resistance training on at least 2 days/week. A history of the individual's physical activity and/or exercise test should be used to produce a plan for activity levels and an individualised exercise prescription.

High-risk patients (e.g. those with recent ACS, revascularization, heart failure) need to be offered medically supervised programmes. Such programmes have been shown to be safe (Franklin et al. 1998; Smart & Marwick 2004) and when offered as part of a CR programme have been shown to slow the progression or partially reduce the severity of atherosclerosis (Niebauer et al. 1997).

Cardio-protective drug therapy

As well as medication given to reach lipid, blood pressure and glucose targets and control ischaemic symptoms, other drugs are used in secondary prevention to reduce morbidity and mortality. A patient's drug regimen will need to be individualised and depend on in-cardiac events, the results of diagnostic tests, procedural interventions and coronary artery disease risk factors.

Antiplatelet agents and anticoagulants

Aspirin irreversibly inhibits the cyclooxygenase enzyme involved in the production of thromboxane, a factor that promotes platelet aggregation. A meta-analysis of about 70,000 patients with cardiovascular disease found that 75–325 mg of aspirin daily resulted in approximately 33% relative reduction in cardiovascular events. Aspirin also reduces mortality (Antiplatelet Trialist's Collaboration 1996; Anti-thrombotic Trialists' Collaboration 2002).

Clopidogrel inhibits platelet activation by blocking the binding of adenosine diphosphate to its site on the platelet surface and clinical trials have indicated that it should be taken for at least 8–12 months by patients with ACS, especially those undergoing PCI (Steinhubl et al. 2002). Clopidogrel should be used in place of aspirin in patients who are intolerant or resistant to the effects of aspirin.

Warfarin inhibits the action of Vitamin K and the action of the proteins and clotting factors involved in the clotting process. Anticoagulation with warfarin should be considered in patients with atrial fibrillation and/or left ventricular thrombus and may be an appropriate first-line therapy in some MI patients (Hurlen et al. 2002).

Recommendations for antiplatelet/anticoagulant therapy are (ACC/AHA 2007):

- Start aspirin at 75–162 mg/day and continue indefinitely in all patients unless contraindicated.
- For patients undergoing coronary artery bypass grafting, aspirin should be started within 48 h of surgery to reduce saphenous vein graft closure. Dosing regimens ranging from 100 to 325 mg/day appear to be efficacious. Doses higher than 162 mg/day can be continued for up to 1 year.
- Start and continue clopidogrel at 75 mg/day in combination with aspirin for up to 12 months in patients after ACS or PCI with stent placement (1 month or more for bare metal stent, 3 months or more for sirolimus-eluting stent and 6 months or more for paclitaxel-eluting stent).
- Patients who have undergone PCI with stent placement should initially receive higher-dose aspirin at 325 mg/day for 1 month for bare metal stent, 3 months for sirolimus-eluting stent and 6 months for paclitaxel-eluting stent.
- Manage warfarin to international normalised ratio 2.0–3.0 for paroxysmal or chronic atrial fibrillation or flutter, and in post-MI patients when clinically indicated (e.g. atrial fibrillation, left ventricular thrombus).
- Use of warfarin in conjunction with aspirin and/or clopidogrel is associated with increased risk of bleeding and should be monitored closely.

ACE inhibitors

Clinical trials have demonstrated that ACE inhibitors are strongly indicated in those patients with a reduced ejection fraction, particularly after an MI (Hunt et al. 2001). The Heart Outcomes Prevention Evaluation (HOPE) trial (2000) has demonstrated the benefit of ACE-inhibitor therapy in high-risk patients with cardiovascular disease without a history of an acute event.

- ACE inhibitors should be started and continued indefinitely in all CHD patients with left ventricular ejection fraction of 40% or less and in those with hypertension, diabetes or chronic kidney disease, unless contraindicated.
- Consider their use for all other patients.

- The use of ACE inhibitors is considered optional among lower-risk patients with normal left ventricular ejection fraction in whom cardiovascular risk factors are well controlled and revascularization has been performed.

Angiotensin receptor blockers

Angiotensin receptor blockers (ARBs) are indicated in secondary prevention only when ACE inhibitors are not tolerated. ACE inhibitors can produce renal insufficiency, cough, hyperkalaemia and angioedema and so having another class of drug as an alternative is useful, although, apart from the cough, side effects for the two drug types are similar. ARBs should be:

- Used in patients who are intolerant of ACE inhibitors and have heart failure or have had a MI with left ventricular ejection fraction of 40% or less.
- Considered in other patients who are ACE-inhibitor intolerant.
- Considered in combination with ACE inhibitors in systolic-dysfunction heart failure.

Angiotensin inhibitors

Angiotensin inhibitors inhibit the effects of aldosterone resulting in increased sodium excretion and reduced potassium excretion.

- Use in post-MI patients who do not have significant kidney dysfunction or elevated serum potassium, who are already receiving therapeutic doses of an ACE inhibitor and beta blocker, have a left ventricular ejection fraction of 40% or less, and have either diabetes or heart failure.

Beta blockers

Beta blockers inhibit the effects of catecholamines on beta-adrenergic receptors and have antianginal, antiarrhythmic and sympatholytic effects. The evidence accumulating from clinical trials has resulted in broader indications for beta-blocker prescription for a larger patient group. Beta blockers have been shown to slow progression of coronary atherosclerosis (Sipahi et al. 2007) and large retrospective review acute MI patients showed that over 2 years there was an overall reduction

in mortality of 40% in those taking beta blockers (Gottlieb et al. 1998). Oral beta blockers are recommended for long-term use (indefinitely) in all patients who recover from an MI and do not present contraindications (European Society of Cardiology 2004). The effect of beta-blocker therapy is greatest in those at highest risk (large anterior infarction with impaired left ventricular function) (CAPRICORN 2001). However, despite knowing the benefits of beta blockers for over three decades (Beta-blocker Heart Attack Study Group 1981) this class of drugs are underused in secondary prevention.

Hormone therapy

Hormone therapy with oestrogen or oestrogen and progesterone should not be initiated to post-menopausal women for secondary prevention after an acute cardiac event. Post-menopausal women already taking hormone therapy in general should not continue taking it unless the anticipated benefits for that individual outweigh the risks. (Roussouw et al. 2002; Manson et al. 2003).

Challenges in secondary prevention

To be effective, secondary prevention needs to be given to those with the most to benefit. However, despite the growing evidence of its benefits, translating the recommendations for secondary prevention into clinical practice is a challenge. There is evidence that such implementation remains suboptimal to the extent that a large proportion of patients in whom therapies are indicated are not receiving them (EUROASPIRE 1 and 11 Group 2001; Smith et al. 2001; Dalal et al. 2004). European surveys highlight that those with known cardiovascular disease continue to have a high incidence of modifiable risk factors and lifestyles that are not conducive to cardiovascular risk reduction (EUROASPIRE 1 and 11 Group 2001).

Effective treatments are frequently not given to those high-risk patients (e.g. the elderly and diabetic patients) who would derive the most benefit (Mukherjee et al. 2005). In particular, the prescription of secondary prevention medication for the sickest patients (such as those who have received coronary artery bypass surgery) has been shown to be less aggressive than for other groups of patients (Ohman et al. 2004).

Cardiac rehabilitation is frequently the vehicle for secondary prevention, and it is known that referral to and uptake of CR services is variable, with some studies identifying only a quarter of eligible patients being enrolled into programmes (Bethell et al. 2001). The reasons for the under-use of services are many and include ineffective links between primary and secondary care; low patient-referral rate (particularly of women, ethnic minorities and the elderly); inadequate resources; organisational factors; geographical limitations to the accessibility of formal programme sites and patient compliance factors. The diagnosis of myocardial damage by troponin estimation is linked to greater reporting of ACSs and a larger potential client base for secondary prevention. This has an impact on the workloads in primary and secondary care with ensuing resource implications and a need for greater specialist knowledge, particularly in primary care (Dalal et al. 2004).

There is a need to develop alternative models for secondary prevention. These include home-based programmes where a nurse acts as the case manager and facilitates and monitors patients' progress (Haskell 2003); community-based programmes (Harris 2003) and web-based programmes (Southhard et al. 2003).

Care settings that manage cardiac patients need to develop strategies to identify appropriate patients, provide practitioners with useful reminders and work with evidence-based secondary prevention guidelines to encourage appropriate intervention. They also need to offer a service that can accommodate individual patient need. Chapter 26 has outlined important strategies in convalescence and models of interventions to promote recovery and adjustment.

Much of the evidence on which secondary prevention is based comes from clinical trial research on atypical patient groups and has tended to focus on drug therapy. Additional studies to clarify the independent and additive benefits of lifestyle modification individually or in combination with other interventions, that include broader population groups and examine cost effectiveness, would provide important information (Franklin et al. 2004; Leon et al. 2005). Providers should have systems in place to audit the provision of

evidence-based intervention to those most likely to benefit. The use of disease registers to support long-term follow-up in primary care is one initiative designed to increase uptake of secondary prevention and the monitoring of its effectiveness.

Conclusion

It is important that the cardiac nurse be aware of current evidence-based guidelines and undertake strategies to implement these. It is also important to recognise that many of these changes require significant adjustment and lifestyle changes. Facilitating access to services, such as CR, that provide support for patients and their families is a critical element of the discharge planning role.

Learning activity

Reflective questions

What are the factors that put a patient at higher risk in the secondary prevention phase?

Reflect on your experiences of discharge planning to date, identify what you consider to be the barriers and facilitators to achieving optimal outcomes in the secondary prevention phase.

Summarise key elements of the nurses' role in facilitating secondary prevention.

References

ACC/AHA (2007). Guidelines for the management of patients with unstable angina/non–ST-elevation myocardial infarction. *Journal of the American College of Cardiology*, **50**:1–157.

Ades, P.A., Balady, G.J., & Berra, K. (2001). Transforming exercise-based cardiac rehabilitation programs into secondary prevention centers: a national imperative. *Journal of Cardiopulmonary Rehabilitation*, **21**:263–72.

AHA/AACVPR (American Heart Association and the American Association of Cardiovascular and Pulmonary Rehabilitation) (2007). Core components of cardiac rehabilitation/secondary prevention programs: update. *Circulation*, **115**:2675–82.

Alberti, K.G. & Zimmet, P.Z. (1998). Definition, diagnosis and classification of diabetes mellitus and its complications, I: diagnosis and classification of diabetes mellitus provisional report of a WHO consultation. *Diabetes Medicine*, **15**:539–53.

Allender, S., Peto, V., Scarborough, P., et al. (2006). *Coronary Heart Disease Statistics*. British Heart Foundation Statistics Database, British Heart Foundation, London.

American Association of Cardiovascular and Pulmonary Rehabilitation (2004). Guidelines for Cardiac Rehabilitation and Secondary Prevention Programmes, 4th edn. Human Kinetics, Champaign IL.

American Heart Association (1994). Cardiac rehabilitation programs: a statement for healthcare professionals from the American Heart Association. *Circulation*, **90**:1602–10.

Antiplatelet Trialists' Collaboration (1994). Collaborative overview of randomised trials of antiplatelet therapy, I: prevention of death, myocardial infarction, and stroke by prolonged antiplatelet therapy in various categories of patients. *British Medical Journal*, **308**:81–106.

Anti-thrombotic Trialists' Collaboration (2002). Collaborative meta-analysis of randomised trials of anti-platelet therapy for prevention of death, myocardial infarction and stroke in high risk patients. *British Medical Journal*, **324**:71–86.

Arima, H., Tzourio, C., Butcher, K., et al. for the PROGRESS Collaborative Group (2006). Prior events predict cerebrovascular and coronary outcomes in the PROGRESS trial. *Stroke*, **37**:1497–1502.

Austin, F. & Closs, S.J. (2007). Cardiac rehabilitation, secondary prevention or chronic disease management. Do we need a name change? *European Journal of Cardiovascular Nursing*, **6**(1):6–8.

Balady, G.J. Williams, M.A., & Ades, P.A. (2007). Core components of cardiac rehabilitation/secondary prevention programmes: 2007 update: a scientific statement from the American Heart Association Exercise, Cardiac Rehabilitation, and Prevention Committee, the Council on Clinical Cardiology; the Councils on Cardiovascular Nursing, Epidemiology and Association of Cardiovascular and Pulmonary Rehabilitation. *Circulation*, **115**:2675–82.

Beta-blocker Heart Attack Study Group (1981). The beta-blocker heart attack trial. *Journal of the American Medical Association*, **246**:2073–4.

Beckie, T.A. (1989). A supportive–educative telephone programme: impact on knowledge and anxiety after coronary artery bypass graft surgery. *Heart Lung*, **18**:46–55.

Bethell, H.J.N., Turner, S.C., Evans, J.A., et al. (2001). Cardiac rehabilitation in the United Kingdom. How complete is the provision? *Journal of Cardiopulmonary Rehabilitation*, **21**:111–5.

British Heart Foundation (2007). *Coronary Heart Disease Statistics 2007*. British Heart Foundation, London.

Brown, B.G., Zhao, X.Q., Chait, A., et al. (2001). Simvastatin and niacin, antioxidant vitamins, or the combination for the prevention of coronary disease. *New England Journal of Medicine*, **345**:1583–92.

Cannon, C.P., Braunwald, E., McCabe, C.H. et al. (2004). Intensive versus moderate lipid lowering with statins after acute coronary syndromes. *New England Journal of Medicine*, **350**(15):1495–509.

CAPRICORN Investigators (2001). Effect of carvedilol on outcome after myocardial infarction in patients with left ventricular dysfunction. The CAPRICORN randomised trial. *The Lancet*, **357**:1385–90.

Chobanian, A.V., Bakris, G.L., Black, H.R., et al. (2003). The Seventh Report of the Joint National Committee on Prevention, Detection, Evaluation, and Treatment of High Blood Pressure: the JNC 7 report. *Journal of the American Medical Association*, **289**:2560–72.

Cholesterol And Recurrent Events (CARE) Trial Investigators: Saks, F.M., Pfeffer, M.A., Moyle, L.A. et al. (1996). The effect of pravastatin on coronary events after myocardial infarction in patients with average cholesterol levels. *New England Journal of Medicine*, **335**:1001–9.

Clarke, A.M., Hartling, L., Vandermeer, B., et al. (2005). Meta-analysis: secondary prevention programmes for patients with coronary artery disease. *Annals of Internal Medicine*, **143**:659–72.

Cushman, W.C., Ford, C.E., Cutler, J.A., et al. (2002). Success and predictors of blood pressure control in diverse North American settings: the Antihypertensive and Lipid-Lowering Treatment to Prevent Heart Attack Trial (ALLHAT). *Journal of Clinical Hypertension*, **4**:393–405.

Dalal, H.M. (2003). Achieving national service framework standards for cardiac rehabilitation and secondary prevention. *British Medical Journal*, **326**:481–4.

Dalal, H., Evans, P.H. & Campbell, J.L. (2004). Recent developments in secondary prevention and cardiac rehabilitation after acute myocardial infarction. *British Medical Journal*, **328**, 693–7.

Daly, L.E., Mulcahy, R., Graham, I.M., et al. (1983). Long term effect on mortality of stopping smoking after unstable angina and myocardial infarction. *British Medical Journal*, **287**(6388):324–6.

De Lorgeril, M., Salen, P., Martin, J.L., et al. (1999). Mediterranean diet, traditional risk factors, and the rate of cardiovascular complications after myocardial infarction: final report of the Lyon Diet Heart Study. *Circulation*, **99**(6):779–85.

Dempster, M. & Donally, M. (2000). Measuring health related quality of life in people with ischaemic heart disease. *Heart*, **83**:641–4.

Dracup, K., Alonzo, A.A., Atkins, J.M., et al. (1997). Working group on educational strategies to prevent prehospital delay in patients at high risk for acute myocardial infarction. The physicians role in minimizing prehospital delay in patients at risk for acute myocardial infarction: recommendations from the National Heart Attack Alert Program. *Annals of Internal Medicine*, **126**:645–51.

EUROASPIRE 1 and 11 Groups (2001). Clinical reality of coronary prevention guidelines. A comparison of EUROASPIRE 1 and 11 in nine countries. *The Lancet*, **357**:995–1001.

European Society of Cardiology (2004). Expert consensus document on beta-adrenergic receptor blockers. The Task force on Beta-Blockers of the European Society of Cardiology. *European Heart Journal*, **25**:1341–62.

Franklin, B.A., Bonzheim, K., Gordon, S., et al. (1998). Safety of medically supervised cardiac rehabilitation exercise therapy: a 16 year follow-up. *Chest*, **114**:902–6.

Franklin, B.A., Khan, J.K. & Gordon, N.F. (2004). A cardioprotective "polypill"? Independent and additive benefits of lifestyle modification. *American Journal of Cardiology*, **94**:162–6.

Frasure-Smith, N., Lesperance, F. & Talajic, M. (1995). Depression and 18 month prognosis after myocardial infarction. *Circulation*, **91**(4):999–1005.

Gluckman, T.J., Baranowski, B. & Ashen, M.D. (2004). A practical and evidence-based approach to cardiovascular disease risk reduction. *Archives of Internal Medicine*, **164**:1490–1500.

Gluckman, T.J., Sachdev, M., Schulman, S.P. & Blumenthal, R.S. (2005). A simplified approach to the management of non-ST-segment elevation acute coronary syndromes. *Journal of the American Medical Association*, **293**:349–57.

Goff, D.C., Brass, L., Braun, L.T., et al. (2007). Essential features of a surveillance system to support the prevention and management of heart disease and stroke: a scientific statement from the American Heart Association councils on epidemiology and prevention, stroke, and cardiovascular nursing and the interdisciplinary working groups on quality of care and outcomes research and atherosclerotic peripheral vascular disease. *Circulation*, **115**:127–55.

Gottlieb, S.S., McCarter, R.J., Vogal, R.A., et al. (1998). Effect of beta-blockade on mortality among high-risk patients after myocardial infarction. *New England Journal of Medicine*, **339**:489–97.

Grundy, S.M. (2004). Atherosclerosis imaging and the future of lipid management. *Circulation*, **110**(23):3509–11.

Hambrecht, R., Niebauer, J., Marburger, C., et al. (1993). Various intensities of leisure time physical activity in patients with coronary artery disease: effects on cardiorespiratory fitness and progression of coronary atherosclerotic lesions. *Journal of the American College of Cardiology*, **22**:468–77.

Harris, D.E. (2003). Cardiac rehabilitation in community settings. *Journal of Cardiopulmonary Rehabilitation*, **23**:250–9.

Haskell, W.L. (2003). Cardiovascular disease prevention and lifestyle interventions: effectiveness and efficacy. *Journal of Cardiovascular Nursing*, **18**:245–55.

Hunt, S.A., Baker, D.W., Chin, M.H., et al. (2001). For the Committee to Revise the 1995 Guidelines for the Evaluation and Management of Heart Failure, in collaboration with the International Society for Heart and Lung Transplantation. ACC/AHA Guidelines for the evaluation and management of chronic heart failure in the adult: executive summary: a report of the American College of Cardiology/American Heart Association Task Force on Practice Guidelines. *Circulation*, **104**:2996–3007.

Hurlen, M., Abdelnoor, M., Smith, P., et al. (2002). Warfarin, aspirin or both after myocardial infarction. *New England Journal of Medicine*, **347**:969–74.

IDF Epidemiology Task Force Consensus Group: Alberti, K.G., Zimmet, P., Shaw, J., et al. (2005). The metabolic syndrome – a new worldwide definition. *Lancet*, **366**:1059–62.

James, W.P., Astrup, A., Finerm N., et al. (2000). Effect of sibutramine on weight maintenance after weight loss: a randomised trial. STORM Study Group. Sibutramine Trial of Obesity Reduction and Maintenance. *Lancet*, **356**(9248):2119–25.

Jesson, S., Farr, D. & Sheedy, M. (2007). Introducing a nurse led service in cardiology encompassing admission, post operative care and discharge. *European Journal of Cardiovascular Nursing*, **6**:38–40.

Joint British Societies (JBS) (2005). Guidelines on prevention of cardiovascular disease in clinical practice. *Heart*, **91**:1–52.

Joliffe, J.A., Rees, K., Taylor, R.S., et al. (2004). *Exercise based rehabilitation for coronary heart disease* (Cochrane Review). Cochrane Library: Issue 1. Wiley, Chichester.

Jorenby, D.E., Leischow, S.J., Nides, M.A., et al. (1999). A controlled trial of sustained-release buprorion, nicotine patch or both for smoking cessation. *New England Journal of Medicine*, **340**:685–91.

Jorenby, D.E., Hays, J.T., Rigotti, N.A. et al. (2006). Efficacy of varenicilin, an $\alpha_4\beta_2$ nicotinic acetylcholine receptor partial agonist vs placebo or sustained-release buproprion for smoking cessation. *Journal of the American Medical Association*, **296**:56–63.

Knowler, W.C., Barrett-Connor, E., Fowler, S.E., et al. (2002). Reduction in the incidence of type 2 diabetes with lifestyle intervention or metformin. *New England Journal of Medicine*, **346**:393–403.

Kromhout, D., Menotti, A., Kesteloot, H., et al. (2002). Prevention of coronary heart disease by diet and lifestyle: evidence from prospective cross-cultural, cohort, and intervention studies. *Circulation*, **105**(7): 893–8.

Lancaster, T. & Stead, L.F. (2002). Individual behavioural counselling for smoking cessation *Cochrane Database Systematic Review*, **3**:CD001292.

Leon, A.S., Franklin, B.A., Costa, F., et al. (2005). Cardiac Rehabilitation and Secondary Prevention of Coronary Heart Disease. An American Heart Association Scientific Statement From the Council on Clinical Cardiology (Subcommittee on Exercise, Cardiac Rehabilitation, and Prevention) and the Council on Nutrition, Physical Activity, and Metabolism (Subcommittee on Physical Activity), in Collaboration With the American Association of Cardiovascular and Pulmonary Rehabilitation. *Circulation*, **111**:369–76.

Manson, J.E., Hsia, J., Johnson, K.C. et al. (2003). Estrogen plus progestin and the risk of coronary heart disease. *New England Journal of Medicine*, **349**:523–34.

Mayou, R.A., Thompson, D.R., Clements, A., et al. (2002). Guideline-based early rehabilitation after myocardial infarction. A pragmatic randomised controlled trial. *Journal of Psychosomatic Research*, **52**(2):89–95.

Mukherjee, D., Fang, J., Chetcuti, S., et al. (2004). Impact of combination evidence based medical therapy on mortality in patients with acute coronary syndromes. *Circulation*, **109**:745–9.

Mukherjee, D., Fang, J., Kline-Rogers, E., et al. (2005). Impact of combination evidence based medical treatment in patients with acute coronary syndromes in various TIMI risk groups. *Heart*, **91**:381–2.

Murchie, P., Campbell, N.C., Ritchie, L.D., et al. (2003). The benefits of nurse led secondary prevention clinics for coronary heart disease continued after 4 years. *British Medical Journal*, **326**:84–7.

National Cholesterol Education Program (2001). Executive Summary of the Third Report of the National Cholesterol Education Program (NCEP) Expert Panel on Detection, Evaluation, and Treatment of High Blood Cholesterol in Adults (Adult Treatment Panel III). *Journal of the American Medical Association*, **285**:2486–97.

Niebauer, J., Hambrecht, R., Velich, T., et al. (1997) Attenuated progression of coronary artery disease after 6 years of multifactoral risk intervention: role of physical exercise. *Circulation*, **96**:2534–41.

Newby, L.K., Eisenstein, E.L., Califf, R.M., et al. (2000). Cost effectiveness of early discharge after uncomplicated acute myocardial infarction. *New England Journal of Medicine*, **342**:749–55.

Ohman, E., Roe, M., Smith, S., et al. for the CRUSADE Investigators (2004). Care of non-ST-segment elevation patients: insights from the crusade national quality improvement initiative. *American Heart Journal*, **148**:S34–9.

Pyorala, K., Lehto, S., De Bacquer, D., et al. for the EUROASPIRE 11 Group (2004). Risk factor management in diabetic and non-diabetic patients with coronary heart disease. Findings from the EUROASPIRE 11 and 11 surveys. *Diabetologia*, **47**:1257–65.

Raftery, J.P., Yao, G.L., Murchie, P., et al. (2005). Cost effectiveness of nurse led secondary prevention clinics for coronary disease in primary care: follow up of a randomised controlled trial. *British Medical Journal*, **330**:707–10.

Roussouw, J.E., Anderson, G.L., Prentice, R.L., et al. (2002). Risks and benefits of estrogen plus progestin in healthy postmenopausal women. From the Women's Health Initiative randomized controlled trial. *Journal of the American Medical Association*, **288**:321–33.

Scandinavian Simvastatin Survival Study (1994). Randomised trial of cholesterol lowering in 4444 patients with coronary heart disease: the Scandinavian Simvastatin Survival Study (4S). *The Lancet*, **344**: 1383–9.

Schwiesow, S.J. (2006). Assessment of compliance with lipid guidelines in an academic centre. *Annals of Pharmacotherapy*, **40**:27–31.

Sipahi, E.M., Tuzcu, K.E., Wolski, S.J., et al. (2007). Beta-blockers and progression of coronary atherosclerosis: pooled analysis of 4 intravascular ultrasonography trials. *Annals of Internal Medicine*, **147**:10–8.

Silagy, C., Stead, L.F. (2001). Physician seeking advice for smoking cessation. *Cochrane Database Systematic Review*, **2**:CD000165.

Smart, N. & Marwick, T.H. (2004). Exercise training for patients with heart failure: a systematic review of factors that improve mortality and morbidity. *American Journal of Medicine*, **116**:693–706.

Smith, S.C., Blair, S.N., Bonow, R.O., et al. (2001). AHA/ACC scientific statement: AHA/ACC guidelines for preventing heart attack and death in patients with atherosclerotic cardiovascular disease: 2001 update: a statement for healthcare professionals from the

American Heart Association and the American College of Cardiology. *Circulation*, **104**:1577–9.

Smith, S.C., Allen, J., Blair, S.N., et al. (2006) AHA/ACC guidelines for secondary prevention for patients with coronary and other atherosclerotic vascular disease: 2006 update: endorsed by the National Heart, Lung, and Blood Institute. *Journal of the American Journal of Cardiology*, **47**:2130–9.

Southhard, B.H., Southhard, D.R., Nuckolls, J., et al. (2003). Clinical trials of an Internet based case management system for secondary prevention of heart disease. *Journal of Cardiopulmonary Rehabilitation*, **23**:341–8.

Spencer, F.A., Lessard, D., Gore, J.M., et al. (2004). Declining length of hospital stay for acute myocardial infarction and postdischarge outcomes: a community-wide perspective. *Archives of Internal Medicine*, **164**:733–40.

Steinhubl, S.R., Berger, P.B. Mann, J.T., et al. (2002). Early and sustained dual oral antiplatelet therapy for percutaneous coronary intervention: a randomised controlled trial. *Journal of the American Medical Association*, **288**:2411–8.

Stratton, I.M., Adler, A.I., Neil, H.A., et al. (2000). Association of glycaemia with macrovascular and microvascular complications of type 2 diabetes (UKPDS 35): prospective observational study. *British Medical Journal*, **321**:405–12.

Taylor, R.S., Brown, A., Ebrahim, S., et al. (2004). Exercise-based rehabilitation for patients with coronary heart disease: systematic review and meta analysis of randomised controlled trials. *American Journal of Medicine*, **116**:682–97.

Timms, F. (2005). A review of the needs of patients with acute coronary syndrome. *Nursing in Critical Care*, **10**:174–83.

The Heart Outcomes Prevention Evaluation (HOPE) Study Investigators (2000). Effects of an angiotensin-converting-enzyme inhibitor, Ramipril, on Cardiovascular Events in High-Risk Patients. *New England Journal of Medicine*, **342**:145–153.

Thompson, D. & De Bono, D. (1999). How valuable is cardiac rehabilitation and who should get it? *Heart*, **82**:545–6.

Thompson, D.R. & Roebuck, A. (2001). The measurement of healthy related quality of life in patients with coronary heart disease. *Journal of Cardiovascular Nursing*, **16**:28–33.

Tofler, G.H., Muller, J.E., Stone, P.H., et al. (1993). Comparison of long-term outcome after acute myocardial infarction in patients never graduated from high school with that in more educated patients: Multicenter Investigation of the Limitation of Infarct Size (MILIS). *American Journal of Cardiology*, **71**:1031–5.

Van Berkel, T.F., Boersma, H., Roos-Hesselink, J.W., et al. (1999). Impact of smoking cessation and smoking interventions in patients with coronary heart disease. *European Heart Journal*, **20**(24):1773–82.

Wannamethee, S.G., Shaper, A.G. & Walker, M. (2000). Physical activity and mortality in older men with diagnosed coronary heart disease. *Circulation*, **102**(12):1358–63.

Yusuf, S., Hawken, S., Ounpuu, S., et al. (2005). Obesity and the risk of myocardial infarction in 27,000 participants from 52 countries: a case control study. *Lancet*, **366**(9497):1640–9.

Useful Websites and Further Reading

In addition to the above-mentioned references and the useful websites and further reading in Chapter 26, the following may be useful.

Corra, U., Giannuzzi, P., Adamopoulos, S., et al. (2005). Executive Summary of the Position Paper of the Working Group on Cardiac Rehabilitation and Exercise Physiology of the European Society of Cardiology (ESC): core components of cardiac rehabilitation in chronic heart failure. *European Journal of Cardiovascular Prevention and Rehabilitation*, **12**:321–5.

Smith, S.C., Blair, S.N., Bonow, R.O., et al. (2001). AHA/ACC scientific statement: AHA/ACC guidelines for preventing heart attack and death in patients with atherosclerotic cardiovascular disease: 2001 update: a statement for healthcare professionals from the American Heart Association and the American College of Cardiology. *Circulation*, **104**:1577–9.

Thomas, R.J., King, M., Lui, K., et al. (2007). AACVPR/ACC/AHA performance measures on cardiac rehabilitation for referral to and delivery of cardiac rehabilitation/secondary prevention services. *Journal of the American College of Cardiology*, **50**:1400–33.

Index